MIND YOUR BODY

MIND YOUR BODY

— 4 WEEKS —
TO A LEANER, HEALTHIER LIFE

10 Core Concepts for an Optimally Balanced You

Joel Harper

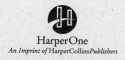

HarperOne
An Imprint of HarperCollinsPublishers

HarperOne

This book is written as a source of information only. The information contained in this book should by no means be considered a substitute for the advice of a qualified medical professional, who should always be consulted before beginning any new diet, exercise, or other health program.

All efforts have been made to ensure the accuracy of the information contained in this book as of the date published. The author and the publisher expressly disclaim responsibility for any adverse effects arising from the use or application of the information contained herein.

FIRST EDITION

Designed by Ralph Fowler / rlfdesign
Page xi photograph by Dylan Coulter
Color photographs by Darren Braun
Model: Ashley Meece

Library of Congress Cataloging-in-Publication Data

Harper, Joel.
Mind your body : 4 weeks to a leaner, healthier life / Joel Harper. — First edition.
pages cm
ISBN 978–0–06–234817–3
1. Weight loss—Popular works. 2. Exercise—Popular works.
3. Self-care, Health—Popular works. I. Title.
RM222.2.H2465   2015
613.7'12—dc23   2014042028

15 16 17 18 19   RRD(H)   10 9 8 7 6 5 4 3 2 1

May this book teach you to awaken and harness the power that lives in you, and help your mind and body work together toward a single purpose, so you can reach new heights in your health, have increased vitality and self-confidence, and achieve all your life goals.

To my parents, Eileen and Michaux,
who gave me both wings and a safety net, so that I could take risks, make mistakes, learn from them, and keep on forging my own path in life.

CONTENTS

MIND YOUR BODY AT A GLANCE

FOREWORD BY DR. MEHMET OZ

Dear Reader,

Much of my time as a doctor has been spent trying to help patients who struggle with the plethora of health problems associated with excess pounds, including high blood pressure, high blood sugar, and high cholesterol. Too many jump at quick-fix solutions that only lead to further frustration and defeat. The yo-yo pattern of weight loss that befalls most dieters is devastating, wreaking havoc not only on the body but also on the mindset of sincere people trying one more time to change their lives for the better.

Thankfully, Joel Harper has crafted *Mind Your Body* as an effective approach to long-term weight loss that harnesses the powerful resources housed in your mind. Joel is my longtime personal trainer, friend, and fitness designer for the best-selling YOU books. He is also my antifluff hero when it comes to healthy, effective fitness.

I first met Joel Harper when I asked him to review the fitness section of my very first YOU book. He was appropriately critical of the initial program and quickly offered an alternative approach that was simple and accessible. Since then, he's been my main fitness collaborator on DVDs and multiple bestselling books. Joel is down to earth, passionate about health, and extremely time-efficient. He helps me and many of the busiest people on the planet come up with programs for fitness and healthy weight that work because he knows how to tap into thinking patterns that promote healthier living.

Joel offers a clear, user-friendly plan for people who have no time to waste. The *Mind Your Body*

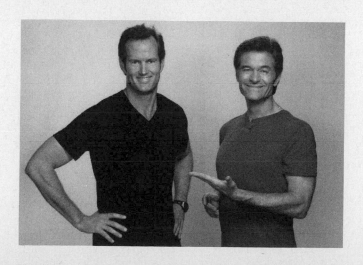

4-week plan clearly outlines what you'll do for a powerful mindset, a quick 15-minute workout, and healthy eating. There's no frustrating flipping back and forth to find which mindset, move, and meal goes with what day. You'll learn how you can lose weight while eating the foods you like prepared the way you like them, thanks to Joel's commitment to coming up with healthy, simple options that fit any lifestyle.

You'll also appreciate Joel's ability to digest and present dense scientific research in a clear, concise, and fascinating fashion that anyone can comprehend and incorporate into their lives. Joel gets the message right, whether he's sharing how his 15-minute workout is as effective as huffing and puffing for twice as long, teaching you how the right foods can eliminate cravings, or illuminating how negative messages can change the neural pathways in your brain to sabotage weight loss and cause weight gain.

In a nutshell, *Mind Your Body* will empower and enlighten you by showing you how, armed with a powerful mindset, you can achieve lasting weight loss, health, and fitness. Joel knows what he is talking about; he has helped countless people get slimmer, fitter, and healthier—and he will help you, too!

Happy reading.

—Mehmet Oz, M.D.
Professor and Vice Chair, Surgery
New York Presbyterian/Columbia
Medical Center

WELCOME

Dear Friend,

I am excited you are here. Just by picking up this book and reading the words on this page, you've shifted into a receptive frame of mind, and in just that flash of openness, your brain's neural pathways have lit up. Your brain is now taking notes, in a manner of speaking, by releasing chemicals and sending electrical signals to represent the information you are digesting. If you pause right now and close your eyes, you'll feel the electricity flowing through your body. Keep reading and following the suggestions in this book, and those signals will become stronger, more empowering, and more permanent. This is just a peek at what I've learned about the powerhouse in your head, and how emotions, thoughts, ideas, and intentions affect your whole being, brain and body.

Whether you are looking to lose ten pounds and feel more energetic or envisioning a deeper and fuller transformation into a whole *new you,* the path to success begins with clearing away outdated messages and embracing the truth you deserve and the success you desire. To do this, you must understand how to harness and change your thoughts. This requires you to be fully awake, aware, and present in your life. The Deserve Level Test will help you master these skills. You'll have the key to your fitness and weight loss goals, as well as all your other life aspirations.

By completing the same test and series of questions that I use with my private clients, you will have the opportunity to intimately explore your unique needs. At this very moment, you are in the right place, and it is the right time for change to begin. If you want it, you can achieve it. You might think you already know where you are, but I guarantee you, you don't. By exploring the ten categories that make up the Deserve Level Test, you'll learn how to truly understand the undercurrents that determine your actions and present situation. You're going to learn how to chisel away unnecessary thoughts, emotions, and actions that

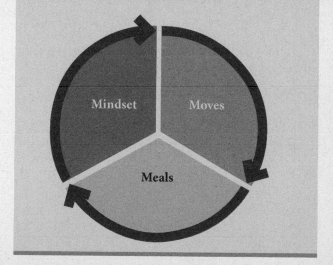

The 3-Step Whole-istic Approach

The following triad gives a general idea of how the *Mind Your Body* method flows and maintains balance to quickly, efficiently, and effortlessly yield successful weight loss, a leaner and firmer body, reduced stress, improved health, increased happiness, and enhanced energy.

Mindset

Moves

Meals

hold you back. With renewed clarity, you'll be able to use your mind as the awesome difference maker it is, and your life will break wide open.

You're going to learn how mindset, meals, and moves—which make up my *Whole-istic* approach—lead to true success. My program works because it consistently and dynamically addresses all the factors involved in sustainable weight loss and behavior change. More than 97 percent of diets, fitness plans, and weight loss programs fail because they only address parts of the problem instead of addressing the needs of your entire being. I'm going to teach you how to trust your gut and never give up, and I will show you exactly what steps to take to become precisely who you want to be—one day at a time.

Thanks to the publicity I've received from being Dr. Oz's longtime trainer and fitness consultant, as well as through the popularity of my DVDs and word-of-mouth recommendations, I'm fortunate to have worked with thousands of people and to have seen what drives them to success—and what doesn't. A personal trainer is like a therapist or a hair stylist—people trust you from the start, and while they are doing sit-ups or push-ups, you get to see how they are wired. I hear about their dreams, fears, and doubts, and I have seen some shocking patterns and themes emerge, some to avoid and some worth emulating. I've spent nearly a decade developing this book, extracting the elements that make people successful, because I wanted to perfect every detail before I shared it with you.

I care deeply about helping you reach your full potential, and my goal is to show you how to tilt your experience and shift your perspective, training your mind and body to see yourself with a new love and appreciation—the sort of love and appreciation that will allow you to look at yourself in the mirror and say, "Damn, I look and feel good," and mean it.

—*Your trainer,*
Joel

Fear says . . .
    no you can't.

Determination says . . .
    yes you can.

Results say . . .
    I told you so.

How This Book Came About

The Skinny Kid

I was a skinny kid. Looking back, I realize now that I was a typical child as far as size and shape went, but for many years I carried around negative messages and beliefs formed in childhood. So even though I had parents who loved me and a small group of friends, was an average student, played sports, and was fair at most of them, inside I was insecure. I felt different.

My leanness was noticeable enough that friends and family often called me Skinny or Twig. My father dubbed me Bones. I despised all those nicknames. (FYI: No guy, young or old, likes to be referred to as "skinny" or even "slim." That's akin to calling an overweight woman "full-figured" or "plus-sized." No matter how good your intentions, what she hears is "fat." Well, we guys translate, too. So please, call us "strong," "cut," or even "lean," but never "skinny" or "slim.")

Later on, I came to understand that no one was out to hurt me. People are largely unaware of the lasting impact words can have on someone's self-image. I'm sure that if the people in my life realized I would carry those nicknames well into adulthood, they never would have used them.

Like most kids, I was mortified at the thought of being different, so I developed my own version of "shapewear." I would wear sweatpants and heavy shirts under my regular clothes to add bulk and padding to hide my "defects." Sometimes I even had to put on two layers under my jeans to get the desired appearance. I can still remember sweat pouring down my back, stomach, and legs on those hot, humid Texas days—all in the name of being "normal."

My Awakening

At seventeen, something happened that would change the course of my self-perception forever: I was approached by a local modeling agency and started doing some local fashion shoots. This was my first clue that my lean physique might actually be an asset. My self-perception began to change. "Maybe, just maybe," I thought, "I am not Bones."

While my experience with modeling helped me break free of my old image and those childhood messages, I was surprised to learn that many models had distorted images of themselves. Some perceived themselves as fat or ugly, or having some other imperfection. These were models working for clients like Versace and Armani specifically because they were perceived as perfect. I remember one stunningly beautiful woman saying, "God, I hate my body. I'm in the worst shape ever! Just look at this cellulite!" She would go to the gym and work out at eleven at night after a full day of intense photo shoots. I watched other models pursue rigid food-restricting regimens or insanely intense workouts.

Many people, not just models and celebrities, suffer from insecurity, anxiety, and sometimes erratic and extreme mood swings that keep them from being whole and happy. These people believe they deserve to be perceived as beautiful—or to lose weight, get fit, earn money—only if they practice almost torture-grade fitness and weight loss strategies, find a magic pill, or employ some other drastic measure. More often, people just don't believe they deserve to lose weight. Instead, they believe that they are overweight because they deserve it at some level. The key here is that what you perceive is what will manifest. You might be beautiful outside but miserable inside, or you may truly struggle with excess weight; either way, what you ultimately believe about yourself will become your truth. And belief lives only in your thoughts. That's why the right frame of mind, attitudes, beliefs, and internal thinking strategies are key to achieving a truly successful, balanced, and emotionally secure life.

Learning That Mindset Matters

When I first started training others, I would often scratch my head, baffled that when I gave two similar clients nearly identical programs, the results could be extremely different. I remember two clients, let's call them Sally and Jane, who each wanted to lose roughly twenty-five pounds, establish a regular fitness routine, and begin healthier eating habits. From the start, I noted that Sally was positive about starting a new path toward improved health, but Jane was pessimistic from the get-go: "I've lost and gained weight so many times, but [*sigh*] I'm willing to give this another try."

Both women reached their goals in a reasonable amount of time, but while Sally found happiness and

fulfillment in her achievement, Jane continually expressed dissatisfaction, barely noticing her accomplishments and complaining increasingly that she hadn't lost enough weight. Jane began to make excuses and miss appointments, even though she was paying for them. Not surprisingly, her weight began to creep back up. "Here we go again," she told me. "Nothing ever works for me." Jane's mind was already made up, and what she was really telling me was that she believed she deserved to fail—and so she did. *When people don't truly and deeply believe they deserve something, they don't make positive choices or take actions needed to reach their goals.* By contrast, Sally sustained her weight loss, felt empowered by her success, and continued to train regularly and improve on her fitness goals. Sally came to me already believing that she deserved better health and weight loss, so she was willing to take the steps to make her dream a reality.

Based on the experiences of Sally and Jane, as well as countless other clients, I began to formulate strategies to help my clients look at their existing beliefs and chip away at negative and self-defeating messages, concentrating on self-belief and self-worth. I saw client after client reap benefits that fell far outside the health and fitness perks: happiness levels soared, relationships grew, and even financial and career paths flourished. It was a ripple effect that happened when the brain was "washed" clean.

As my client base continued to grow, I started training celebrities, elite athletes, Broadway actors, and famous musicians. I've been deeply blessed to be able to work with people from all walks of life. I've sought feedback from my clients about the strategies I teach, so I can say with resounding confidence that no matter who you are, how much money you have, or

> Doesn't work: Meals + Moves
>
> **Works:** Mindset + Meals + Moves

Jane		Sally	
Age: Forties **Weight:** 160 **Goal:** Lose 22 pounds		**Age:** Forties **Weight:** 165 **Goal:** Lose 25 pounds	
Regimen			
Do weekly no-equipment total-body workouts; walk whenever possible		Do weekly no-equipment total-body workouts; walk whenever possible	
Attitude			
• Jane was pessimistic from the get-go, saying, "I've lost and gained weight so many times, but *[sigh]* I'm willing to give this another try." • Jane wasn't expecting this to work, and she made that a self-fulfilling prophecy.		• Sally came in smiling and excited about starting a new path toward improved health. • Sally had a success story in mind and knew why this effort would help her in life.	
Results			
Lost 4 pounds; regained all of it		Maintained a 25-pound weight loss	

what resources are at your fingertips, the key to true success is learning to transform mental belief systems to empower you to break out of your comfort zone and succeed.

I train Dr. Oz, his wife, Lisa, and his daughter, Daphne. While some clients need more help than others in changing their attitudes, the Oz family came to me already equipped with an abundance of positivity. They have a way of being completely in the moment and doing the work in front of them. These are people who know they deserve happiness, so it manifests with abundance—and this gift is also available to you!

By the time you complete this book, you will be your own trainer, coach, and mentor. I've watched as countless women and men came to their first appointment feeling doubtful and dissatisfied. Over time, by practicing mindset, moves, and meals, they become inspired, empowered, and enthused. They achieve their dreams and become more and more balanced, whole, and complete. All that and more is in store for you, too!

Why This Book Now?

You may have sincerely tried to follow the advice given to you by your doctor, other health professionals, diet groups, books, personal trainers, even your friends and family. I continue to see dreams of slimming down go up in smoke for good people who have spent years, often decades, of their lives sincerely investing in one weight loss strategy after another. The problem is that the existing solutions bypass the actual cause of excess weight, the one area that doesn't get proper nourishment or the right sort of stimulating exercises:

the brain. You fail because the control center of your being is ignored, misused, or left out of the weight loss equation.

My clients often first come to me feeling frustrated, cynical, and defeated but willing to hear what regimen I have in mind for them. Maybe you expect, as they often do, that I'll tell you how many squats to do or how many slices of bread to eat each day. While that's part of what I do, it's not what I have in mind at all. What I have on my mind is the mind—or, more accurately, *your mind.*

A Program of Balance

Happiness is not a matter of intensity, but of balance, order, rhythm, and harmony.

—THOMAS MERTON

I know that the starting point, not just for weight loss but for transforming any area of your life and living out your wildest dreams, is right between your ears. And if you are an I-need-to-see-it-to-believe-it type of person, then you'll be happy to know that astonishing advances in brain research have produced mountains of scientific evidence to validate this point of view (I'll refer to this evidence throughout this book). I say that your brain is a starting point because without incorporating the physical body, you won't get much done. The human body is biologically designed to constantly seek a state of equilibrium. *You are meant to be a balanced being*—in your muscles, your outlook, and all the other categories that make up a happy life. Imbalances happen all the time, and they occur in the mental, physical, and nutritional realms. A pessimistic attitude, a bad back, or a high-sugar diet are examples I see all the time.

With the brain-imaging techniques now available, we can literally see how the brain affects the body in a myriad of ways, and vice versa. Your entire being is made of feedback loops with the body sending signals to the brain, the brain responding, the brain sending signals to the body, and the body responding. For example:

- What you eat sends signals and triggers to your brain, your muscles, and your fat stores, and they respond by telling you to eat more or less, to store or burn fat, and more.

- Your brain sends out signals in the form of chemical messengers, based on the nutrients you consume. For example, if you eat sugar, your brain sends out insulin that tells your body to store fat and crave even more sugar.

- When you move your body, it sends signals to your brain requesting more energy, and your brain responds by releasing feel-good endorphins and neurotransmitters. When you burn calories through exercise, your brain also releases chemicals that tell you to eat to replace the calories you just burned.

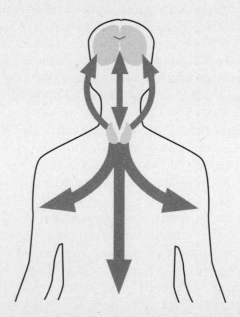

What you eat, how you move, and what you think signals channels of information from your brain to your body, and from your body to your brain.

Your brain is the control center of your being. It is responsible for triggering and releasing chemical messengers that largely dictate your behavior and your beliefs. Simply put, if your brain is out of balance, your body will be out of balance, and the opposite is also true. Fortunately, when you start the *Mind Your Body* way of life, you will learn that as soon as you correct one imbalance—a negative mindset (a mental imbalance), for example—you will begin to see a positive ripple effect. When negative people begin to practice affirmations, they start to lose weight because they are no longer partaking in emotionally triggered eating (a nutritional imbalance), suddenly they aren't avoiding exercise (a physical imbalance), and so on. And the benefits just continue to multiply: it becomes easier to sleep restfully, to be more productive at work, and even to attract romance. What this means is that any step you take in opening the door to positivity will pay you back with abundance.

Mind Your Body ties it all together by dynamically incorporating how you think, the way you move, and how you nourish your body to make lasting changes that will help you shed weight, get fit, and improve your entire life. *Independent studies also show that incorporating a mind-and-body routine over the course of one to three months can quadruple weight loss, improve effective exercise by 85 percent, and boost happiness and energy more than 40 percent, compared to those who follow the typical weight loss or fitness plans on the market today.*

My Final Words

I hope to awaken the enlightened journey that lives deep inside you. We are all unique, but we are the same when it comes to accessing these positive results. You have the tools; I just need your willingness to show up. I'm going to teach you how to get in touch with every muscle in your body and show you how to achieve optimum levels of mental, physical, and nutritional balance using a mindset that can't fail. You're going to learn how to be consistently surrounded by happiness, clarity, intense focus, love, and serenity that will put you in charge of your mind. I'm going to teach you everything you need to achieve happiness in every area of your life.

My deep certainty in the power of the mind to change your body and your life came first from my own experiences, then from observations of the world around me, and finally from working closely with clients. The more I help people balance out with positive mindful practices, effective and efficient exercise plans, and mindful eating guidelines, the more I see my clients succeed in all areas of their lives. Now I want to help you flourish. Take the test on the next page to see how close you are right now to being who you want to be.

Are You Who You Want to Be?

What you think about yourself and how you describe yourself affects both your body and your mind. Take this quick test to assess your current state.

From the list below, circle the five words that you feel best describe you. Don't overthink this, just choose what speaks to you first.

unflappable	honest	outgoing	knowledgeable	inventive
moral	confident	organized	rich	creative
powerful	sexy	fit	beautiful	enthusiastic
funny	humble	passionate	empathetic	reliable
supportive	trustworthy	skilled	exciting	coordinated
scattered	introverted	lethargic	disheveled	anxious
successful	easygoing	personable	caring	rational
fashionable	gentle	conventional	wise	musical
athletic	encouraging	strict	authentic	smart
capable	unconventional	independent	attractive	dependable
leader	shy	cold	quiet	angry
fearful	clumsy	disorganized	calculated	invisible
awkward	boring	hurried	entertaining	neat
faithful	artistic	watchful	spontaneous	inspiring
high achiever	graceful	optimistic	famous	clever
married	single	caring	nurturing	assertive
inhibited	testy	melancholy	curious	lovable

Now go back through the list and put a checkmark next to the five words (they can be the same as the ones you circled or different) that describe the person you ideally want to be.

Scoring. Tally up how many words you chose both times. If none, then your score is 0; if all, then your score is 5. *Interpreting your number.* 0: You are not the person you want to be. The good news is that *Mind Your Body* will show you how to reach the ideal you. 2–3: You are on your way to becoming the you of your dreams, but you have work to do. This book will show you how. 4–5: You have the right mindset and are well on your way. You're about to learn even more about perfecting your mindset.

PART ONE

GET READY

The Foundation for Optimal Success

I

How to Use This Book

What you are going to learn in the following chapters will give you the power to summon your most potent resources in an instant.

In part 1, you'll be introduced to the 10 Core Concepts for Optimal Success. Over the years, I have found that these ten guidelines are essential to reaching your full potential in every area of your life—from where you live to your hobbies, to your innermost dreams. Then, in chapter 3, you'll take the 10 × 10 Deserve Level Test, which will give you the insight to internalize, practice, and sustain the 10 Core Concepts with passion, empowerment, and potency.

In part 2, you'll be introduced to the Whole-istic approach that *Mind Your Body* is based on. Each chapter in this section will separately address the mind, exercise, and nutrition designs of *Mind Your Body*, as well as the tools you'll incorporate to make the Core Concepts an automatic part of your life.

In part 3, you'll begin the 4-week plan. Each day will be clearly detailed with activities for those twenty-four hours, including a prescription for mindful exercise, the 15-minute workout, and your meal plan. Then we'll look ahead to weeks 5 and beyond, and we'll address how to move forward in your life with the *Mind Your Body* method.

The *Mind Your Body* toolbox is found in part 4; each chapter in this section contains detailed instructions contained in the 4-week plan.

Finally, be sure to check out the appendix where you will find easy-to-use charts that help you quickly identify commonly experienced emotions and physical imbalances, and show you easily accessible solutions you can use to instantly get relief, and more.

To make this book extremely user friendly, make copies of pages 148–49, 150–57, and I-6–I-7.

STARTING LINE!

Are you tempted to skip ahead?

**Do you think it would be better to jump right into the program
and skip the mindset section?**

Think again.

Within the next pages, you'll learn how to gain clarity about your deep-seated thinking and behavior patterns, and how they might be holding you back subconsciously or consciously. You'll find the information you need to gain clarity, cultivate budge-proof motivation, and learn fundamental techniques for unstoppable success. If you flip forward without the foundation you need, you won't understand how deep-seated thinking and behavior patterns hold you back from long-lasting change. Grab a blank notebook or journal and keep it handy. I want you to take notes, jot down ideas, and answer questions.

Mandatory: There are several intensive self-assessment tools that you must experience to open your mind up to a transformative way of thinking and being to keep you on the road to success. I promise that taking the time to fully participate in the exercise and ideas that precede the 4-week plan will reprogram you to create a crucial state of mind that's ripe for change. You will learn to think outside the box, take fear out of the picture, and dream big. Plus, you'll establish your starting point, understand exactly what you want for your life, and know how to employ fundamental tools for optimal success. The rest of the *Mind Your Body* framework will build on these ideas. It's all about *you,* and you'll be guaranteed to have the passion and tenacity required to reach and maintain your most sought-after goals.

2

The 10 Core Concepts
for Optimal Success

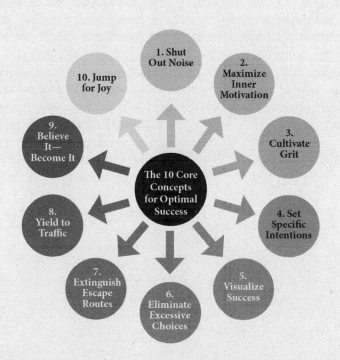

To grow a prize-winning blue-ribbon watermelon for the county fair, farmers know that they have to adhere to certain steps when caring for their melon crops. They aren't just growing your average plant, they're looking to produce a superior product, so they follow strict rules to give their plants the right amount of water, sunshine, soil, fertilizer, pruning, and weeding, as well as to protect their crops from adverse weather and pests. You and your goals are no different. If you want to succeed, you need to follow the rules to achieve your goals.

Think of the 10 Core Concepts for Optimal Success described in this chapter as an unshakable foundation that will lead you to blue-ribbon success! These concepts consistently keep you in the present moment, fully awake and alert, living with the unquestionable truth that you deserve everything you desire.

1. Shut Out Noise

Noise is my way of describing the constant stream of negative thoughts or defeating distractions that plague many people. Before anything else can be accomplished, it is essential that you be able to constructively filter your thoughts, so that you can discern and shut down disruptive mental static. I've put this

Shut Down Physical Noise, Too

Noise can play out in physical ways, too. When I first started working with Adrienne, she couldn't stop playing with her hair. She'd pause several times during our sessions to mess with her locks, so I told her she needed to wear a headband, and we made a deal. If I caught her playing with her hair, she'd have to do thirty extra Towel Runs (page I-48). Now she has laser focus during her training session, and it's rare for Adrienne to think about her hair while exercising.

rule first because noise does far more harm than just making you grumpy. It is the most persistent obstacle to your goals. I can immediately pinpoint people who will struggle to make changes based on the noise they carry around in their heads. Some of my clients have so much dialogue going on in their heads during training sessions that when I tell them the next exercise, they look at me but it doesn't register. I ask them what I just said, and they have no idea. The chatter in their heads is at such a high volume that nothing else can get through. Noise can also play out in the person I like to call the Jokester. This is the client who always needs to make jokes or tries too hard to be liked. A jokester constantly babbles and tries to distract me to avoid doing exercises.

Automatic mind messages—the stream of self-talk you have in your head—can be positive or negative, but research indicates that we humans tilt toward pessimism. According to the Laboratory of Neuroimaging at the University of Southern California, we have up to 70,000 thoughts per day. Consider what that would mean if just 10 percent of our thinking was negative? That would still leave 7,000 negative thoughts a day. That's nearly 300 gloomy thoughts per hour.

This pessimistic trait may be a leftover from our ancestors. They had to be vigilant about scanning their world for threats, so having the brain constantly on alert for saber-toothed tigers made sense. Today it limits thinking. Your brain has blinders on when you are negative (higher-order areas of the brain shut down to let the instinctual fight-or-flight areas take over), so your ability to think actually narrows, which means you have difficulty seeing the best strategy and are easily frustrated.

People who let mental or verbal chatter overwhelm them tend to struggle more with poor health and obesity because stinking thinking blocks their ability to change behavior. In the research arena, this is called the nocebo effect, which happens when you describe negative side effects of a medication but then give the person a placebo (sugar pill). In one study, described in a recent Harvard University article, people who thought they were getting chemotherapy but were really getting saltwater lost their hair and felt nauseous! The lesson? What you believe matters. In a study from the University of Pittsburgh, researchers found that pessimistic thinking led to increased hostility, worse health, and a shorter life compared to optimistic thinking.

2. Maximize Inner Motivation

Self-motivation is fueled by an intimately personal and deep-rooted desire for change. If your reasons for losing weight are grounded in other people—a loved one who is pushing you to slim down or a doctor who monitors the scale's latest readout—then you might be setting yourself up to become demotivated when times get challenging. Scientists who study motivation call this *controlled motivation,* as opposed to autonomous motivation. Researchers from the University of Kentucky define controlled motivation as coming from an outside source, while autonomous motivation is what lights your inner drive. Determining your personal and emotion-driven reasons for wanting to change is what will sustain your motivation long term. For example, according to recent research from Portugal that looked at the exercise behavior of more than two hundred women, ages thirty to forty-five, those who had the most internal motivation lost more than four times as much weight and exercised 85 percent more than those who were not self-motivated.

3. Cultivate Grit

In the scientific community, the concept of grit is all the buzz with researchers who study the psychology of success. Grit is the ability to try and try again; it is exhibiting passion and perseverance. It's the ability to say, "I can do whatever it takes to accomplish my goals, no matter what." University of Pennsylvania researchers, who did the groundbreaking work on grit, found that having it could improve success rates for almost any type of goal by more than 30 percent. The big news

here is that it really isn't about a high IQ or how much money you have; what matters is resilience, resourcefulness, and self-belief. I will teach you to have this stamina, endurance, and tenacity in your core so that you will never give up, no matter what. Period.

I've come to the realization that once you lose the weight, you don't suddenly get happy. Sure, it's easier to put on clothes, but I've lost the weight so many times thinking, "Oh, if I just weighed this much, I'd be so much happier." I know now I still have to work on that other stuff that has nothing to do with weight.

—VALERIE BERTINELLI

---

4. Set Specific Intentions

Clearly knowing what path you are on will help you remove distractions and self-defeating habits from your life. Establishing extremely detailed daily goals and a plan of action that resonates with the unique vision you have for yourself can result in twice as much weight loss compared to those who don't have any planning in place, according to an English study. Researchers from the University of Sussex and Warsaw University had women eighteen to seventy-six write out detailed plans for handling temptation triggers, such as drinking herbal tea instead of giving in to nighttime sweet cravings, or keeping healthy snacks in their purses to avoid the vending machine or fast food joints when they got rushed at work. After eight weeks, the planners had lost more than nine pounds compared to just over four pounds in the no-planning group. In another study, Israeli researchers found that of 632 women and men, ages thirty-five to fifty-seven, those who had a plan of action for dealing with temptations and challenges lost 40 percent more weight than those who didn't. The researchers referred to this as having an "implementation intention," or an "if-then" strategy. You'll learn techniques for setting effective goals in chapter 7, as well as the importance of having a specific deadline.

5. Visualize Success

Using images is a powerful way to get a clear picture of what you want in your life. When you feel your willpower wane, or if you start to succumb to negative or self-defeating thoughts and feelings, picturing

Inner Motivation Wins Outright

Emily, a client of mine, came to me wanting to lose weight so she'd look fabulous for her twentieth high school reunion. She confided in me that she'd always felt she wasted her high school years because she had such low self-esteem and set herself up for rejection. "There's no good reason why I should have been asked out back then. I wouldn't have asked me out if I'd met that girl I was. I would have run the other way," she said.

Emily told me that she'd recently reread her diary, and she couldn't believe how self-defeating and sad she was. "I used to really justify how lazy and unmotivated I was, and I stayed that way into my adult life," she said.

Emily said that she could understand why her work as a travel agent wasn't up to par. Her agency had just hired another woman who was also lazy, and Emily told me how annoying this co-worker was. "It's like looking in a mirror and really seeing my reflection for the first time. I could see that it wasn't who I wanted to be," she said. "Seeing how I really am makes me want to go back and change my story right from the beginning. I want to alter how others see me. I want to show them the real me, not this sad sack I've been. I know I can change," she said with fire in her eyes.

Putting Wood on the Motivation Fire

What Emily wanted most was to rock a pair of jeans and to feel comfortable wearing them. I gave her some assignments. First, I told her to hang the affirmation "I love the way I feel both on the inside and outside; I am stunningly beautiful" in her house where she would see it frequently, and to stop and repeat it to herself every time she passed it. Next, I ordered Emily to buy the actual pair of jeans she saw herself wearing to the event, even though they wouldn't fit yet. Finally, I asked her to try these jeans on every day before getting dressed in the morning.

In the meantime, Emily and I got to work on exercise and nutrition. We met three times a week, and she followed my videos two days a week. After nine weeks, Emily burst into a session to tell me that the jeans she'd been trying on every week were now too loose. She ended up having to buy a smaller pair for the reunion. She had lost two pounds every week since we'd started our work together.

What Happened?

Emily explained to me that the physical act of trying on those jeans each morning provided a regular reminder of her goal and how much she wanted to get those jeans over her hips, be able to zip them up, and walk outside and breathe freely in them. Saying the affirmation helped her change her thought patterns and encouraged her to believe in herself. Trying on the jeans helped Emily live in reality, and repeating the affirmation helped her shift her reality to the person she wanted to be.

As Harvard University social psychologist Amy Cuddy points out, this is "faking it till you make it," and it works.

positive images will increase your ability to stick to your goals. And it's versatile: you can do it when you are riding on the subway, driving your car, waiting in line at the grocery store, delayed at the airport, or on hold on the phone.

Studies show that mental imagery stimulates areas of the brain linked to higher-order thinking, self-regulation, and impulse control that are associated with increased motivation, confidence, and self-belief. Scientists who study visualization have some theories for why this works. First, mentally seeing your future develops a visual layout in your brain. This works like a blueprint or a road map that shows you how to get to where you want to go. Repetitive practice of visualization is a powerful exercise, speculate researchers, because it lays down actual physical frameworks via neural connections in your brain. Second, mental practices have been shown to be physically effective because they engage your muscles even when you are sitting still, and increase muscle mass. The more specific your mental image, the more specific your results will be. In chapters 4 and 9, you'll learn how to create crystal clear visualizations, and to make them work for your mind and body, so you can experience the release of empowering chemicals to engage your brain, tap your passion, and reinforce your resolve and resiliency. Visualizing success is like a reservoir of hope. It's having the ability to tap visual

What Is Willpower?

The basic definition of willpower (also called self-control, self-discipline, or self-regulation) is the ability to control one's emotions, desires, and actions. Recently there's been a wealth of research on willpower, and the evidence shows that in many ways, willpower works like the muscles in your body.* Each of us has a given amount of willpower per day. It is a limited quantity that fluctuates from person to person. For some people, willpower is freshest in the morning (early birds), while others feel that their willpower switches on later in the day, peaking in the evening hours (night owls). But whatever type you are, your willpower, like your muscles, depletes as you use it but with the right exercises you can also build your willpower stamina.

What Drains Willpower?
Self-control is diminished by more than tempting foods. Your willpower can be drained by many things—lack of sleep, controlling your temper (suppressing emotions), forcing yourself to laugh at an unfunny joke (expressing false emotions), sitting through tedious meetings (practicing patience), or pushing yourself to keep working when you are tired. These struggles will deplete your self-control temporarily, but practicing them in the right amounts has long-term benefits.

What Strengthens Willpower?
Willpower is increased over time by exposure to stress, just like a muscle. For example, turning down the doughnuts at morning meetings may temporarily drain you self-control, but over time, exercising resistance strengthens your resolve, making it easier to turn down future temptations. You can extend and replenish your willpower with a restful night of sleep, with a nap, by practicing meditation, by going for a walk, with breathing exercises, and with positive self-talk.

* R. F. Baumeister, E. Bratslavsky, M. Muraven, and D. M. Tice (1998), "Ego Depletion: Is the Active Self a Limited Resource?," *Journal of Personality and Social Psychology* 74(5), 1252–65. R. F. Baumeister, M. Gailliot, C. N. Dewall, and M. Oaten (2006), "Self-Regulation and Personality: How Interventions Increase Regulatory Success, and How Depletion Moderates the Effects of Traits on Behavior," *Journal of Personality* 74(6), 1776–1802.

resources that allow you to see new possibilities that crystallize success.

6. Eliminate Excessive Choices

We are blessed in this society to have literally hundreds of food choices, but when you're trying to lose weight, too many options can backfire. When you need salad dressing at the store, you find rows and rows of products—what should you choose? Going out to eat? Will it be Chinese, Thai, Indian, Mexican, Argentinian, American, fusion, family style, Italian, or your neighborhood diner? Variety may be the spice of life, but it can also be overwhelming. Making decisions depletes willpower (see "What Is Willpower?" page 9), according to research. Having at least one planned meal per day can help make healthy eating automatic, which you'll master with the *Mind Your Body* meals in chapter 7. Researchers from Swarthmore College have found that too many choices add stress and drain willpower, making it more likely that you'll make a snap decision to have a less healthy meal because you aren't thinking clearly. Eliminating excessive choices is about making a shift from zoning out to zoning in.

7. Extinguish Escape Routes

Having the tenacity to stick to goals requires that you clearly know and be deeply passionate about what you want—to lose thirty pounds, to lower your blood pressure, to fit into size 8 jeans, or whatever your goal is. When you have this level of intensity, excuses for veering off track vanish. Peter came to me after years of yo-yo dieting. He lost weight, but he could never seem to keep it off. During one of our early sessions together, I commented that it must be expensive to have to keep buying clothes in different sizes.

"I don't do that," he said, "I keep my fat clothes because I know my pattern is to regain the weight."

Keeping larger clothes was Peter's way of maintaining an escape route. He agreed to let me come to his apartment and help him clean his closet of clothes that were too big. Escape route—extinguished! Mission accomplished! Now Peter only keeps and wears clothes that fit—and the happy news is that they are smaller sizes than before.

Other common escape patterns are the people who say, "If I don't do my exercise at noon, I can do it tonight" or "I'll get back on track tomorrow; I'm going to eat the ice cream now." These are classic escape patterns—better known as procrastination. Anything that delays your goal or lowers your standards can take you so far off course, you'll never get back on track. Close those side doors and focus only on the path that leads to success.

8. Yield to Traffic

Learning to yield to traffic means having grace under pressure, going with the flow, and making on-the-spot adjustments. You do this by accepting that there are times in life when things won't work out exactly as you had planned—and making sure you enjoy the process anyhow. When you're stuck in traffic or have a tailgater on your bumper, you have choices. You can give in to road rage, or sit and stew, feeling your blood pressure spike through the roof—or you can accept the fact that some things are just out of your control, and you can surrender. When trying to lose weight, you carefully plan your meals, and have your healthy dinner all prepared, when your husband announces that he's taking you out to dinner. You know you should feel thrilled, but instead you panic; then you remember to yield to traffic—and you accept that you can go with the flow. You smile and grab your jacket, and when you get to the restaurant, you stay true to yourself by choosing healthy options from the menu. Yielding means knowing you can gracefully merge with the traffic and enjoy yourself in the process.

9. Believe It—Become It

Your beliefs about who you are and who you can become determine exactly who you will be. Cutting-edge research, previously used in academic settings

Exercise: Look in the Mirror

One of the most common mistakes I see people make is jumping into a new diet or exercise program without a plan in place. Clients also often describe waking up in the morning having a deep and sincere intention to exercise and eat healthy all day, only to find themselves unconsciously noshing on a doughnut an hour later, and then throwing in the towel on their exercise plans.

How do you get to your desired destination without getting sidetracked? It starts with knowing your starting point. Simply put, you must know point A before you can get to point B. When you get diverted from your goals, it's a sign that you are unclear about where you are standing in your life path. The following exercises will help you gain clarity and perspective, and will allow you to break destructive patterns, so you can move forward with open and loving eyes. You'll be able to find answers to small questions, like "Am I hungry?" as well as big ones, like "Am I happy with my body and myself?" or "Does my marriage work?" And anything in between.

Here are two variations on Look in the Mirror exercises.

Look in the "Reflective" Mirror

Stand in front of a full-length mirror (you can keep your clothes on). Be fully present in your mental and physical self. Imagine that you are getting ready to make your New Year's resolution (yes, even if it is April or August). Begin by focusing on your breath. Feel each inhale and exhale. Peacefully take in your reflection. Look into your eyes and examine your body. If you find your gaze wandering, take a few breaths and bring your gaze back to your image. Imagine what you look like to the outside world, to your friends, family, and loved ones—even your dog or cat. Look at your skin, your face, and the rest of your body. What messages have you heard about your appearance? What have you always wanted to change? After a few breaths, while looking into your eyes, ask yourself, "What do I want for myself? What do I want in my life? How would I like to change?" Continue focusing on your breath while you wait for insight.

If your response is "I want to lose weight," meditate on that—sit with the thought and take it further. Why do you want to lose weight? What are you willing to do to lose weight? How will it change your relationships with the people in your life? How will it change who you are? Feel the feelings that come up without resistance. Now grab a pen and paper, and without analyzing your thoughts, write what came to your mind while you were looking in the mirror. Answer the following questions:

1. What do you want to change?
2. What are you willing to do to achieve it?
3. What else came up during the exercise?
4. Are you 100 percent ready to commit to yourself?

Look in Your Mind Mirror

This exercise is an on-the-spot check that you can do any time you are unsure about a decision you are facing—if you aren't sure what to eat, how you feel, what you need to do next in your day, and so on. Wherever you are, pause and take a moment to close your eyes and visualize yourself in your mind's eye. Let your thoughts pass by as clouds in the sky. Say or think, "I love my body, and my life is always changing." Repeat this several times. Then ask yourself, "What do I see? What do I want? How am I feeling?" The answers will come if you give yourself quiet, calm, and loving respect.

to improve grades and test scores among students, is now showing that what you believe influences your ability to lose weight and keep it off long term. The theory that what you believe will become your reality isn't new; it's been around in research circles since the 1970s. What is new is the understanding that you can set yourself up with a belief system that produces dramatic differences in your health. According to an Israeli study published in 2007, if you have self-confidence in your ability to succeed at weight loss, it can triple the amount you'll lose compared to those who doubt themselves.

On the flip side, if you don't truly believe you can do it, you will sabotage your best attempts. I find that people who carry defeating thoughts learned in child-hood manifest exactly what they don't want in their lives. I get my clients to talk out loud while they are working out to expose these misperceptions. Some-times they don't even know why they say what they say when I ask them questions like "Why do you think you are uncoordinated?" or "Why do you think you have awful balance?" The answer I get many times is "I don't know. That's something my parents used to say when I was a kid." You'll learn how to identify and discard outdated internal messages as they relate to your emotions, exercise, and nutrition, and how to re-place them with empowering beliefs to become the person you've always wanted to be.

Just believe in yourself. Even if you don't, pretend that you do and at some point you will.

—VENUS WILLIAMS

---

10. Jump for Joy

Taking the time to recognize your accomplishments is what builds skyscraper-tall levels of self-worth, which determines how successful you're going to be. When University of Connecticut researchers put women on

The Core Concepts—Recap

1. Shut Out Noise
2. Maximize Inner Motivation
3. Cultivate Grit
4. Set Specific Intentions
5. Visualize Success
6. Eliminate Excessive Choices
7. Extinguish Escape Routes
8. Yield to Traffic
9. Believe It—Become It
10. Jump for Joy

a twelve-week diet and offered half of them a weekly chance of receiving small rewards if they lost a pound, those who received rewards lost twice as much weight. Taking the time to reinforce your adherence to goals by celebrating your successes can similarly boost your motivation.

This used to be one of my biggest challenges. I'm better at it today, but I still have a tendency to accom-plish something, and without pausing, I'm on to the next thing, forgetting to congratulate myself on a job well done. Just like you, I have areas to improve on. For example, I never went to my college graduation. I had put in hour after hour of studying and doing the work, and without even thinking about it, I simply didn't go. I deeply regret not going, and I can't go back. It taught me a valuable lesson.

Nowadays, when I finish a project or complete a race, I take the time to congratulate myself by getting a massage, taking in a Broadway show, or spending a special evening with friends. A reward doesn't have to be a trip to the Caribbean; it just needs to bring a smile to your face. Jumping for joy means remembering the importance of taking time to celebrate today's successes, to love and appreciate what you're doing right now, and to acknowledge each moment fully.

Final Words

Now that you are armed with the foundational guidelines to the *Mind Your Body* method, it is time to turn your attention to the next chapter with the groundbreaking 10 × 10 Deserve Level Test. Grab a pen or pencil and your notebook, and let's explore and discover the real you. This investigation will reveal the areas in your life that you can't see from your current vantage point—the areas that are begging for attention and change. Your commitment and honesty in completing this deep self-assessment tool will anchor you in the 10 Core Concepts for Optimal Success by clearing away the debris and excuses that have kept you stuck in your life. For the first time, you'll see what's been holding you back, and how to fix it once and for all.

3

The 10 × 10
Deserve Level Test

The greatest revolution of our generation is the discovery that human beings, by changing the inner attitudes of their minds, can change the outer aspects of their lives.

—WILLIAM JAMES

To follow, apply, and sustain the Core Concepts for Optimal Success described in the last chapter, you need a clear understanding of the overall quality of your life right now. That's where the 10 × 10 Deserve Level Test comes in. This intensive self-assessment tool—made up of 10 essential categories, or deserve levels, and a simple rating system—will provide you with the answers that are necessary for effectively practicing and sustaining the 10 Core Concepts for Optimal Success.

Author Louise Hay popularized the concept of "deservability," describing it as the idea that if you believe at your innermost core you don't deserve to have what you wish for, then you block it from manifesting. The flip side is that if you *do* believe at the deepest level that you deserve something, then you will do what it takes to make it happen, and it will manifest. I've taken this concept and paired it with a quantifiable rating system to provide a quick and effective way for you to see the level of your deservability in any area of your life—your deserve level.

You become what you think you deserve to be.

Joel's Jargon

A **DESERVE LEVEL** is a rating of self-worth, self-respect, and self-esteem for a given category in your life. It's the blessing or permission you give yourself based on what you believe you deserve in your life.

Desiree and the Deserve Level Concept

In 2010, Desiree, a successful business owner, came to me wanting to improve her health and lose weight. At the first session with a client, I start by having a conversation to collect a history. (Since training sessions are limited to an hour, there is no time to have clients complete a full test—that is an added benefit of *Mind Your Body*.) I began by asking Desiree about her work and daily schedule. Desiree told me that she frequently traveled for work, and since she was dedicated to working out and performing optimally on her job, she took pains to find five-star hotels with fitness centers. Desiree never skimped on giving herself a comfortable, cozy, rejuvenating place to stay. Desiree stuck to her luxury-sleeping environment and steady workout schedule because she believed unequivocally that they enabled her to perform at her best, and that she and her business deserved nothing less. Interestingly, when I turned the conversation to food, the discussion soured.

To say that Desiree had subpar nutritional habits would be like saying deep-fried Twinkies are a little bad for your health. Desiree's daily diet included sugary sodas, fast food meals, vending machine snacks, and quick-mart chips and candy bars. The kicker was that she also smoked cigarettes. These actions clearly stated that Desiree didn't deem her body worthy of healthy, nutritious, and sustainable foods (or fresh air).

I saw immediately that Desiree's deserve levels were all over the map. Desiree made sure to get in a workout no matter where she was traveling, but she sabotaged any healthy fitness gains with fattening empty foods and smoking. I could see that the first step in our training would be to enlighten and educate Desiree as to how her goals to lose weight and get healthy became snagged on the contradictions in other areas of her life. I introduced her to the 10 × 10 Deserve Level Concept and explained how to use the 1-to-10 rating system to identify her deserve levels.

I first asked her, "How important is it for you to have a comfortable place to relax and sleep at night?"

"10," she said.

"And how important is it for you to exercise?"

"10. I never miss my workout," she said.

Next I asked, "How important is it for you to lose weight?"

Again "10" was the response.

Then I asked, "How healthy did you eat yesterday?"

"2," she mumbled.

We discussed what she'd been eating, and her deep-down reasons for why she was eating this way, and she agreed that her typical eating plan put her at a 1 or 2 in the nutrition category, which was an obstacle to losing weight and improving her health.

When I pointed out the extreme imbalance in her habits, she was truly surprised. I asked her if she thought she deserved to eat healthy to reach her goals. "Absolutely!" she said.

Seeing the numbers helped Desiree clearly understand the discrepancies. She realized she wasn't nurturing her insides by eating healthy, which was much more important than 1,500-thread-count sheets. This awareness, along with other techniques to improve awareness, empowered Desiree to change her value system about nutritional habits, and she increased her nutritional deserve level to a 9. She still stays at plush hotels, but today Desiree has ditched the sodas and smokes, and now prioritizes eating healthy foods just as much as exercise. Not surprisingly, Desiree is now at a healthy weight and full of energy and passion for her life!

Think about it: if I had told Desiree to focus on fitness before addressing her nutritional and health issues, she would have remained out of balance, and any weight loss wouldn't have been sustainable. All the exercise in the world couldn't counteract the effects of smoking and the junk-food-junkie lifestyle she was leading. When you don't address what is out of balance, you can't make changes stick. Desiree might have seen short-term results in her fitness if I had focused on improving her exercise technique or given her eating tips, but by addressing the mind-set underlying *why* she ate the way she ate and why she smoked, her motivation became much stronger, and she was empowered to take control of her life and health.

Your deserve level is the conviction with which you say, "I deserve this!" in response to the questions in the test. Deeply believing that you deserve something is where true budge-proof motivation comes from; it's what makes possible incorporating and achieving the 10 Core Concepts.

The quiz is broken into 10 categories that are intimately intertwined with your level of mental, physical, and nutritional health. Each plays a critical role in making the difference between a miserable or a magnificently balanced life.

What You Need

You'll need to set aside at least forty-five minutes of uninterrupted time to complete the test. And since you'll return to this test repeatedly throughout the program, you may want to make copies of the pages. Have a notebook and a pen handy in case you want to jot down any creative thoughts. Remember that there are no wrong answers. The aim of the 10 × 10 Deserve Level Test is to shine light on areas where you excel, as well as on areas that need nurturing, attention, and development. There will be fluctuations. You will rate high in some categories and low in others. Everyone has strengths and weaknesses; this is normal. Right now you are just determining a baseline. Answer the questions from the perspective of what a good friend or someone with whom you are close would say. If you come upon a question that you can't immediately answer, pause, take a few deep breaths, and quiet your mind. Let the answer come to you. Then proceed.

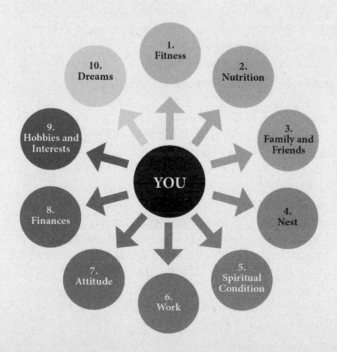

How to Rate Deserve Levels

Numeric rating scales are useful because they are an objective way to quickly and clearly communicate what areas of your life most need attention. A rating of 10 is perfect, as good as it gets, or of extreme importance, while a 1 is the worst it can get or extremely unimportant.

Rate each question or statement on a scale of 1 to 10:

10 = Absolutely yes! Always or absolutely the strongest or most important.

1 = Absolutely no! Never or absolutely never, zero, zilch.

Rating	Your Level	You Might Say
1 to 3	Extremely low deserve level	• "It's probably not going to happen for me." • "It's not something I think about." • "It's so bad that I block it out."
4 to 6	Low deserve level	• "I'll definitely get to it, but I'm not going to do it today." • "I'll do it tomorrow for sure." • "When I have the time I'll do it."
7 to 8	Moderate deserve level	• "I'm doing a great job, but I don't want to break too far out of my comfort zone." • "I meet my goals 75 percent of the time." • "I feel good about this."
9 to 10	High deserve level	• "Success is mine! I'll accomplish it without a doubt." • "I'm doing amazing with this." • "I love this area of my life." • "I deserve all the good the universe has to offer."

Important Note

I've included Desiree's ratings in the first two categories to give you an illustration of how to do your own scoring. See how much higher she scored in fitness than in nutrition? You can see how imbalanced these two categories are—and how she needs to optimize her nutritional deserve level to begin to see more success in her life. You can also see the importance of looking for lower ratings *within* each category by looking at Desiree's fitness deserve level.

See how Desiree rated a 7 on variety and a 6 on stretching? This tells me that she needs to work on these areas to reach her optimum fitness level.

Remember, you don't just want to have all 10 categories as balanced as possible; you also want to optimize within each category and strive for all 9s and above.

1. Fitness

Having a strong deserve level in regard to fitness doesn't necessarily mean that you always look forward to your workout. There may still be days when it's hard to get started, but when you have a strong fitness deserve level, you deeply desire what exercise gives your body and brain. You move, and move often, because you clearly understand that exercising your body will ultimately make you feel better, mentally and physically. The questions here will address how you feel about exercise, how often you do it, and what types of exercise you do.

I can physically do whatever it takes to accomplish my goals. I know my body is strong.

Rate Your Life

A quick and effective way to take the temperature of how you are doing with just about anything is to use a 1-to-10 rating system. For example: How tense are you? How hungry are you? How bored are you? How happy? How sad? How tired? Just be aware that the rating scale will need to be adjusted depending on what you are asking. For example, if you ask, "How tense am I?" and the answer is 10, then your goal is to lower it. On the other hand, if you ask, "How happy am I?" and your answer is 1, then you'll want to raise it. So sometimes a 10 is good, and sometimes it indicates that a change is needed. Adjust the scale to work for you. Ask what rating you'd like to reach, and think of action steps you can take to get there. When you get in this habit, everything you experience, think, or feel is within your control.

Fitness Deserve Level	Desiree's Ratings	Your Ratings
How strong is your desire to improve your body?	9	
How good do you feel about the quality and variety of your workouts?	7	
How confident are you that you can avoid injury in your workouts?	8	
How strongly do you feel that fitness improves your overall health or feeling of well-being?	10	
How important is strength training to you?	9	
How easy is it for you to balance on one foot?	9	
How important is stretching to you?	6	
How important is cardiovascular exercise (workouts that get your heart pumping) to you?	8	
How successful are you at consistently working out each month, including this past month?	8	
When you exercise, how hard do you work, motivate, and push yourself?	8	
Total (add up all 10 ratings) 9+7+8+10+9+9+6+8+8+8=	82	
My fitness deserve level (divide above total by 10): 82/10 = 8.2 (round to 8)	8	

2. Nutrition

Eating should promote health, but it should also be a pleasure as well as a mindful activity. Someone who scores a high deserve level for nutrition is sensitive to what hunger, satiety, and fullness feel like, and respects the body's hunger signals. A high-deserve-level eater doesn't let emotions dictate eating and, equally important, doesn't let eating dictate their emotions. What you put into your body influences how you think and feel, and can certainly hamper or help your energy level and your desire to exercise.

Today I will . . . eat healthy,
feel healthy, be healthy.

Nutrition Deserve Level	Desiree's Ratings	Your Ratings
How important is healthy eating to you?	7	
How successful are you at eating nutritious food?	2	
How successful are you at drinking the right amount of water each day?	3	
How are you about making time for meals and eating at a relaxed pace?	7	
How easy is it for you to prepare nutritious meals?	2	
How confident are you in your knowledge of healthy foods and your eating habits?	3	
How confident are you about stopping when you feel full?	2	
How strongly do you feel about nutrition's ability to improve your overall health and feelings of well-being?	9	
How often do you eat well-balanced meals?	2	
Do you avoid skipping meals on most days?	4	
Total (add up all 10 ratings) 7+2+3+7+4+2+3+2+9+2 =	41	
My nutrition deserve level (divide above total by 10): 41/10 = 4.1 (round to 4)	4	

3. Family and Friends

These are the people who offer you emotional support and comfort, warmth and nurturing, protection and security. Research shows that both family and friends can improve your health, reduce mood disorders such as depression and anxiety, and increase your life span. Having a group of people you trust—people you can laugh with, share difficult times with, and who are there for you—is essential to living a balanced, happy life. Supportive friends and families encourage your dreams, and you encourage theirs. How fulfilled and satisfied you are with your friends and family situation will determine your deserve level for this category. Acknowledging your current situation is a starting point for making changes and getting the support you need. Sometimes your family is incapable, and that is okay. You can find friends who become your family.

You are an average of the five people you surround yourself with.

Family and Friends Deserve Level	Your Ratings
How important is family to you?	
How would you rate your connection with family today?	
How would you rate your friends and family's support for your life choices?	
How satisfied are you with the quality of your relationships with friends?	
How good do you feel about how many times you saw or talked to your family and friends this past month?	
How happy are you with the status of your top five relationships?	
How encouraged do you feel when talking to loved ones about your goals?	
How free do you feel to express your troubles to family and friends?	
How free do you feel to be yourself with family and friends?	
How satisfied are you with the quality of your relationships with family and friends?	
Total (add up all 10 ratings)	
My family and friends deserve level (divide above total by 10)	

4. Nest

Your home is meant to be your haven, a place you look forward to coming home to. A high-deserve-level home feels like a sanctuary, a peaceful place you can retreat to, a relaxing environment in which to rejuvenate and recharge. Your bedroom should be restful, dark, and serene, a place where you can rest. A healthy neighborhood is one where you feel safe, where you're comfortable taking strolls, where you know your neighbors at a friendly level. You'll assess how refuge-like your habitat is, and you'll become clear on whether you need to make improvements.

It's not about the size of your house—it's about the happiness in your home.

Nest Deserve Level	Your Ratings
How important is it for you to have a living space that lifts your spirit and makes you feel fabulous?	
How walkable and friendly is your neighborhood?	
How satisfied are you with the quality of water and air in your home and neighborhood?	
How true are the following statements?	
I can't wait to go home; I love it there.	
I spend less than two hours a day on a screen (computer, iPad, smart phone, or television) at home.	
I use my bedroom only for sleep and intimacy, and it is a tranquil, nurturing haven.	
My house is clean and clutter-free; when I look for something, I can find it easily.	
I have a personal sanctuary in my home where I can unwind and find peace.	
My home inspires creativity; it's rejuvenating and inspirational.	
I have a peaceful and respectful relationship with my neighbors.	
Total (add up all 10 ratings)	
My nest deserve level (divide above total by 10)	

5. Spiritual Condition

Spirituality is an intensely personal and sensitive issue for some people, so let me begin by saying that I'm not touting any specific religion or belief system. I use the word *spiritual* because I find it to be an accessible and user-friendly word for many people. You can replace it with any term that fits for you—God, Buddha, Allah, higher power, presence, being, nature, Mother Earth, the divine, and so on.

The core of a high spiritual deserve level is the ability to believe in something larger than yourself—a higher power or higher perspective, a set of morals or beliefs that propels you toward being your best self. Some believe that their higher power is outside themselves, others feel it is inside, and still others believe it is both—there are no wrong answers here. For many this includes identifying, applying, incorporating, and ultimately living by your primary values. Some people describe this as living on a higher path by honoring integrity, honesty, respect, love, tolerance, kindness, serenity, courage, and grace. For some, attending a spiritual group, church, or temple fits the bill, while others find spirituality by communing with nature or listening to music.

Being spiritual means being in touch with something larger than you—inside and out.

Spiritual Condition Deserve Level	Your Ratings
How important is it for you to have a connection to something larger than yourself?	
How comfortable do you feel when discussing your spiritual ideas with others?	
How often do you sit quietly and let your thoughts freely flow (go to a house of worship, pray and meditate, commune with nature, go on retreats)?	
How successful were you at nurturing and practicing your spirituality this past month?	
Do you experience a genuine connection to your spirituality as you understand it?	
How important is it to you to build your character and live by a moral code?	
How true are the following statements? I feel secure and satisfied with my spirituality.	
I know clearly in my heart what my relationship is to my higher power or God as I understand it, him, or her.	
I have a strong and clear code of spiritual or moral values or guidelines.	
I find the world and existence to be full of wonder and mystery.	
Total (add up all 10 ratings)	
My spiritual condition deserve level (divide above total by 10)	

6. Work

How you spend your days, what your interactions with other people involve, and your level of stress and demands can all play a role in how you feel in your life. If you have a work deserve level of 10, then your place of business is a nurturing, invigorating, and inspiring environment where you look forward to spending your days, and you work with people you find enjoyable, stimulating, and helpful. If this isn't the picture of your work life—if your work leaves you feeling exhausted, without enough time or energy left over to exercise or cook healthy meals, or if demands from an overbearing boss have you feeling stressed and defeated, then at some level you have accepted that this is all your work life has to offer. The questions here will help you identify how satisfying your work life is right now.

If you can't figure out your purpose, figure out your passion, and it will lead you to your purpose.

—BISHOP T. D. JAKES (PARAPHRASED)

Work Deserve Level	Your Ratings
When you wake up in the morning, how much do you look forward to going to work?	
How stimulated do you feel at your job?	
Do you feel that you are becoming increasingly knowledgeable about your work duties?	
Are you working at the level you deserve? (Have you advanced or received promotions you sought?)	
Does time fly while you're at work?	
Do you get to tap into your "best self" at work?	
How much do you enjoy the people you work with?	
How much do you respect your co-workers?	
How true are the following statements?	
I never fantasize about another career or job.	
My job is exciting and stimulating. It rarely produces anxiety.	
Total (add up all 10 ratings)	
My work deserve level (divide above total by 10)	

7. Attitude

Your mindset is your mental perspective, the general flavor that makes up your viewpoint, but that still doesn't encompass all that makes up your way of thinking. A high attitude deserve level is positive, proactive, and grateful. I've discovered a fantastic way to get a quick read on a person's mental frequency: I ask, "What were the top five feelings you experienced most this past week?" I find this instantly produces an accurate picture of a person's demeanor. The questions here will help you get a core understanding of this deserve level. The good news is that your temperament can change lickety-split with the right tools.

Everything we do is infused with the energy with which we do it. If we're frantic, life will be frantic. If we're peaceful, life will be peaceful. And so our goal in any situation becomes inner peace.

—MARIANNE WILLIAMSON

Attitude Deserve Level	Your Ratings
How would you rate your self-worth?	
How happy or optimistic would you say you are?	
How much control do you feel you have over your temper?	
How much do you enjoy the flow of your thoughts and emotions?	
How often do you have fun and laugh?	
How true are the following statements?	
When a new opportunity arises, I am happy and excited.	
I rarely worry about making choices or decisions. I easily make decisions, and I can make changes happen.	
I rarely feel agitated or anxious.	
I am rarely numb, paralyzed, or on autopilot.	
I'm not easily swayed by the emotions of others.	
Total (add up all 10 ratings)	
My attitude deserve level (divide above total by 10)	

8. Finances

I would like to say that money is not important, but it does offer options. The more we have of it in this society, the more freedom we have to make choices. This can be a good or a bad thing. If you have an abundance of money that comes to you without a lot of stress or anxiety and meets your needs effectively, then you have a high deserve level in this area. This is a subjective measure. What matters here is having enough money for you. If you are constantly worried about paying your bills or accumulating debt, you may need to look closely at this deserve level.

I am constantly manifesting growth and change, and increasing my awareness of abundance.

Finances Deserve Level	Your Ratings
How financially secure would you feel for the next ten years if you had to stop working?	
How easy is it for you to pay your bills on time?	
How satisfied are you with your retirement plans?	
How easy is it for you to save money automatically each month?	
How organized are your finances?	
How true are the following statements?	
I don't worry about having enough money.	
I'm satisfied with my earning capacity and financial status.	
I don't have any debt to worry about.	
I have enough money to do what I want whenever I want to do it.	
Money comes to me easily.	
Total (add up all 10 ratings)	
My finances deserve level (divide above total by 10)	

9. Hobbies and Interests

When people spend time doing things that make them feel good, it activates areas of the brain that improve the way they feel about life in general and make them feel happier. Having an enjoyable interest not related to work or responsibility enhances creativity, memory, and focus. Regularly making time for leisure activities can improve brain chemicals involved in memory, motivation, mood, and impulse control, such as serotonin, norepinephrine, and dopamine. All this gives you more energy for exercise and eating right. Plus, a boost in serotonin has been shown to reduce sugar or carb cravings.

Hobbies are how we adults "play," and you can gain benefits from just about anything—knitting, gardening, playing tennis, volunteering at an animal shelter, drawing, playing or making music, surfing, fishing, golfing, playing cards, learning to dance, cooking, scrapbooking, mentoring a child, visiting museums, garage sale shopping, going to concerts, hunting, archery, learning to do magic, origami, meditation, yoga—even keeping chickens.

Hobbies and Interests Deserve Level	Your Ratings
Rate how quickly and satisfyingly you can finish this statement: I can't wait to get better at . . .	
How true are the following statements?	
I am comfortable with how I spend my free time.	
When someone asks me what I do outside of work, I am comfortable answering.	
I am always wanting to try something new.	
I always have plenty to talk about at social gatherings.	
I weekly make time for certain leisure activities.	
My hobbies are relaxing and rejuvenating.	
I implement my creative passions and desires.	
My regular schedule includes time for my hobby every week.	
I can easily tell you what my hobbies are.	
Total (add up all 10 ratings)	
My hobbies and interests deserve level (divide above total by 10)	

10. Dreams

Having an abundance of hopes, goals, desires, and aspirations is a sign that you value yourself because it shows that you prioritize what you want for yourself. Having a bucket list of things you want to do before you leave this blue and green globe is a sign of great physical and mental health. This category's questions will give you an indication of how much value and intention you give to your goals. I believe we are all unique, beautiful beings with a divine purpose. I find it troubling when I see talented people not nurturing or sharing their gifts with the world and those they love.

A happy person is not a person with a certain set of circumstances, but rather a person with a certain set of attitudes.

Dreams Deserve Level	Your Ratings
How easy is it for you to implement goals?	
How successful are you at living out your dreams?	
When you have new thoughts, do you often act on them?	
How satisfied are you with the last week in terms of living out your dreams or doing something on your bucket list?	
How often do you think outside of your comfort zone?	
How important are your dreams and goals to you?	
How much value and effort do you put into making your dreams come true?	
How much progress have you made in accomplishing your dreams in the last two years?	
How true are the following statements?	
When someone else talks about their dreams, I get excited and support them.	
I can easily tell you what my dreams are.	
Total (add up all 10 ratings)	
My dream deserve level (divide above total by 10)	

Calculating Each Deserve Level Category

You should have finished answering all 10 questions in each of the 10 categories. Now, take a moment to add up the ratings within each category and divide by 10. This will give you an average deserve level for each category (you'll find sample numbers for the first two categories on pages 19 and 20). If you get a number with a decimal, round your score up or down (round 8.5 up to 9, 8.4 down to 8). These numbers reveal your personal strengths and those areas needing attention, so you can create a plan for a well-balanced, fulfilling life. I encourage you to be entirely honest when answering the questions to get the best results.

Calculating Your 10 x 10 Deserve Level Test Score

1. Input each category deserve level

Now I want you to transfer your deserve level ratings for each category to the box at right in the column titled Average Rating. This shows all your deserve levels in one place, which begins to reveal how you need to prioritize your program. In Desiree's sample column, you can see that she needs to work first on nutrition and then, since they are a tie, on her spirituality and hobbies.

2. Calculate your adjusted ratings

Now, before you go any further, I want you to knock down each deserve level rating by one point. Input these numbers into the right-hand column labeled Adjusted Rating. Why would I be so cruel? I find that most people exaggerate scores. They tell me they drink tons of water, but when I examine them closely, I find they could actually drink a few more glasses. When they tell me they eat a healthy diet, they often leave out the Snickers bar they grabbed at the gas station on the way home. So, to get really real, subtract one point from each score. This is your true score for each category.

3. Figure out your overall deserve level

It's now time to get an overall average. As you will see, Desiree has a 6 as her overall score. Add up your ten ratings next to Desiree's sample ratings in the column labeled Average Rating and divide by 10 to arrive at your overall deserve level. Now do the same for the Adjusted Rating column. This is your overall adjusted deserve level. These two averages provide a picture of what you presently feel you deserve in your life.

Category	Average Rating		Adjusted Rating (Subtract 1)	
	Desiree's Sample	Yours	Desiree's Sample	Yours
Fitness	8		7	
Nutrition	4		3	
Family and Friends	7		6	
Nest	9		8	
Spiritual Condition	5		4	
Work	9		8	
Attitude	7		6	
Finances	8		7	
Hobbies and Interests	5		4	
Dreams	8		7	
Average	70/10 = 7	/	60/10 = 6	/

You Can't Change What You Refuse to Confront

I have a longtime client I'll call Barry who is tremendously successful in the movie industry. When he decided he wanted to hire a fitness trainer, he had "his people" set up our first appointment. Little did I know at the time, but it would take two more attempted appointments before we connected face-to-face.

I arrived at the first appointment, was greeted by Barry's assistant, and was led directly into his personal office, where I sat and waited. And waited. While I sat, I looked around the room at walls and shelves that were covered from ceiling to floor with trophies, awards, and pictures of my new client with some of the most popular celebrities in the trade. Thirty minutes went by before the assistant returned, apologizing that Barry was stuck in meetings.

After more than two decades of training people, I've learned to tell when someone is playing games, and I knew right away that Barry was a master game player. Not with me, mind you. Barry was playing games with himself.

I knew that, as successful as he was, if he really wanted to get out of a meeting, he'd get out of the meeting. Obviously, he wasn't really and truly ready to get started with training.

On our third attempt, Barry did arrive at the meeting, fifteen minutes late. He apologized and then started talking in a rush of run-on sentences about why he was overweight, how it was so uncomfortable when his legs rubbed together, how embarrassing it was when he went to get fitted for clothes, how he always thought people were looking at him like he was "a big fat pig," how he didn't have time to exercise, and how he was worried about his health.

I'm not a big talker during sessions. And I have a rule that clients are allowed to talk only while they are exercising. I'm there for action, so that I can provide results in a time-efficient manner. After about five minutes, I stood up. I had heard all I needed to hear. He had confirmed something I'd already suspected: he was out of shape for a reason—too much talking, not enough action. I could tell that Barry was out of his comfort zone. He was used to being the boss, in charge of all interactions.

After a few more minutes of rambling talk, I stopped him and let him know that I'd heard him by summarizing his lengthy monologue. Next, letting him know that I valued his time, I suggested that we get going on the workout, but first I looked him square in the eyes and asked, "Do you have the body you want?"

"No, I don't," he said.

I explained to Barry that his choices had helped create his current physique, and I told him that I was going to show him how to uncreate it.

"Do you feel like you deserve to be in amazing shape?" I asked.

"Yes," he answered.

I told him to stand up and copy my warm-up movements, explaining my rule about talking only while moving.

Then I talked to him about his work category and asked him where it was on a scale of 1 to 10. I thought he'd say 10, but he surprised me by telling me that it was 100! So I asked about how he'd rank his deserve level for fitness, nutrition, and overall health. He told me that he didn't want to die.

"So you only want to change your habits enough so that you don't die?" I asked.

"That's right," he said.

I explained to Barry that this would translate into a 1. I explained that we needed to get his deserve level above this minimal level or he wouldn't see any lasting change.

He sat with a perplexed look on his face.

"Does your wife like your body?" I asked.

He dropped his head, and with the first real emotion I'd seen, he said, "*No!*"

"Well, it sounds like you enjoy making your wife unhappy by being overweight and not doing anything to change it," I said.

He immediately said that his busy schedule never gave him time to think about his weight, but I countered that I have many clients who are just as busy.

Then I lowered the boom. I told Barry that if he meant what he said about having no time to work out, we should stop now instead of wasting each other's time. I explained my deserve level concept, adding that if he wanted to change his health, he would have to believe that he deserved to change his health by making it a priority, just like his work. I explained that he had plenty of wiggle room with his work deserve level, since it was at 100 (an unhealthy high). I knew Barry could afford to give up a few points to fitness and nutrition, but the decision was up to him. He said he couldn't.

"What do you want from me, Barry? Why am I here?" I asked.

He didn't answer. I told him that we could start with one session a week, and he needed to be on time or he'd owe me $1,000 for the missed appointment, since it would be taking time away from someone who really wanted it. He agreed.

It took some time for Barry's deserve levels for health to move from a 1 to a 2, then from a 2 to a 3. It is still slow going, but at least he is seeing positive change. And a 3 is definitely better than a 1.

Recently, I asked Barry what fitness rating he'd like to reach, and he said that a 4 would be good. When I asked why he didn't want to take it higher, he told me that he felt it was all he could do. Barry wouldn't budge even after I explained that this would be like a gym rat whose job is in jeopardy because he refuses to stop taking long lunches at the health club.

We all get to define, expand, or limit our own reality, so Barry's change is slow and plodding. It's sad because he can't see that his work life would actually improve if he took time to exercise, because he'd have way more energy, a better outlook, and a lot less stress—and his work would never even fall close to a 10.

Don't be a Barry. You can let some of your overachieving categories come down so that you can raise up areas of your life that are depleted.

I still work with Barry. At each session we chip away at his deeply ingrained thinking, but it's a challenge. Sometimes being the best of the best at something can detract from other important areas of your life. That's why *Mind Your Body* is all about finding overall balance along with overall success.

Final Analysis: Self-Reflection

Now that you have all your numbers in order, I want you to take a break. Go get a glass of water, do a few stretches, or take a short walk around the block. Come back after fifteen minutes with your notebook and a pen, when your senses are fresh and revived.

Good. Now, go back and review your numbers, then answer the following questions in your notebook.

1. Your overall score

Take a look at your current overall adjusted deserve level scores. You want to have a 9 in each category, and ultimately, by the end of this book, a 10. If you are lower than that, and it's rare that someone starts at the high end, it tells you that you have some work to do. I'm not trying to be a downer; raising awareness is the first step to successful change. Knowing is a good thing. Usually the pressures of life don't allow time to step back and reflect. By looking at all these dimensions of your life at once, you can see if you are in balance or if some areas need more attention. Take a moment to reflect on how you feel about these scores and how you'd like them to change. Write your thoughts in your notebook.

2. Your three bottom scores

Do you see any extreme fluctuations in your scores? For example, if your work is a 10, but family and friends are a 2, it indicates that there is some balancing to be done.

A. Take the three lowest-scoring categories and write them in the first column. In the second column put the rating for each category, and in the last three columns write down the top three feelings you have about these scores. If other feelings come up, you can add them below or on a separate sheet of paper.

Lowest Categories	Rating	Feeling	Feeling	Feeling
1.				
2.				
3.				

B. Now ask yourself, why do you want to feel these feelings? You can't say, "I don't" because *you and only you* allow your scores to be at this level; this is your choice. So dig deep and analyze your feelings to figure out how you are feeding them. Jot down any thoughts in your notebook.

Important note: While we are in control of the vast majority of our feelings, thoughts, and behaviors, some situations and medical conditions call for professional help. This book is not intended to be a substitute for professional therapy or needed medical attention. If you have or suspect that you are suffering from any serious emotional, medical, or physical issues, including major depression, severe anxiety disorder, alcoholism, abusive relationships, untreated diabetes, heart disease, or other symptoms, I encourage you to consult your physician or health care provider to obtain professional medical advice.

C. Do you get attention from others in some way that is actually hurting you in other ways? If you work long hours, for example, maybe it is because you get kudos from the boss, even though it is zapping your home life.

D. Do you honestly believe you deserve better in these areas in your life?

E. On a scale of 1 to 10, how motivated are you to change these scores?

F. If not a 10, why not? Remember, if you don't prioritize your goals or believe you deserve change, chances are good that you won't attract change to you.

G. Write three simple actions you can do now, one for each category. These should be small actionable steps that you can take *today* to improve your numbers in these areas. You might say, "I will leave work at six P.M. today so I have time to exercise or spend time with the family."

1. **Category**   **Action**

_____

2. **Category**   **Action**

_____

3. **Category**   **Action**

_____

H. How likely is it, on a scale from 1 to 10, that you will take these actions today?

I'm not suggesting that you fix every low score today, but this is a beginning to how you can address areas of your life consciously and mindfully each morning, each day, and each week of your life. When you choose to take control, you'll be amazed at how quickly you see positive changes flow into your life.

3. Your Three Top Scores

Now let's take the same steps with your highest adjusted categories by writing them in the first column after this paragraph. In the second column, put the adjusted rating you scored for each, and in the last three columns write down how each of these scores makes you feel. If other feelings come up, add them.

Highest Categories	Rating	Feeling	Feeling	Feeling
1.				
2.				
3.				

A. Again, consider why you want to feel these feelings. Figure out why these ratings are where they are. Do you get attention from others for these categories? In what way? Do you believe you still deserve better in these areas of your life? For example, maybe your fitness rating is an 8, but you'd still like to see it move up.

B. On a scale of 1 to 10, how motivated are you to pump these scores up even higher than you thought possible? Why?

C. Write three actions (one for each category) that you can take *today* to improve your numbers or attention in these areas.

D. How likely is it, on a scale from 1 to 10, that you will take these action steps today? Write down three ideas for how you will make these actions happen.

1. **Category**   **Action**

_____

2. **Category**   **Action**

_____

3. **Category**   **Action**

_____

Be a victor, not a victim. Lose the wishbone and get a backbone.

_____

4. Your Four Middle Scores

After you've reviewed your highest and lowest categories, you will be left with four categories. These are your middle scores.

Write three actions (one for each category) that you can take *today* to improve your numbers or attention in these areas. Write them in your notebook.

1. **Category**   **Action**

   _____

2. **Category**   **Action**

   _____

3. **Category**   **Action**

   _____

5. Final Step: Post Your Intentions

You now have 10 action steps for your 10 categories. Prioritize your actionable steps from easiest to hardest (this is supposed to be subjective). In your notebook, list what you think will be least challenging ("I can do this in a few minutes") to most challenging ("This is really out of my comfort zone").

Easiest

1. _____
2. _____
3. _____
4. _____
5. _____

6. _____
7. _____
8. _____
9. _____
10. _____

Hardest

Write a short version of these on a sticky note, and put them in a row on your desk. For example, if the first item in your list says, "Cleaning stacks of papers off my bedroom floor," then your sticky note would say, "Clean stacks."

When you have all 10 sticky notes in a row on your desk, put this book down and start doing your tasks. After you do the first one, throw away the sticky note, until all 10 notes are in the trash. Throwing away each note gives you a sense of accomplishment and helps you move forward feeling less weighed down, so by the time you have gotten to the hardest one, you have built up confidence and have a flow going. Don't come back until all 10 are off your desk.

Final Words

Now that you've established where you are and where you'd like to go, it's time to get into the design of *Mind Your Body*. We're going to start on the next page by diving into the murky waters of your mind. I'm going to show you the traits of a successful mind and the tools to get one of your own. Put on your thinking cap and turn the page.

PART TWO

GET SET

The Design for Optimal Success

Knowing and putting the following into practice will build up your ability to internalize and adopt the 10 Core Concepts for Optimal Success.

Mindset:	Moves:	Meals:
The Mental Edge Plan	The Enlightened Exercise Design	The Mindful Eating Method
The 10 Traits of the Mentally Fit		
The 10 Brain-Boosting Tools	*The 10 Rules for the Physically Fit*	*The 10 Rules for the Nutritionally Fit*
	The 7 Components of a Successful Workout	*The 10 Tools of the Nutritionally Fit*

4

Mindset
The Mental Edge Plan

Master your mind and re-create your reality,

—SONIA RICOTTI

At the heart of *Mind Your Body* are mental strategies and exercises that will empower you to make true long-lasting changes in all 10 deserve level categories. Yes, I said *all* categories. Even if you already rate high, at an adjusted 9, in some areas, you can still improve, unless you are like Barry (see page 30) and you have an extremely high rating in one category and an extremely low rating in another—then you would focus on the low number to foster balance. If you're thinking that it's impossible to do better, hold on. I used to think this way, too, then I had a better-than-the-best-peach experience, and it changed my frame of mind. Let me explain.

Some time ago, I visited a friend's house, where I saw a bowl of peaches sitting on her dining room table. My friend noticed my eyes resting on the bowl and offered me one, saying, "These are the *best* peaches *ever.*"

"I bet they aren't better than the one I had at the Golden Door Spa in Escondido, California," I thought. "*That* was *the* best peach ever."

However, not being one to turn down free food, I took a bite, and you know what? It *was* a better peach. That experience got me thinking. When I work with elite athletes, they never tell me, "Hey Joel, I just wanted to let you know that I'm the best, so I won't need to train anymore." Never happens. Instead, top-tier athletes always work to improve their game. Similarly, the better-than-the-best-peach taught me a valuable lesson: *You can never really say you've reached your upper limit because there are always greater dreams to dream and better-than-the-best goals to reach.*

One of the reasons we did "adjusted deserve levels" is because of this concept. Even if you think you are at the top of your game in a certain area, I guarantee you that there are always ways to improve.

With that in mind, we'll begin this chapter by considering how your deserve level scores can be improved from the mental angle. Then we'll take a close look at how successful minds function so you'll have a clear model to follow. Finally, you'll learn the essential tools that boost the 10 Core Concepts for Optimal Success that we discussed in chapter 2. You will know how to change how you feel in a matter of moments in order to make the changes necessary to get the results you desire—and you'll feel energized, not deprived, as you work toward your goals.

Improving Your Mental Edge

You have taken your Deserve Level Test and have your 10 deserve level scores, one for each of the 10 categories, as well as an overall deserve level. If you scored below 9 in any of the categories, this is where you will learn how to get your brain on board so you can improve your scores and stabilize the mental imbalances that are keeping you from improving.

If your test produced wildly fluctuating scores—an 8 for work but a 2 for family and friends—you'll want to focus on bringing up that 2 before boosting your 8 any higher. In Desiree's case (page 29), she rated an 8 in fitness but a 4 in nutrition, so we focused on nutrition first. Giving lower ratings more attention by using some of the skills you have in high areas will give you faster results in all areas. When Desiree began to eat healthy, she had more energy to ramp up her fitness. Sometimes, clients are concerned that a high score might drop (that work deserve level might go from an 8 to a 7), but that rarely happens, and if it does, it's only temporary. The benefits you gain from improving a low deserve level will eventually boost your high levels back up to where they were, or even higher. I call this phenomenon *spreading*, because you *spread* the traits of success from a high-scoring category to

a low one. Eventually both scores improve and you balance out overall. The result is a happy, successful, well-adjusted life.

The 10 Traits of the Mentally Fit

In chapter 2, you learned the 10 Core Concepts for Optimal Success, which are central to reaching your goals. To see how this looks in real life, it helps to take a close look at success-oriented people.

Those who thrive in their lives have internalized a deep inner drive that keeps them glued to taking actions that always move them closer to their goals. That doesn't mean they don't encounter setbacks, bump into obstacles, or come upon challenges. Life is still life for all of us, but these people have the passion and self-love it takes to keep on even when times are tough. These are the elite athletes and celebrities who have worked hard to get to the top, as well as the other high achievers in life—you know, those moms, neighbors, and colleagues who seem to glide through without the snags, messiness, or troubles the rest of us seem to have.

Why don't they ever seem to feel hopeless, fearful, or filled with doubt? These are people who live and think in an integrated *Mind Your Body* way, so when the road of life gets bumpy, they have an automatic reaction that quickly gets them back into smooth waters. While these traits may exist more naturally in some people, these are all skills that you can and will internalize by following the *Mind Your Body* program.

1. Follow-Through

People with follow-through say what they mean, mean what they say, and do what they said they would do. People with the follow-through trait practice self-control and spend a lot less time struggling with temptation or decision making. They pick the best plan to reach their goal, then follow through with the actions that will deliver the results they are after.

You don't have to be born with this skill to develop it, but practice is essential. It comes from having a clear objective and steady, reliable habits that support your actions. I should know. I put this trait at the top of the list because it was one of the hardest for me to learn. Today, it is one of the skills I value most.

I attended a Montessori school when I was young, and I was, as my mother used to say, "a mentally floaty child," meaning that I was easily distracted and had a difficult time staying on track. The Montessori school was a good fit because it allowed me to choose what I wanted to learn first, but I still had to learn how to stay on track and study properly to avoid getting bad grades. My parents let me take a summer study program when I was fifteen, which helped tremendously, but it wasn't until I moved from Texas to California to go to college that I really learned the importance of follow-through. Once I got to college, I saw how expensive tuition, books, and classes were, and that got my attention. I wasn't going to waste a dime on bad grades. That's when those study skills became priceless. They paid off. Today, friends and family often compliment me on my self-discipline, and they are surprised when I explain that this trait didn't come naturally, but is a result of dedication and practice.

Making a commitment is serious business. Successful people realize that sticking to a decision, making a commitment, or setting a goal sometimes comes with sacrifices. Being willing to make sacrifices is the flip side of follow-through. Sometimes you have to forgo other opportunities if you want to keep promises. Part of being good at follow-through is remembering to review what's already on your plate. When you practice follow-through, you treat your commitments with the respect they deserve, which earns you trust, admiration, and a stellar reputation.

2. Perfectly Imperfect

A person who is perfectly imperfect is someone who is entirely comfortable with being a flawed human being. They don't take themselves too seriously or think they are better than anyone else.

I frequently attend lectures, and when I do I almost always pick up on a slipup during the presentation. It isn't that the best lecturers don't make blunders—they do, but they trust the free flow of life and have confidence that their minds work just fine. The result is a fluid, resourceful mind that isn't limited by anxiety. A mistake disrupts the flow of the talk only if the lecturer is insecure. Sometimes lecturers flub a word or lose their train of thought—it's a great opportunity to see the different ways minds work. Some speakers freeze up and have a difficult time getting back on track, and you can feel the audience squirm. Other lecturers laugh at themselves, or just pause and take a breath, while still others are so well trained that if they do notice the error, they don't let on. As long as the presenter is comfortable with imperfection, the audience remains engaged. The ability to accept that making mistakes is part of the process of being human allows you to stay calm under pressure. If you tell yourself that *something* is going to happen and it's no big deal—"I'm going to say something wrong and stumble over my words"—it takes the power out of it and allows you freedom to express your most creative self.

The pessimist complains about the wind; the optimist expects it to change; the realist adjusts the sails.

—WILLIAM ARTHUR WARD

---

3. Realistic

Successful people are positive, but they don't live in a fantasy world. They know that changing habits and achieving goals take real work, and they welcome the effort because they know the payoff is worth it. Being an optimist is a great starting point, but if you think things are going to magically change simply because you'd like it to happen, you'll be disappointed. That's not how real life works. You need both optimism and realism to make dreams come true. You have to take both strengths and weaknesses into account, and understand that to accomplish something truly remarkable—swimming the English Channel, for example—takes some serious preparation. You're going to learn all about being an optimistic realist by the time you finish this program.

4. Curious

The curious person is extremely inquisitive, loves to ask lots of questions, and listens with immense interest to the information received. I meet a lot of famous people, and I can tell you that celebrities come in different categories. There are those who feel that they "have arrived," and have nothing left to learn, and there are those who are always hungry to learn more. In my experience, the latter group is the most successful, because they remain teachable. Many actors are in this group; they are like sponges, ready to soak up new information. It's essential to their craft to be adept at morphing flawlessly into ever-changing roles. They are seekers, always inquisitive and trying to see life from a new perspective.

Being curious helps you try new things. You can tap into this trait by being willing to explore a place you've never been or try a new activity. This helps you detach from your regular routine, and to fully recharge, rejuvenate, and grow. The truly prosperous individual understands that curiosity is a key component of personal expansion.

5. Empathetic

It's instinctual to see only one side of an equation—your own! But it takes real skill to recognize the emotions another person is feeling, especially during a heated conversation. People who lack empathy can alienate others and be perceived as arrogant. When you are able to step outside yourself and look at how others are feeling, everyone wins.

If being empathetic doesn't come instinctively, that's okay; it just means you need to practice until it becomes as reactive as sneezing when you smell pepper. This ability can be even more powerful when you apply it in a situation where it isn't *your* responsibility, something I learned firsthand recently.

Not long ago, an appliance repairman came to my weekend house to fix my new stove, grill, and dishwasher. I had been trying to arrange an appointment for more than four months with this man and had been extremely detailed about the make and model of my appliances, giving meticulous information about the problems that I was having with them. Still, when this man arrived at my house, he took one look at the appliances and began complaining that he was missing needed equipment. As I listened, I could feel the pressure building, and as brains will do, mine produced the following thoughts: "You have to be kidding me! This should have been finished *four* months ago! *I* am not being treated fairly! These are new products."

When another person makes you suffer, it is because he suffers deeply within himself, and his suffering is spilling over. He does not need punishment; he needs help.

—THICH NHAT HANH

Had I expressed my sentiment, I'm sure the only thing that would have happened that day would have been a shouting match. Instead, I paused and took a breath. I tried to imagine what it must be like to be this repairman and how frustrating it would be to arrive without the proper equipment. Then I visualized my appliances completely repaired. I pictured myself grilling, boiling water, and running the dishwasher later that evening. I could feel my energy shift from exasperated to empathetic. When the handyman was done talking, I was able to respond with compassion. "Wow, that sounds frustrating," I said, letting him know that I could see the situation from his side. "I am so glad you are here to help me fix these issues," I finished, showing him how much faith I had in him.

Then I waited and trusted. Suddenly, the repairman looked more hopeful. He told me he thought he might have some saved parts in his truck that would work—and he did. Being empathetic toward this man by showing him that I knew the position he was in helped him return the same sentiment to me. He tried harder to find a solution—and we both won.

6. Team Players

Having a team means you have people in your life you can rely on, and vice versa. Having others to lean on is essential to the human animal, and being able to give to others is a trait of the happiest humans. (It gets you out of your own head, for one thing.) People who have close friends, belong to a support network or church, or have close ties to family are all at lower risk for depression and anxiety, and tend to have better health than those who claim to be an island.

7. Always Prepared

This is the person who thinks through everything from every possible angle and imagines all conceivable scenarios—they are *always* prepared. A client I work with is a hugely successful interior designer. Recently, in the middle of a training session that she had squeezed in a few hours before hosting an important dinner party, she got a call that might have upset some of the most unflappable people I know. The cleaners were calling to tell her that the tablecloths were not ready for the event. She didn't miss a beat. She calmly told her staff to tape newspapers to the table and worked it into the decorations. Later I learned that the papers were such a hit that several guests, who were restaurant owners, started using them as a theme at

their establishments. Not only were they economical, the papers were environmentally friendly. Brilliant!

8. Exceptional Recall

Quick and highly capable minds amaze me, which is why I'm always impressed after I spend a session training Dr. Oz and his wife, Lisa. Here's how a typical afternoon at their house goes:

First I work with Dr. Oz. While we are exercising, we're constantly talking, and he always has a bunch of ideas for me. He'll say, "You need to meet this person" or "You must write an article on mindfulness" or "I think you should read this book." When we finish, it's Lisa's turn for a workout. When their training is complete, I go to pick up my backpack from the foyer, and there, next to my bag, is the book Dr. Oz mentioned during our session. By the time I get home and check my e-mail, there's a message from Dr. Oz that details every idea we discussed that day, including phone numbers and links necessary to complete his suggestions.

9. Forgiving

This is the ability to let go of resentment or a wrong that was done to you. The forgiving person isn't someone who denies, minimizes, or justifies a wrong—but they aren't held hostage by it either. They have the ability to let it go, and by doing so, they gain peace and freedom. Studies show that people with highly forgiving personalities tend to rate their lives as highly rewarding, while those who harbor grudges live in mindsets of negativity. Being forgiving boosts your health, according to a study from the *Journal of Behavioral Medicine* that found forgiveness to be as-

---

Holding on to anger is like drinking poison and expecting the other person to die.

—EMMET FOX

---

sociated with lower heart rates and blood pressure, also reducing chronic stress. When you are unable to forgive, you pay the price of sheltering bitterness, and you can pass these negative emotions on to others. The forgiving person grasps that resentments stimulate a state of perpetual toxicity that keeps you trapped. The only way to be truly free and to live in the present moment is to forgive.

10. Presence

Having the ability to live fully in the present moment is a true sign of wisdom. I have had the absolute honor and pleasure of knowing Clive Davis, the American music executive, for more than a decade, and besides having the best memory ever—at eighty-three, Clive can remember the name and exact location of a restaurant we went to years ago in some small European city—he also lives entirely in the present moment. I find it remarkable that Clive is always intensely awake and aware of all that is going on around him; you can feel his electrified energy. When he talks to you, you believe you are the most important person in the room. When people come up to him to take a picture, give him a demo CD, or ask for his autograph, he's never inconvenienced. Clive responds with kindness and grace, asking them, "Where are you from?" or "Who is your favorite artist?" This is the quality of presence in action. Clive realizes that life really is play when you stay in the here and now. He has taught me again and again that love always sells better than hate. This is a skill that will teach you to live fully in the present moment.

This is the real secret of life—to be completely engaged with what you are doing in the here and now. And instead of calling it work, realize it is play.

—ALAN WATTS

The 10 Brain-Boosting Tools

Each of these tools will help you develop the skills needed to internalize the mindset part of the Wholeistic approach. Here you'll find the descriptions of 10 powerful mental strategies to help you maximize success in all areas of your life.

In chapter 9, I'll provide specific, detailed, and doable daily prescriptions for mind-stimulating exercises, as well as some general ideas and themes to focus on each week. For example, on week 2 you'll focus on motivation, and for each day that week you'll do mental exercises that focus on increasing your drive, enthusiasm, and resilience.

Note: How you eat, drink, and move also influence your mental edge. The essential nutritional and physical tools for success will be addressed in the following two chapters.

1. Writing

The act of putting pen to paper is something most of us do every day, from making a simple grocery list, putting a reminder on a sticky note, or leaving a message for a roommate, child, or spouse, to keeping a daily food diary, journal, or exercise log. Writing can help you clarify your thoughts, remember what you did yesterday, and help you get done what you need to accomplish today.

I find writing therapeutic because it helps me get clear on the patterns in my life, and I use to-do lists every day to keep me organized, manage my time, and help me remember those little things that I might otherwise forget. It doesn't take fancy journals or expensive pens. I write my daily list on a used envelope each morning, and at the end of the day I recycle it. The process of throwing away my task list at the end of the day gives me a feeling of satisfaction and accomplishment. It not only keeps clutter out of my house, it keeps it out of my head as well.

I make pro-and-con lists whenever I am in conflict and can't make a decision about a person, opportunity, or circumstance. Taking a few extra minutes to analyze the good and bad on paper provides me with crystal clear direction, and all confusion evaporates.

I also use writing to formulate and keep track of ideas. I've learned from practice that I can have a great idea, but if I don't write it down somewhere I usually forget it, and then something that could have been life changing is lost. I also do this when I wake up in the middle of a dream, even if it is midnight. Dreams often give insight on how to solve a problem or clues about what we want in our lives, but if we don't write them down, dreams quickly fade into the subconscious.

Putting your goals into writing creates commitment. Even if your journal is completely private, it still keeps you accountable because writing by hand taps into complex neural pathways. Handwriting seems to be more powerful than two-handed computer keyboarding because writing requires more fine motor skills than tapping on keys, according to researchers from the National Center for Reading Education and Research in Norway. The researchers believe that writing helps you focus deeply, leading to greater commitment. Many of my clients feel that their commitment to exercise is more concrete when they put it in writing.

Here's a sampling of how writing can benefit your life.

- Enhances problem solving, judgment, and focus.

- Improves mental and physical health.

- Increases self-awareness.

- Enables better goal achievement.

- Clarifies priorities.

2. Meditating

A little dose of doing nothing each day helps improve impulse control, self-awareness, self-control, and stress management. Meditation is the act of focusing on an anchor (often the breath, but also sights,

Joel's Jargon

FLOATING. My term for meditating. When I float, I allow myself—my thoughts, my feelings, and my physical being—to drift by like clouds in the sky. I drift without focusing on any one thing, just letting my thoughts wander where they want. I visualize my mind as a river, and the leaves and twigs floating by are my thoughts. I let them follow the stream. I'm often rewarded with inspiring thoughts and intuitive ideas.

sounds, activities, and so on) and releasing attachment to thoughts, feelings, and distractions. It's a simple practice but not always easy. I love meditating. It helps me quiet the thoughts and opinions of others and myself. Meditation is a great way to shut down the useless mental static that so often runs amok in our heads. It helps me take responsibility for my thoughts, feelings, and actions.

Simply taking a few minutes to watch thoughts and emotions "float" by helps me realize the true nature of what is going on, and that helps me let go. At the very least, I gain clarity and am less likely to automatically or unconsciously react on an emotion that could have unpleasant results.

Sometimes when I meditate, I'll notice a cyclic thought that my mind keeps repeating. I refer to this as "the conveyor belt." These are thoughts I can't seem to get out of my head. After I meditate, I'm able to consciously understand what is underlying the thought. That allows me to let it go.

How can meditation benefit you? Here are several examples:

- Builds willpower.

- Releases negativity and improves mindset.

- Boosts weight loss.

- Magnifies brainpower and memory.
- Reduces stress.

3. Visualization

Visualizing is like previewing directions in Google Maps before driving to a new location. After you've looked at the route, it is easier to find the actual place because you've mentally practiced driving there. Using your imagination to walk through various scenarios does the same thing. Visualizing yourself succeeding at something you'd like to do—losing weight, running a marathon, effortlessly passing up tempting treats—is rehearsing the situation in your mind. Thanks to brain-imaging studies, we know that it works! Remember my designer client who had the trait of being "always prepared" (page 41)? She was able to effortlessly substitute newspapers for the missing tablecloths because she had played out the scenario in her head before it happened.

Mentally picturing or imagining a future event fires off the neural pathways in your brain that light up when you are actually doing the activity. For example, if you close your eyes and see yourself nonchalantly waving off a tray of fried wontons at that upcoming work party next week, then when the actual event rolls around, you'll effortlessly bypass the tempting morsels because your brain believes you already did! In other words, your brain already laid down the tracks for what you want to do, so it takes less effort to stay on track. It's like walking in the footprints of the person in front of you on a snowy day—it's easier because a path has been already prepared.

Athletes from Michael Phelps to Billie Jean King swear by visualization exercises as being central to why they win. Visualization has long been an essential training tool of elite sports. The United States took nine sports psychologists to the Sochi Winter Olympics to practice mental imagery with their athletes.

To get the best results, you must focus with as much detail—sounds, visuals, smells, and feelings—as possible, which you'll learn in chapter 9. It might be all in your head, but using your imagination can bring a plethora of benefits to your life:

- Lose weight.
- Build strength and shed fat.
- Improve self-discipline.
- Curb cravings.
- Reduce pain.

Nothing is either good or bad,
but thinking makes it so.
—WILLIAM SHAKESPEARE

---

4. Affirmations

These statements that you think or say aloud to yourself are designed to change how you feel about yourself, your world, other people, and your perspective in general. They are also used to motivate and energize, to reinforce goals you wish to stick to, and to decrease negative thought patterns. Self-affirmations were popularized by French psychologist Émile Coué in the 1920s in his book *Self-Mastery Through Conscious Autosuggestion*. Coué believed that people could heal themselves by using such statements to mobilize the imagination to reprogram their brains. His most famous affirmation, "Every day in every way, I'm getting better and better," is still used as a common affirmation today. How do affirmations work? The scientific thinking is that when you say, for instance, "Exercise is an inherent, effortless, and enjoyable part of my day," repeating it several times, you create a grooved pathway in your brain (by affirming this thought to yourself) that makes believing the affirmation and committing to it automatic and effortless. In addition, when you fill your mind with positive thoughts, they lead to positive feelings and actions. Your thoughts cause chemical reactions in your brain and body and influence your behavior. If the thought is negative, so is the chemical reaction, which leads to negative feelings and behaviors, and vice versa; positive thoughts yield positive chemical reactions, which lead to positive feelings and behaviors.

I use affirmations constantly for myself and prescribe them to every client during every session. I choose phrases that focus on the most important goals, values, and aspirations you have for yourself in your life. If you want to lose weight, statements that support and reinforce this goal make sense. If it is stress relief and relaxation you are after, use statements about maximizing serenity and tranquillity. Affirmations work because your brain remodels itself based on what you ask it to do, and positive, self-affirming statements do just that—they create neural pathways in your brain that reinforce positive messages. You can use these little magic bullets at right on almost anything because they tap into your unconscious and make it a conscious working part of your mind.

- Improve mood: *"Divine energy flows through me, and I am filled with happiness."*

- Decrease negative thoughts: *"I know that the positive energy of the universe is flowing through me and revitalizing my being." "I accept only positive energy into my mind, body, and life."*

- Increase self-worth: *"I love myself just as I am." "I am lovable and worthy of love."*

- Rev up energy: *"I am radiant, shining, with an abundance of energy." "My body is vibrant, glowing, shimmering with energy."*

- Foster resilience: *"The challenges and obstacles I face are gifts of learning and growing."*

- Promote healthy eating: *"I love nutritionally dense foods that invigorate, strengthen, and energize my body and soul."*

Spreading Affirmations

Affirmations are magic little nuggets of self-nurturing you can give yourself anywhere. When you practice them enough, they become automatic and spread to all areas of your life.

I've learned that one of the best ways to implement affirmations is right when a negative thought arises. I hear plenty of negative thoughts as I'm training my clients because people feel insecure about their performance and voice how they are feeling. For example: "I can't do that, I'm too uncoordinated." "That's too hard for me." "I can't do any more."

My response is usually "I know you can do this. Let's go, and while you're doing five more leg pendulums, please repeat after me, 'I have amazing coordination. I can easily do any and every exercise. I

have an abundance of energy. I can do whatever I want whenever I want to do it.'"

I was working with my client Sylvia recently, who has used these affirmations several times, and she said, "I have to thank you. I was unexpectedly called into a big meeting at work the other day, and my mind immediately started telling me that I wasn't prepared. My chest got tight, and I started to sweat profusely, but then I heard your voice telling me to repeat the affirmations. So I walked down the hall to the meeting repeating to myself, 'I can do anything at any moment in time.'"

Sylvia said she felt great during the meeting, and her boss piped up at the end, boasting to her co-workers, "Do you see why she is on my team? She's a rock star!"

- Improve body image: *"I love my amazing body and all that it does for me." "I am filled with beauty."*

- Set intentions: *"Today I have a plan for living my life passionately and with purpose."*

5. Spirituality

One thing is a sure bet: being spiritual in whatever way works for you equates with success, happiness, ease, and confidence, according to scientific research.

What I have found by nurturing my own spirituality is a deep appreciation for the uniqueness and beauty, the specific purpose, of each of us. Acts of compassion and selflessness or altruism, and the experience of inner peace are all characteristics of spirituality. Taking time to nurture your own spirituality provides physical, mental, and nutritional benefits.

Though neuroscience still can't fully explain it, spirituality seems to stimulate many areas of the brain in beneficial ways. The evidence doesn't give any guidelines about believing in one sort of God over another. Rather, it's just having a belief in something—a deep reverence for life, a feeling of wonder about art, or a deep respect for impermanence, as Buddhists believe. Simply believing in something that is more powerful than little old you helps people make changes, improve health, and overcome obstacles:

- Improves mood.

- Promotes better outcomes after surgery.

- Increases life span.

6. Socializing

When I talk about socializing as a tool, what I mean is the process of cultivating and fostering your social network. This includes family and friends, as well as members of a shared support group, church, or other social group (a knitting circle, Zumba class, or your golf buddies). It also includes acquaintances you make each and every day. This tool refers to any and all opportunities to socialize; while every individual has different needs when it comes to interacting with others (depending on whether you are an introvert or extrovert), it is still important that we all have the maximum deserve level quota of social support.

The beautiful thing about socializing is that there are tons of opportunities to do it every day, and if you do it right (especially when you don't feel like it), you will feel happier, more energized, and more motivated than if you isolate yourself. While it's important to have a regular social network of loved ones, family, friends, and acquaintances, you can also derive much benefit each time you come into contact with any other human being. This can be especially powerful if you are able to share a little kindness or a smile with someone who is grumpy or sad.

Humans are social beings, and there's no paucity of research on the benefits of social interaction. Here are some examples:

- Double your weight loss.

- Boost your brainpower.

- Get sick less often.

- Be happier, less lonely, and more empowered.

- Ease stress.

7. Sleep

Sleep is endlessly fascinating to scientists, probably because no one has yet been able to determine exactly what happens when we sleep. Nonetheless, you know what you feel like after a lousy night of tossing and turning. Your face is puffy, and you feel foggy, crabby, and fuzzy. You can't muster up energy to do your exercise, and you give in to the doughnuts at work that you'd usually pass up. What is known for sure is that when you don't get enough ZZZs, your body and brain don't function effectively. This is partly because when you're tired, your cells don't absorb glucose from your bloodstream as well as they should, then fatigue zaps your self-control and leaves you feeling anxious, irritable, and, of course, exhausted.

Most sleep scientists believe that slumber is a restorative and rejuvenating time for your brain, sort of similar to a computer set to automatically run consolidating functions, debugging programs, and updates at night. Obviously your body does get a mini-hibernation during each night's rest, but your brain is busy consolidating the happenings of your day, playing out scenarios of future hypothetical events, and replaying unresolved past experiences. You also get a chance to replenish your reserves because during sleep the cells in your body and brain rejuvenate and repair themselves.

Unfortunately, we are living in the midst of an insomnia epidemic. As many as 70 million Americans report trouble sleeping, but there is good news. It's fairly easy for most of us to improve our sleep schedules and get the seven to nine hours a night that we should be getting.

If you're still not convinced that you need to change or improve your sleep habits, then review the benefits that healthy rest yields:

- Lose weight and curb hunger.
- Strengthen your immune system.
- Reduce anxiety and depression.
- Increase happiness and energy.

The Sleeping Beauty

I train an actress, Renee (not her real name), who came to me complaining of feeling blah during the hours she most needed energy. When I asked about her sleep schedule, she admitted she was sleeping only four or five hours a night. I asked what her monthly budget was for moisturizer and facial creams. "Hundreds, but I don't know exactly. Cost doesn't matter for my looks. It's worth it," she said.

"Without proper sleep, you can't rejuvenate your face. You are doing more damage than any moisturizer or concealer can fix. You are cutting your career short by prematurely aging yourself," I said. There was no way of being subtle about it. Sometimes you have to be a flying brick to get attention.

My blunt comment did the trick. Renee set herself a curfew and made it happen. She began bringing friends to workout sessions instead of staying up late talking on the phone. The change wasn't immediate, but within a month I could see a noticeable difference. Her eyes went from glazed over to sparkling, and her energy soared. When Renee linked sleep to her looks, she was able to prioritize rest hours.

8. Music

Making, playing, and listening to music does something magic to your brain. Studies have found that when we listen to harmonies, compositions, and songs we love, it helps us exercise longer and harder, and we enjoy it to boot. I have clients pick music to fit their mood that day, and it always helps get a workout pumped up to the maximum level. Each person is different, and everyone has personal preferences. I've had clients that get pumped up listening to sad, melancholy music, others who love big band productions, and still others that love metal rock. It doesn't matter as long as the music "speaks" to you in the moment. It's also important to update your music each time you work out. What sounds good to you on one day may not work at all on another.

Fact: Music is one of the few activities that activates, stimulates, and uses the entire brain.

Thanks to an ingeniously designed study from Germany, we know that making music also increases endurance and strength. The researchers designed gym workout machines to produce music based on how hard people worked out. The harder participants pumped the machines, the louder the music got. Compared to traditional exercisers, the music-enhanced exercisers worked out much harder and longer. Researchers speculate that it may be similar to the way fieldworkers or people on chain gangs sang as they worked. Music seems to trigger the emotional part of the brain, which is mostly unconscious, so your efforts seem diminished but returns are increased. Here are some other scientifically proven benefits music can bring to your mind:

- Work out longer and harder.
- Reduce negative emotions and physical pain.
- Change your mood.
- Make exercise feel effortless.
- Improve sleep.

Although someone else could wash your physical body, only you can cleanse your own soul; you are responsible for polishing it.

—RYUHO OKAWA

---

9. Breathing

Naturally, breathing keeps you alive, which certainly makes it an important tool, but what I'm talking about is using your breathing properly to derive multiple benefits. Yes, it is something you do unconsciously, but most people do it incorrectly most of the time. Breathing exercises can be used in various ways to increase energy, decrease physical pain, reduce anxiety, improve impulse control, increase relaxation, lower heart disease and blood pressure, and enhance serenity. Here are just a few of the benefits of inhaling and exhaling:

- Reduce stress and depression.
- Increase heart health.

- Protect the lungs.
- Increase energy.
- Improve emotional balance and stability.

10. Self-Reflection

This is a tool you have inside your brain that allows you to process and evaluate experiences that result from the outside world combined with your feelings, thoughts, and behaviors. This tool takes the nine strategies to the next level because it teaches you to be, in a very real sense, your own coach. Practicing the first nine strategies as outlined in this book, especially following the daily prescription given in chapter 7, will hone your ability to be your own motivator. That said, I'm not saying that any of us, except those who actually have gone to school to be a therapist, are indeed therapists. I am pointing out that you will gain a wealth of extremely healing knowledge about yourself by learning and implementing this tool. Each of you has the ability to tap an internal wisdom that will guide you to the answers that are right for you, and self-reflection is how you tap this inner wisdom.

Many people aren't aware that they have this tool inside them, while others use it all the time without even realizing it. Using self-reflection means being able to look at your life from a distance to see what change is needed and what patterns are keeping you from your goals. Having awareness is key to taking action to remove obstacles. It is learning to ask the right questions for you and for your growth. You will see the freedom and power that comes from accepting responsibility for yourself and being accountable. Being skilled at self-reflection means that you are able to tell yourself 100 percent of the story with absolute honesty—with all the dark dusty corners revealed. You won't just look at the parts of your life that paint a pretty picture, and you won't go looking for the answers you want to hear. This is about being truthful and looking at the whole picture. It's about becoming fully self-actualized, and that means having the courage to face strengths and weaknesses alike. This is about living life on life's terms and taking the needed action so that you get the results you want in life.

Here are the benefits of self-reflection:

- Improve self-motivation.

- Provide accurate and loving self-awareness.

- Eliminate unhealthy attachments.

- Reduce the need for approval.

- Boost emotional intelligence.

- Promote positive, empowered thinking.

- Increase honesty and clarity.

It is important to examine our thoughts as if they were in a transparent glass box and to consider whether we would be embarrassed if those thoughts were revealed to others.

Final Words

By using the tools and strategies outlined in this chapter, you will come to exemplify the traits of a highly successful person. You will know your limits and honor healthy boundaries. You will be confident, trustworthy, and action oriented. You will know how to have fun and how to laugh freely. You will be optimistic and forgiving, and you will set realistic goals and know how to stick to them. Finally, you will discover strengths you never knew you had, you'll uncover others that have been hidden away, and you'll learn how to put them to use.

The Good Side of Stress

Usually when you hear about stress, it's a bad thing; it makes you sick and can cause high blood pressure, depression, and heart disease, according to many health professionals. It's hard to open a magazine without seeing an article about the harmful effects of stress, but there's a brighter side to your body's natural fight-or-flight system. It is actually your beliefs about stress that determine its effect on your health, according to Kelly McGonical, health psychologist at Stanford University.

According to studies from Harvard and the University of Wisconsin, if you believe stress is a good thing—that it is your amazing body's way of preparing you to meet an upcoming challenge—then you actually trigger positive physiological responses in your brain and body that help you live longer and achieve your goals.

One of these positive responses is the hormone oxytocin. Oxytocin is called the cuddle hormone because it is also released when you hug or are hugged by someone, as well as by other sorts of pleasant social contact. Oxytocin has been shown to protect your heart from the negative effects of stress—and it is triggered by social contact, which means that whatever negative effects might come from stress, you can create stress resilience by helping someone else or letting someone else help you, by having fun with others, or by engaging in other social interactions.

So the next time you feel your heart racing or notice that you are breathing faster, pause and remember that your heart is preparing you for action, your lungs are getting more oxygen to your brain, and hormones such as oxytocin are being released, which will encourage you to take positive action, protect your heart, and help you live longer.

5

Moves

The Enlightened Exercise Design

Fitness is not about being better than someone else.
It's about being better than you were yesterday.

—UNKNOWN

Now that you've read all about brainy matters, let's get physical. It's time to take you through what I do with Dr. Oz and tell you what my private sessions are all about. My 15-minute philosophy of fitness will help you lose weight, tone up, and improve your overall health. You'll also learn how to use time wisely, avoid common blunders, and eliminate muscle imbalances and unnecessary pain. You will become your own expert on the essential components of exercise—proper warm-ups, strength, stretching, balance, breathing, and endurance—and how to incorporate them for maximum benefits.

Improving Your Fitness Deserve Level

In chapter 3, I explained how the goal for all deserve levels is optimization and balance. Turn back now to

My Goal for You

At the end of each workout, I want you to feel energized and tension free.

page 19 and review your fitness deserve level. I find that we can always find room to improve, areas to enhance, and ways to pump up a workout to the next level. The trick is to find your unique needs in regard to fitness. When a client comes to me, I ask a series of questions:

1. How much water have you had in the past twenty-four hours?

If you haven't had enough, it could affect your workout. (If you don't know, see nutrition rule 1 on page 68.)

2. Are you experiencing any tension or discomfort?

If you are having shoulder, neck, knee, hip, or other pain, it needs to be addressed before moving on (for directions for doing this, see pages 209–11).

3. What is your energy level on a scale of 1 to 10?

If you are at a 4 or less, you need to start off slowly and give yourself additional time to warm up. If you push too fast, you can cause injury or deplete your energy before you get to your workout.

4. What is your goal in working out today?

I find that every day and every workout is different. Sometimes it might be about sticking to healthy goals, getting fit, or losing weight; other days you might be looking for an outlet for anger or hoping to feel less sad, anxious, or depressed. Checking in with how you are feeling will guide how gentle or intense you need your workout to be.

The 10 Rules for the Physically Fit

To change your body, you first need to master the following 10 behaviors. For success to be guaranteed, it is essential to ingrain each one into your way of thinking and your daily life.

1. Connect Mind to Body

Your body sends signals and speaks to you, just as your brain uses emotions to alert you about imbalances and manufactures thoughts to suggest options and spur behaviors. The successfully fit person knows to automatically check in with the signals the body gives on a day-to-day basis, and understands that every day will be different. I want you to learn to listen to the signals that your body gives until it becomes instinctual.

By scanning your body from head to toe, you'll learn that you can diminish any discomfort, physical stress, or tension you are experiencing. Since your

The 15-Minute Secret

How can you get done what you need to get done in fifteen minutes? When you do the workouts in this book, you'll understand firsthand how you can address all aspects of your fitness in a quarter of an hour. The other reasons I've chosen fifteen minutes as your baseline exercise program is because everyone can find fifteen minutes a day. I work with extremely busy people, and while they work a full hour with me, I often prescribe the 15-minute workout for off days because I know it is extremely effective. It takes just fifteen minutes of strength training to get all the muscle burning you'd get in thirty-five minutes, according to an Australian study. In another study, from the *Journal of the American Medical Association*, researchers found that doing small bouts of exercise, about ten minutes at a time, improved long-term weight loss, compared to women who exercised for one forty-minute session. I encourage you to move your body more than just during the 15-minute workout, but as far as strength training, stretching, balance, and a good start on aerobic activity go, this is the workout for you.

mind and body create much of what you experience as reality, you also have the power to uncreate it. Whenever something is bothering you, pause and take the steps necessary to fix it immediately (see "Enhance Body Awareness" on page 60 to see how to do this). This is very important to do before exercise to prevent injury. I'm not saying that all physical forms of pain can be simply dismissed, but many can be relieved or greatly diminished.

2. Don't Compare

Every person I meet with has a unique body and an individual goal—as do you. Sometimes a person's goals are realistic and self-respecting, but other times—not so much. If you are five foot one, there's nothing I can do to make you five foot seven. I can show you amazing yoga poses to elongate your body, but you still wouldn't grow half a foot. I can also teach you how to maximize your strength and tone, but if you have a naturally curvy physique you will maintain your curves, as you should. There will always be someone who is in better shape or someone who has more talent in some area. There will also always be someone worse off. My point is that comparing yourself to others is a waste of energy. Period. Stop doing it. Comparing yourself to someone else may temporarily motivate you to try harder, but if what you want isn't realistic or doesn't fit who you really are, it will only be a short-term, flimsy fix that won't last. It is not about who you are *not*. It's about who you *are*.

Comparison is the thief of joy,
—THOMAS EDISON

Whenever I teach people in groups, I see this play out firsthand. Some people are extremely flexible but not very strong, while others are just the opposite. And age or body shape doesn't always matter either. My mom, who is in her seventies, can do some moves that my twenty-something clients struggle to maintain. Does my mom work out more than fifteen minutes a day? Nope. She didn't exercise at all before I got her into doing my short workouts, and now she is more fit than many people decades younger.

Comparing is also just plain bad for your soul. It creates an incredibly judgmental mindset, and if you get in this habit, you will think others are looking at you in the same way. It is an extraordinarily self-defeating attitude, which creates an endless negative cycle that ultimately defines who you are—in a bad way. Free yourself by listening to thoughts as they come up and then letting them float away. Actually watch them drift off into the clear blue sky, gradually getting smaller and smaller until you can't see them, hear them, or pick them back up.

I told you at the beginning of this book how I used to hide because I thought I was too skinny. I was living in a comparing mindset—how could I be "too skinny" without comparing myself? I learned to free myself from that mindset by letting go of comparing. Our society teaches us to believe in a very narrow view of beauty, and I invite all of you to join me on the bandwagon for a more open-minded opinion. We can all strive to be our most beautiful selves. As Oscar Wilde said, "Be yourself; everyone else is already taken."

3. Make Exercise Automatic

We all brush our teeth daily (I hope), and many of us do this multiple times each day. We can't brush our teeth only on Sundays and expect to keep them strong and healthy, right? You've been doing this for so long that's it's probably a well-established habit. I bet you do it without even thinking. Not brushing your teeth isn't an option. Exercise is something to view in the same no-option way. I want physical activity to be a habit that is so automatic you won't even have to think about it. Why? The benefits of exercise are countless. It has been shown to work as effectively as medication to increase fitness and diminish excess weight, depression, heart disease, blood pressure, anxiety, fatigue, cancer, insomnia, and so on—you just can't beat

I have a client named Meghan who is a highly successful photographer. Meghan loves to exercise and especially enjoys the rejuvenated, energized way she feels after stretching. Her story shows how a seemingly unrelated issue can be dealt with during exercise by using questioning, retelling of your story, and exercise to "spread" skills from one area to another to create balance.

Step 1:
Identify the Problem by Listening to Your Body

During a recent session with Meghan, she started telling me how tight and tense her neck was feeling, like the weight of the world was on her shoulders. When I dug a little deeper, Meghan told me about her highly critical and demanding boss. She rattled off a whole laundry list of bad feelings that were triggered around him: jittery, anxious, tense, edgy, agitated, distressed, paralyzed, afraid, and so on. These feelings were signals that wanted to be heard.

Step 2:
Gain Clarity and Perspective

I pointed out that the negative experience was something Meghan could change: "You have the power to delete those negative thoughts and translate those feelings into positive, empowering emotions. It's time to stop unnecessarily giving your boss your power. It's time to take it back," I told her. "Your feelings create loaded thoughts, but you have the choice to buy into them or not."

I went on to explain that all human beings are made with minds that construct thoughts based on what we experience. Most people don't know that they have the power to choose which thoughts to discard.

Step 3:
Dissect the Issue

"But he's always rapid-firing questions my way, and even though I can answer 95 percent of his questions, there's still 5 percent that I can't," she countered.

I pointed out that 95 percent was quite high, and maybe she was being too hard on herself. Meghan agreed that most of the issues she couldn't respond to related to photo shoots that hadn't happened yet, so she couldn't possibly have had the answers.

Step 4:
Investigate Positive Possibilities and "Tell a New Story"

Next I had Meghan investigate her boss's intent. Meghan told me that being a photographer for a major paper in New York was an intensely deadline-driven job. After giving it some thought, she admitted that her boss was probably just trying to be efficient and that his brusque style wasn't personal. "I guess he is just respecting how busy I am and trying to rapidly fire off questions to save time," Meghan told me. We decided that this would be the "new story" she would adopt. Meghan responded that she could already feel her stress dissipating.

Step 5:
Spread the Physical to the Mental

By this point you might be asking yourself, "What the heck does this have to do with exercise?" Remember I mentioned at the beginning of Meghan's story how great she felt after stretching? This physical sensation can be "spread" to the mind-based experience she has with her boss.

Meghan and I agreed that the next time she met with her boss, she would schedule a few minutes before the meeting to do stretches.

Step 6:
Follow Through

(Remember that follow-through is one of the essential traits of the mindfully fit person, described on page 39.)

The following week, I checked in with Meghan to see how her new tools were working. "We had a meeting yesterday, and just as we discussed, I reminded myself that my boss's intention was to not waste my time, to be efficient, so I took five minutes and did the stretches we agreed on, *then* I headed to his office. Bam! He fired off questions just like always, but I remained calm, cool, and confident throughout. I wasn't distracted by my shoulders and neck tensing up, so it freed my mind. And I even heard myself offering suggestions and answers before he had thought to ask about them. I could tell he was impressed and pleased. And I even raised some issues he hadn't thought to address," she said.

Meghan had quickly learned to identify the relationship between body pain and mental tension, and she was able to shift her perspective by tapping into her mind's ability to tell a new story. Meghan also learned to use stretching to relax mental tension and prevent future body tension. Incorporating these skills helped her increase her resilience and empowered her. At later sessions, we were able to move to more advanced work because we had resolved the true cause of her neck and shoulder issues.

it. Once you make exercise an automatic part of your life, you'll have one of the Core Concepts—number 7, Extinguish Escape Routes, page 10—nailed down.

4. Release Tension Immediately

Whenever you feel tension in your body, you need to get rid of it immediately. You don't deserve it. You wouldn't go around with food stuck in your teeth. You'd floss the debris right out. If you didn't, bacteria in your teeth would lead to larger issues such as cavities, gum disease, or root canals. It's the same with your body, but many people ignore warning signals such as stress, tension, strain, or tight or painful muscles or tendons, and they end up with serious injuries that can lead to surgery, disability, or both. Body tension, like mental tension, is a sign of imbalance that should never be ignored. Once identified, tension needs to be addressed immediately and dispersed. If it isn't addressed, a muscle imbalance will eventually throw your whole body off, and what may have started as a small twinge in your lower back will trickle to other areas, perhaps causing severe hip, back, knee, neck, shoulder, or ankle pain.

People come to me all the time looking for a solution to pain and tension. About 95 percent of the time, these complaints turn out to be muscle imbalances. Many people who complain about back pain are really experiencing hip tension that is throwing their back off, while most people who experience neck tension actually have tight shoulders (see page 210). Got achy knees? Most likely muscle imbalances in your quads, calves, and shins are pulling on your knee joints. Think of the old song, "Your hip bone's connected to your thigh bone; your thigh bone's connected to your knee bone," and it makes sense. If one area is hurt, it will affect other parts of your body. The key is to find the source and correct the imbalance.

5. Get Plenty of Sleep

We've talked about the importance of sleep for maintaining a healthy mind, but getting your rest is just as important for your physical body. Unless you have a times you can change your hand position slightly to target different parts of the same muscle. Seemingly minor adjustments make huge differences. The workouts in this book are designed to do just that. I also schedule workouts so that you are targeting different body parts on different days, so your muscles can repair themselves with time and proper nutrition. Strength training tears down muscle fibers, and your body responds to this fatigue by rebuilding with more and stronger muscle fibers. That's one reason you can get so much done in just a quarter of an hour.

Balance is another benefit to working your body from a variety of angles. This also helps prevent injury that could result from repetitive routines. The workouts provide pain release and tension relief because they are designed to correct body parts that are out of balance. For example, you can't have a strong, pain-free back without strong belly muscles; that's why we work abs and back, not just one or the other.

newborn baby, nothing is worth sacrificing sleep. As discussed in chapter 4, you won't have the energy to stick to your goals, especially to exercise, without getting your quota of sleep. The guidelines say to aim for seven to nine hours a night, but if you are a napper, you may be able to make do with a six-hour night and an hour nap. Whatever your sleep cycle is, respect it and stick to it. You can't catch up on sleep once you've lost it. Trying to make up for a week of no sleep by sleeping in on Saturday is like trying to brush your teeth for twenty extra minutes to make up for not brushing for three days straight.

6. Work Every Muscle from Every Angle

To have a truly sculpted and sleek body, be careful not to just work a muscle from one side or work the same muscles repeatedly. When you do a bicep curl, for example, you work the front part of your upper arm, which is good. However, to have a truly sculpted upper arm, you need to vary the angle from which you target your upper arm muscles. Sometimes this comes from moving your arms in different patterns; other

7. Mix It Up

Your muscles have a memory, and if you do the same exercises all the time, your body and mind get used to them, and you start to burn fewer calories. When you start an aerobics class, for example, and you feel uncoordinated, that is actually a good thing. Not knowing what you are doing engages more muscles and burns more calories than doing an exercise routine that your body is accustomed to. Variety is the key to challenging your muscles; that is how you get maximum results.

I want you to get it in your exercise mindset to crave doing something different every time. I've made this easy by incorporating plenty of variety into the daily workouts in chapter 7, but I want you to break the mold in other areas as well.

8. Be Your Own Cheerleader

I teach my clients to be their own cheerleaders. Yes, a rah-rah-rah, get your pompoms on type of cheerleader. I want to share my message and train lots of people, but ultimately I want to put myself out of a job. I want you to be 100 percent motivated and invested

Recipe for a New Habit

Scientists who study habits now understand that while you can never truly eliminate a habit, you can effectively reshape a bad habit into a good one. The trick is in applying the time and effort to analyze the existing behaviors that make up an undesirable habit, identifying what makes it happen, and then replacing key elements to change undesirable behaviors into desirable ones. Here's how:

At the core of every habit is what neurological scientists call a loop that consists of three parts:

1. A cue: what tells your brain to start the pattern

2. A routine: the pattern of behavior or habit you are creating

3. A reward: what makes your brain learn to crave the routine

To create a new habit—making sure you do the 15-minute exercise *routine* as prescribed in chapter 7, for example—you need to choose a *cue*, like laying out your workout clothes and this book, with the page for tomorrow's workout marked, the night before. Then pick a *reward,* like spending thirty minutes on Facebook, watching a new episode of *Game of Thrones,* or eating a square of dark chocolate. Choose something you can do immediately after exercising so you feel the connection between the two. After several days, when you see your workout clothes laid out, your brain will start craving the reward (choose the one that works best for you). After a week or two, you can start to phase out the planned rewards, because simply doing the routine and feeling the benefits of the exercise will be reward enough.

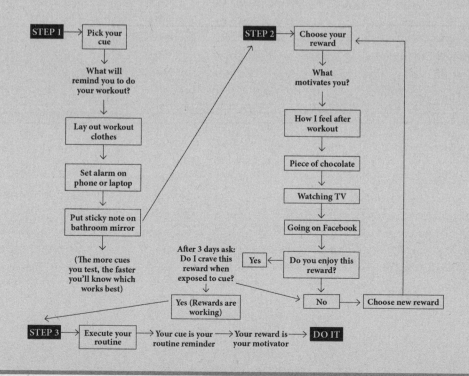

The Other Twenty-Three Hours and Forty-Five Minutes

While the bulk of your workout will be done during the 15-minute routine prescribed in chapter 7, that doesn't mean I'm giving you permission to sit on your butt for the rest of the day. To see the best results—and to see them happen fast—you need to get in the habit of including daily behaviors that add up to at least an hour of moderate-intensity activity. This doesn't have to be exercise in the formal sense, but if you enjoy doing aerobics, running, swimming, biking, hiking, tennis, and so on, fantastic! Otherwise, you can find tons of ways to move your body for at least sixty minutes a day. Consider the following:

Just Sit Less

There are tons of ways to do this, and all of them reduce your risk of heart disease, diabetes, cancer, and obesity. Be on the alert for any time you can get moving. Ideally you should get in 10,000 steps a day. If you'd like to see how you are doing, pick up a pedometer to track your steps or buy an app that will do so on your smart phone. Here are just a few ideas:

- Be a pacer. Whenever your phone rings or you make a call, get up and move. Even if you are just walking back and forth in your office, you'll more than double the calories you'd burn while sitting in your chair.

- Make appointments to move. Ask colleagues if they'd consider having a moving meeting. This is especially creative if you tend to work at your desk during lunch. Lace up and stroll while you talk strategy. If you think your boss might be hesitant, point out that moving meetings have the benefit of increasing circulation to brain neural pathways, which increases mental acuity and makes you more productive overall.

- Walk your errands whenever possible. Take an extra-long stroll to the post office. Just need a few items from the grocery store? Strap on a backpack and hit the pavement—or, better yet, get a basket or saddlebags for your bike and go on bigger trips, too.

- Always choose the farthest parking spot, and never use the elevator.

- Move once an hour. The human brain cannot concentrate for more than forty-five or fifty-five minutes, so take advantage and stretch or stroll once an hour. Get up and drink a glass of water, walk to the farthest restroom, or go talk to a co-worker instead of sending an e-mail.

- Create active family time. Instead of watching a movie, take an after-dinner stroll. Walk the dog together, go for weekend family bike rides, play Frisbee or catch.

- Whenever your computer spins its wheel or goes to its screensaver, or if your foot falls asleep, use it as your cue to walk into the other room and have a glass of water.

in training yourself, because this will give you the motivation you need to push yourself to the next level. When, for example, I've prescribed a set of twenty-five crunches but you are only feeling the intensity at a 6 (on a scale of 1 to 10), I want you to adjust to thirty-five reps or more, until you feel the effort at a 10 (see "The 1-to-10 Burn Scale" on page I-4). That's how you keep improving.

I'll teach you how to play mind games like this one, which I play with clients who try to shortcut exercises. If I catch someone trying to stop short of what I've prescribed and what I know they can do, I count in the opposite direction. (I always count down so there is a finish line. It seems like a small thing, but trust me, with finish-line counting you get a feeling of accomplishment and can always go farther than if you count up.) So if a client stops at 3, I start counting up until she or he starts doing the exercise again. When I see the client moving, I go back to finish-line counting. Try it and you'll see that you can always do more than you think you can. When you begin to see that you *can* do more, you'll push yourself for more, not less.

9. Reward Yourself

All winners know to reward themselves for a job well done. Remember the tenth Core Concept, Jump for Joy, is all about the importance of celebrating your successes. Rewards are a great way to reinforce that

The Best Time of Day to Exercise

People are always asking me about the best time of day to exercise, and my answer is always the same: the best time is the time that is right for you.

What does that mean? Each of us is different, and no person, magazine, or newspaper article should tell you what time of day to exercise. You are your own best expert, and you can learn what's best for you by listening to your body and mind. It's pretty simple: exercise when you feel best and are most successful at following through on your fitness goals. Here are a few examples:

- I have a client named Anthony who works out in the morning because he knows this is when he is most energetic. "It invigorates me, gets my blood pumping, and it sets the pace for the rest of my day," says Anthony. A couple of times, Anthony had to reschedule to an evening training session. I could tell immediately that he was out of sync. He was sluggish and couldn't wait for our session to be over, and later he told me that he hadn't been able to sleep. Lesson learned—morning exercise is best for Anthony.

- Another client, Samantha, is a sunset exerciser. Samantha knows that she needs to start her day off at a slower, more relaxed pace. "My job is super fast paced, and at the end of the day I'm wound up and overstimulated. After I leave the office, a workout is the perfect way to settle down and transition into my evening. I arrive home in a relaxed state of mind and can go right to sleep," says Samantha.

- While most people lean toward either morning or evening workouts, there are also people I call "floaters," who have schedules that vary from day to day. They are able to successfully exercise by evaluating each day's schedule and fitting in a workout whenever their gut tells them it will work. Floaters like spontaneity and variety, and they enjoy not exercising on autopilot.

What type are you?

you are worth effort and time. Put rewards on your calendar once a week. However, remember that rewards come only after you do the work. While this might seem obvious, I have a family member who will give himself the reward even if he skips his workout. Not surprisingly, he never gets around to doing the exercise—and sadly, he's unable to lose his excess weight. With this in mind, only treat yourself *after* you've put in the time.

My personal favorite reward is a massage. It's the perfect way to give a gift to yourself for moving your body consistently. When was the last time you got one? Your muscles need it, and I recommend one every other week. In fact, I insist. Many health insurance companies now reimburse for massages, so take a moment and check. If money is not an issue, get one every week. Choose what stimulates, rejuvenates, and relaxes you.

10. Be Consistent

This is the most important rule because it ties together the previous nine, not to mention the third Core Concept for Optimal Success, Cultivate Grit. You must be steady with your workouts and exercise, or your progress will be much slower than you desire. I can't stress enough how essential this is. One reason you can get the results from *Mind Your Body* in just fifteen minutes is consistency. You must make every minute of the fifteen count. Doing otherwise would be like expecting to become fluent in Spanish but only studying sporadically. *Perseverance is not a long race; it's many short races one after the other.*

Keep Your Eyes Up

Whenever you are walking, make sure you keep looking above eye level. When you let your gaze drop, your shoulders tend to follow. Most people have bad posture because when they look down, their shoulders and back slump. Look toward the horizon to immediately fix your posture.

Enhance Body Awareness

Before and during workouts, I want you to get in the habit of doing a quick body scan to get a feel for where you might be out of balance. People get hurt when they aren't aware of imbalances and tension. *You might not even think you have any imbalances* until you do this. This short exercise creates body awareness. Your goal is to have zero tension 24/7. Here's how to scan your body:

1. Sit up straight in a chair with arms and legs uncrossed, and act like a string is pulling the top of your head away from your tailbone, elongating your spine. You can close your eyes if it helps you focus.

2. Take a few deep breaths, and then, starting at your head, begin to scan each body part.

3. Bring your attention to your head and face. Feel any tension in your facial muscles, your forehead, the top of your head, the back of your head. Take a deep breath and release any tension as you exhale. Visualize tension flying out of your ears.

4. Now bring your attention to your neck and shoulders. Turn your head from side to side, bring your ear to the right shoulder, then to the left, do a few shoulder circles forward and back, and shrug your shoulders up and down. Take a deep breath and release any tension as you exhale.

5. Moving down your body, bring your attention to your upper and lower back. Notice any pain or tightness there. Breathe deeply through this area and allow your muscles to relax. Feel the tension releasing and flying away.

6. Focus your attention on your stomach. Pay attention to how it moves as you breathe in and out. Release any tension as you exhale.

7. Turn your attention to your hips, butt, and thighs. Tense up all the muscles in this area, then relax. Repeat this by contracting muscles when you inhale, then releasing all tension as you exhale.

8. Now, bring your attention to your calves and shins. How do they feel? Visualize breathing air into these areas and then exhaling out any tension.

9. Finally, bring your attention to your ankles and feet. Circle your feet to the left and then to the right. Flex and point your feet and toes. Wiggle your toes. Release any tension.

10. If you noticed any areas of your body that were painful or overly tense, take time to do a few extra stretches for these areas. Turn to the workouts insert for stretching suggestions for your whole body.

The 7 Components of a Successful Workout

Now that you've got the 10 rules for achieving your maximum levels of fitness, let's take a look at what you'll need to build a successful workout. I believe there are seven essential components to full body fitness: warm-up, strength, flexibility, balance, coordination, breathing, and heart strength. In chapter 7, you'll find a prescription for exercise that will incorporate all this, but I'm sure you want to know the reasoning behind the exercises you'll be doing. Plus, I want you to be empowered to put together a top-notch workout all on your own. I model all workouts after my highly successful training sessions, so let me explain how I attend to critical areas to make each workout amazing.

To do this, you must completely understand what the word *burn* means when I apply it to working out. When you are working a muscle and you feel it getting warm but not hurting, that is the burn. If something is painful, hurting, clicking, or aggravating, *stop*. It's never good to be in pain while working out. Every body is different, and as I've previously mentioned, you must always listen to your body. If a move doesn't feel right to you, you need to stop and figure out why, fix it by adjusting, and only proceed if you feel the proper burn, not pain. Burning means toning, firming, and strengthening the muscle. In my sessions, clients often remark, "Wow, this hurts," and I always check in to make sure they are experiencing heating or burning, not pain or irritation. If it is the latter, we stop, fix, and then proceed. Sometimes this means making a slight adjustment to the move, grabbing a towel for a cushion, or other solutions (you'll see suggestions in the workouts insert).

1. Warm-up
Giving your body time to transition from being stationary to being active is crucial before every workout because it gives your body time to increase circulation, warming joints, tendons, and ligaments, and because everyone has muscle imbalances. Often you don't know you have a tight or tense area or imbalance until you start moving your body. If you jumped right into a challenging exercise without limbering up, you could cause serious injury. Warming up gives you time to stretch out these areas and connects your body to your mind (rule 1 for the physically fit, page 52). Since shoulders and hips are common areas of tension in most people, I suggest doing arm rolls and hip rolls during every warm-up to get the blood flowing. These are especially important if you are a side sleeper and work out in the morning, or if you work at a computer all day long.

2. Strength
The moves I include to build strength do not build bulky muscle. First of all, muscle is much more compact

and sleek than fat, so it really isn't a worry for most people. Muscle is also a benefit because it burns more calories than fat, it gives you more energy so you can do more during your day without feeling fatigued, and it helps your body protect itself from injury.

3. Flexibility

I am a big believer in incorporating stretching into each workout because I see and experience firsthand the benefits of opening up and elongating the muscles immediately after they've been fatigued. Stretching reduces immediate soreness and keeps flexibility maximized so you stay limber and protected from injury and imbalance. The workouts in the "Moves: Your 15-Minute Workouts" insert incorporate stretches with strength moves for this reason. Doing exercise in this sequence leaves your body open, free of tension, and energized. Plus it uses time wisely by not compartmentalizing stretching at the end of a workout.

Stretching should always feel good. A stretch should be gentle and feel invigorating; never force a stretch. When people force a stretch by pushing farther and faster than their body is ready for, it causes muscles to lock and may cause damage. For all stretches except dynamic ones, you'll get into the position and then concentrate on feeling the tightest area in the stretch, breathing deeply into it while visualizing a huge balloon, and releasing the tension. This encourages you to bring oxygen into the area, which increases fresh blood circulation (full of nutrients and oxygen), and encourages the muscle to gradually open. Stretching should always feel good. Think of it as a way of massaging your muscles from the inside out.

There are four types of stretches: passive, dynamic, active, and resistant. The first two stretches can be done before or during your warm-up, whereas the latter two are safe only after your body has been fully warmed up.

- Passive stretching uses your body and gravity, so you put yourself into the position and relax by using your body's weight. The goal is to release tension and melt into a passive stretch.

- Dynamic stretches are popular in warm-ups used in sports. They are active movements of muscle that bring forth a stretch but are not held in a stationary position. In dynamic stretching, you are continuously moving to gently target and improve your range of motion.

- Active stretches, or as I call them, crank poses. There is a point where you can pull or push (a crank) and intensify the stretch. These are best done when you are warmed up. The goal is to relax into an active stretch.

- Resistant stretches are those that use some sort of resistance (a wall, another person, or yourself). You press against it for fifteen seconds, then release and gently go deeper into the stretch for twenty seconds.

4. Balance

The older we get, the more likely we are to lose our sense of balance. Being young is no guarantee you have good balance either. I work with teens and young adults all the time who have poor balance. I even work with a Broadway dancer who has poor balance. *I'm talking about a Broadway dancer.* You would think she would have mastered balance. Not so. Some of my simpler poses are tricky for her. So it's something that everyone needs to practice. I've incorporated balance exercises into each workout so you will get all the practice you need in your 15-minute workout. I also encourage you to practice balance by standing on one foot or on your toes whenever you are talking on the phone or standing in line. While doing these exercises, turn your head to look to the left and then to the right. Your goal is to get to where your body doesn't wobble. The more you practice balancing exercises, the better you'll be.

5. Coordination

Remember trying to pat your head and rub your belly as a kid? This is the classic exercise that many gym teachers use in elementary schools to tap and train coordination. Coordination exercises recruit and trigger complex motor pathways, which is good for your brain and your body. Complex movements build neural connections through your entire being, which help make you sharper and more agile in the way you think and move. Coordination exercises also develop faster reactions so you can self-correct when you trip or begin to lose your balance. And they're fun. I incorporate coordination into all workouts, with moves that have body parts doing different things simultaneously (one hand making an arc, the other making circles, for example).

6. Breathing

I've never worked with someone who has perfect breathing. The problem is that people think breathing should happen automatically, and they don't realize that you can control and improve how you breathe to get the results you want. Many people also hold their breath during exercise, which is extremely dangerous and spreads tension to many areas of the body (see "How to Breathe Properly During Exercise," page I-5). The key is to keep your breath flowing so you become the master of the movement being prescribed. You control your breathing; the movement doesn't control your breathing. When I find that clients are holding their breath, I tell them to count the reps out loud, because you can't count and hold your breath at the same time. If you notice that you are straining or holding your breath, try counting.

7. Heart strength

What you call cardio, aerobic, or cardiovascular exercise, I refer to as "heart strength," because it more ac-

curately describes the benefits you'll derive from any heart-pumping activity. Your heart is a muscle just like your biceps; it needs to be exercised. Any exercise that gets your heart rate up helps shed overall body fat and improves fitness, but it also is the best sort of exercise to strengthen and improve heart health, not to mention lungs and overall circulation. And when you get your heart rate up, all parts of your body benefit, including your brain. You move the larger muscles of your body when you do cardio—jumping jacks, jumping rope, fast walking, swimming, tennis, running, and so on—which demands more oxygen, making your breathing increase and your lungs work harder. Your body demands more oxygenated blood, so your heart must beat faster to supply this needed blood. So, while it feels like you are exercising the outside of your body, you are actually exercising your insides just as effectively, and this improves fitness rapidly because you nourish your entire body, inside and out.

Spend just thirty minutes taking a brisk walk, riding a bike, or going for a run, and you'll pump extra oxygen-rich blood to your brain, delivering nutrients that improve memory, problem-solving ability, and decision-making skills. Translation? You'll have more mind muscle to stick to your goals. Exercise also increases the mood-boosting brain chemicals serotonin, dopamine, and norepinephrine, which help with focus, impulse control, and motivation.

Final Words

Now that we've got your mind and body plans down, it's time to add the final piece of my Whole-istic approach—the nutritional plan. In the next chapter, you will receive all the nutritional guidelines, mindful eating strategies, and rating scales for hunger that you will need to gain more energy, feel more balanced, and lose weight steadily and effortlessly.

6

Meals

The Mindful Eating Method

Tell me what you eat and I will tell you what you are.

—JEAN ANTHELME BRILLAT-SAVARIN

Food. We need it to survive. Food is fuel. The saying "You are what you eat" is so true. You can see how people eat by their level of energy, by their attitude, and by physical features such as eyes, skin, hair, and weight. I often hear complaints from people who exercise strenuously and frequently at the gym that they aren't seeing the results they want, and my first thought is "I wonder what that person eats?" (Remember Desiree? See her story on page 16.) What you put in your mouth is key to how you feel, how you look, and what you accomplish. I can't stress enough how vital a healthy diet is to your overall balance and success.

In this chapter, you'll learn to listen to what your body is saying about how and what you eat. The mindful eating method is designed to give you maximum enjoyment and help you lose excess weight. You will learn to make some new meals, so give yourself time to adjust. You will make changes that might feel challenging at first, but don't fret. Remember that making changes often triggers a little discomfort. That's perfectly okay. You are not alone. If you feel frustration, just take a few deep breaths, relax your eyes, massage your temples, and be assured that this plan is designed to uncomplicate your life, to leave you feeling satisfied, confident, peaceful, and centered. You're also about to discover how changing this one area of your life will spread and improve many other deserve level categories.

Your Nutritional Deserve Level

Now let's revisit the nutrition deserve level rating you gave yourself in chapter 3 (page 20).

How did you do? Write your rating here_____. If your end score was an 8 or lower, you need to look closely at this area. Where do you feel you could improve? What are the top three changes that could be made to your nutrition? I have a client Farah who needed to address eating times to increase energy and decrease hunger so she didn't overindulge in the evenings. We focused on dinner and snack planning strategies to improve her nutrition and help her lose weight. Problem solved!

People tend to underestimate their unhealthy eating habits, so this is an area where I really dig for the truth, and I encourage you to be ruthlessly honest with yourself as well. I always tell my clients, "You've got goals—let's accomplish them," and I say the same to you! Time is a limited resource, and most of us have jam-packed schedules. This isn't about judging, humiliation, or shame; this is about getting an honest and accurate picture of your eating habits so you can quickly address what is tripping you up.

In your notebook, write down the three areas you'd most like to improve. For example, staying out of the candy dish on your co-worker's desk, corking the nightly glass of wine, or clearing the freezer of mint chocolate chip ice cream.

This is part of living in reality. Now you have identified three ways you'd like to change, so you can be your own best coach. With this in mind, write in your notebook three ways that you can change these habits. Think about this as if you were giving advice to a really

Why You Should Eat Organic

Eating organic is where it's at. In almost every way, research now shows that not only are foods without additives, toxins, or pesticides better for the environment but they are the only thing you should be putting in your body. Consider the following findings shared by researchers from the agricultural division at the University of Minnesota, University of Washington researchers, the president's 2010 Cancer Panel Report, Washington State University, and the United States Department of Agriculture:

- Organic foods are higher in levels of beta carotene, cancer- and heart disease–fighting antioxidants, essential minerals, good fats, and vitamins C, D, and E.

- Organic products are produced and processed without synthetic fertilizers, growth hormones, artificial ingredients and preservatives, or genetic engineering.

- A diet composed of organic foods instantly and dramatically eliminates exposure to pesticides known to cause neurological damage in developing infants and children.

- Organic foods cut in half the incidence of some forms of cancer.

- Organically grown tomatoes are nearly 80 to 100 percent higher in various cancer-protecting antioxidants and bioflavonoids.

- Organic grapefruits are higher in health-promoting ascorbic acid and flavonoids, and lower in cancer-causing nitrates.

- Plants grown organically are exposed to water that is 60 percent lower in nitrates.

good friend who needed help. What would you tell a friend who was struggling with these food issues?

To help my clients establish mindful eating, which is at the core of healthy eating for a balanced mind, body, and weight, I usually ask my clients within the first five minutes of our first training session to rate how well they eat on a scale from 1 to 10 (1 meaning awful and 10 being perfect). This quickly gives me an idea of what sort of work clients need to do to balance their eating patterns and nutrition deserve level. It tells me how they feel about their nutrition and whether they take ownership of what they put in their mouth. I want you to learn to do this, too.

For example, if a client rates her eating as a 6, we know we have work to do. It's the same for you. If you gave yourself a 6, think about it in terms of a school grade. A 6 would translate to a 60, which is a failing grade in school. If you want to stay at an F for food, then you won't change anything.

I want you to carry this 1-to-10 mentality with you all the time. It will help you stay on track around food. If you are at a dinner party, for instance, you can use the 1-to-10 game plan there by rating foods on the buffet table. The almonds, hummus, and veggies all get a 10, while the cookies and brownies get a 1. Aim to average out your 10 choices to maintain a 9 or above. That means you can eat only one food at a 1, and the rest must be at the top end of your game plan. Ideally you'll skip the 1 altogether, but if you've planned a treat, you can consciously decide to indulge while still staying true to your nutrition deserve level.

The *Mind Your Body* Menu and Recipe Design

I have designed my recipes to offer variety that packs a nutritional punch. Most people tend to find foods they like and then stick with them, perhaps adding something unhealthy because they think low fat or healthy is bland. But you'll soon see this isn't the case.

It's great to eat what you enjoy, and I support that, but I also want you to get the variety it takes to maximize the vitamins, antioxidants, and nutrients your body needs to function optimally.

I'll teach you how to mix it up without messing it up. For example, whenever you are at a restaurant, scan the menu and order a healthy option that you don't normally have or cook at home, which will work to increase your satisfaction and your need for variety. In my recipes, you'll find a wide spectrum incorporated into the design so you don't have to think about it. It's essential to delight in what you eat. If you don't enjoy it and it doesn't taste good, why bother? Life is too short. As you'll see in chapter 10, I have concocted recipes that are of the finest nutritional quality, quick and easy to prepare, and designed to last for many meals. Plus, you'll be introduced to items you may have never tried before. Before you decide you aren't going to like something, try it first—you may surprise yourself. When I was experimenting in the kitchen for this book, my mom saw the Vegan Chocolate Mousse (page 204) and said, "This sounds awful, I'm definitely not eating that." But she gave it a taste. Turns out she loved it and has made it for my dad several times since then. You'll love it, too—trust me.

As long as you keep an open mind, I know you're going to fall in love with the unique dishes you'll learn to make, both for their nourishing substance and because they are easy to make and taste delicious.

As far as the daily composition of your food, you'll get around 30 percent of the leanest, healthiest protein, 30 percent healthy fats, 40 percent healthy carbohydrates, and at least 30 grams of fiber per day.

The 10 Rules for the Nutritionally Fit

The following rules are eating and drinking guidelines that I follow myself and prescribe to all my clients. While no one is perfect, my most nutritionally successful clients tend to feel the best, reach their goals faster, and have the most energy. They allow themselves some room for error but always aim to maximize healthy and minimize unhealthy. For the next twenty-eight days, I want you to follow these rules exactly.

1. Hydrate Right

Drink a sixteen-ounce glass of room temperature water when you wake up every morning. Keep it next to you on your nightstand. Drink up within the first ten minutes of consciousness.

Why?

Most people I know don't drink enough water. By starting off your day with 2 cups (16 ounces) of water, you'll begin to reap the benefits of right hydration. Staying hydrated is essential to a healthy body and mind. More than half the human body is water. As babies, we start out being around 75 percent water, and by the time we reach our golden years, that falls to around 55 percent.

The Power of Hydration

Water is good for you in so many ways. Here is a sampling of the importance of proper hydration:

- **Eases headaches.** Did you know that 85 percent of migraines are caused by dehydration? It makes sense when you realize that your brain is 73 percent water. Not getting enough water can trigger headaches and migraines, according to British researchers from Loughborough University and the City of London Migraine Clinic. The Migraine Clinic also found that you can get headache relief in as little as thirty minutes from drinking a glass of water (taking a couple of painkillers takes about forty-five minutes).

- **Protects your heart.** When you are dehydrated, your blood thickens, which puts more demands on your heart because it has to work harder pumping dehydrated blood through your veins. Getting in the habit of starting off your day with water will help ease the demands on your heart.

- **Balances body temperature.** Being properly hydrated is central to how your body maintains a safe temperature. The human body regulates its temperature by sweating (loss of water and salt) when you heat up, because of the outside temperature or your activity level. When you are highly active and sweating, your body can lose over eight cups of water in one hour. Having your morning water will jump-start your hydration.

- **Improves thinking.** When you drink water, it increases your alertness, according to British researchers from the University of Bristol. In another study, Ohio University researchers found that dehydration diminished alertness, decreased the ability to concentrate, and reduced short-term memory. Starting your day by hydrating will turn on your brain so you can make better decisions all day long.

- **Keeps kidneys healthy.** Proper water consumption is essential to healthy kidneys, and proper kidney function allows your body to rid itself of waste. By having 16 ounces of water first thing in the morning, you'll help your body start off with enough fluid to feed your kidneys.

How Much Water Should You Drink a Day?

It used to be easy enough to follow the old eight glasses of water a day rule, but fresh research has revealed that it isn't that simple. Older studies that established the eight-to-ten-glasses-a-day rule didn't take into account other beverages or foods that contribute to hydration. Coffee, tea, and other drinks have water in them, and the foods we eat also have some water in them, making up around 22 percent of the water you get in a day. Plus, you have to take your activity level into account: the more you exercise or sweat, the more fluids you need to replace. Thanks to these new findings, the answer about how much you really need to drink per day is still floating around. That said, I have a simple formula that seems to work pretty well. Divide your weight in half and drink that amount in ounces each day. So if you weigh 160 pounds, you need 80 ounces of water per day or eight glasses of water. To account for activity, add 5 ounces of water for every thirty minutes of exercise or activity (raking leaves, shoveling snow, etc.). Also, don't wait until you feel thirsty to drink. When your mouth is dry and you feel thirsty, you are thirty minutes too late. Start checking in with yourself throughout your day and rating how well you are hydrating on a scale from 1 to 10.

2. Always Eat Breakfast

It's important to start your day off with a high-fiber, filling breakfast. You're going to love the easy, nutrition-packed breakfasts on the *Mind Your Body* 4-week plan—you'll never again wonder what to have to fuel up right. Mom was right. Breakfast is a meal for champions, and research backs it up.

Why?

Scientific studies on breakfast eaters and skippers find that those who eat breakfast have better-functioning brains, more emotionally balanced lives, and more energy. They are also less likely to be overweight.

3. Eat Fruits Solo

If you eat fruits with a meal or with other fruits, you'll probably suffer from bloating, indigestion, or other digestive discomforts. Eat fruit one hour before or after a meal.

Why?

The theory here is that our bodies use different enzymes when digesting fruits and that fruits are the most rapidly digested foods we eat. When you eat other foods with fruits, the fermentation can upset your digestive system. Fruits are rich in simple sugars and need time to be completely absorbed by your body without interference from other foods. When fruits are consumed solo, your stomach can more effectively digest the nutrients, minerals, fiber, and natural sugars. The good news is that this makes fruit the perfect snack for between meals.

4. Chew Food Thoroughly

Chew each bite of food twenty to forty times, until it is at a consistency that you could feed to a baby.

Why?

Most people think digestion starts in the stomach, but you actually begin the process of digestion when you put food in your mouth. This first stage is called ingestion, and it is where chewing happens. Your teeth break down the food and mix it with saliva, and this action triggers chemicals that begin processing your meal. Your saliva stimulation also triggers gastric juices in your stomach to prepare for the arrival of food. If you don't take the time to chew about twenty times for each bite, as most nutritionists recommend, your food can arrive bulkier than it's meant to and without proper incorporation of the salivary enzymes, which means more work for your stomach and possible discomfort or indigestion. Also, when you chew your food properly, you make it easier for the nutrients to be absorbed. Plus, without proper chewing, you risk overeating because it takes about twenty minutes for the satiety signal to tell you that you are satisfied.

5. Eat Beverage-Free

I recommend holding off on water or other liquids when you eat. And stay dry for about forty-five minutes after your meal.

Why?

Drinking during meals dilutes the digestive acids in your stomach. We are fortunate to have such an amazing digestive system. It actually understands what you are eating and releases gastric juices accordingly. If you add too much liquid to the mix, it alters the balance of the digestive mix, which focuses on taking out the water while the other nutrients sit. What ends up being left is thicker than the food you started with. Why is this bad? It throws off a beautifully balanced

Understanding Carbohydrates

Carbohydrates' reputation has swung from good to evil over the last several years, but it's important to understand that there are different sorts of carbohydrates, and some are essential to your health. Carbs can be both good and bad. You'll notice that my recommendations and recipes feature the highest-quality whole grains, fruits, and vegetables, all of which are carbohydrates. These are the heroes of the carb world because they are full of fiber, minerals, antioxidants, and vitamins that are absorbed slowly by the body to nourish and fill you up. I don't include highly processed or refined carbohydrates, such as white sugar, white rice, white bread, crackers, chips, and so on, because these simple carbohydrates damage your body and increase your risk of disease, including diabetes, heart disease, and cancer. Plus, these villains of the carb world zap you of energy, causing you to overeat and to crave more and more sugar.

Here's what you need to know about simple versus complex carbohydrates:

Simple Sugars
These are made up of glucose and fructose; they include fructose, high-fructose corn syrup, maple syrup, honey, agave nectar or syrup, brown sugar, malted barley extract, evaporated cane juice, malt syrup, date sugar, and so on.

Fructose
This simple syrup makes up 50 percent of most sugars and 55 percent of high-fructose corn syrup. The special problem with fructose is that it must be sent first to your liver to be converted into fat and glucose, which puts a heavy burden on your body. It has been shown to increase rates of diabetes, fatty liver, obesity, and heart disease. While fructose is the main sugar in fruits, fruits also come with a large amount of minerals, fiber, and other nutrients that reduce the impact and improve the benefit for your body.

Complex Carbohydrates
As the name suggests, these are sugars that are complex, meaning that they are made up of several chains of sugars and starches. Starchy vegetables, such as potatoes, are fairly high in sugars, while others, such as broccoli, kale, tomatoes, carrots, and other vegetables, while still high in sugars, have high amounts of fiber, minerals, and antioxidants.

system, which can trickle into other areas, including your intestines, your blood system, and even your skin. The result can be slow digestion and cramping in some people. Initially, this may take some effort, but it quickly begins to feel normal. If you absolutely can't eat without water, then I suggest a very small glass and only taking the tiniest of sips as needed. Also, make sure the water is room temperature, because cold water interferes more with digestion. Better yet, have a glass of water thirty minutes before the meal.

6. Lunch Like a King

Eat your largest meal in the middle of the day, and dine light at night.

Why?

This is a matter of common sense. Generally speaking, people are most active during the middle of the day. It is the time when you use the most energy and burn the most calories, so it makes sense that you would need to refuel around midday. It will also help you lose weight more effectively, according to a recent Tufts University study of 420 women placed on a twenty-week weight loss program. The researchers found that those who ate their largest meal early in the day lost more weight than those who ate their larger meal later in the day. The women who ate later also were more likely to skip breakfast, which is a no-no.

7. Don't Eat Before Bedtime

Aim to eat your last bite of food at least three hours before you go to bed. If you waited too long for dinner or are feeling famished close to bedtime, have a small cup of soup, such as the Parsnip Soup on page 166, and call it a day.

Why?

Eating too late at night can leave you with too many calories to digest and interrupt your sleep. Unfortunately, evening hours are when many people fall off

Why Fiber Is Your Friend

I would be surprised if you didn't already know that fiber was good for you—it's touted constantly on the news, in magazines, even in commercials, but most people don't know that you don't have to eat foods that taste like dirt to get plenty of fiber. In fact, even though fiber is the part of food that your body can't digest, you can find plenty of it in delicious berries, dark green veggies, sweet potatoes, whole grains, apples, beans, and almonds. You can also use a powdered supplement (I like psyllium husk mixed in drinks or water to ramp up the daily quota). Aim to get 30 grams per day to reap fiber's benefits, which include lowering blood pressure, reducing the risk of obesity, diabetes, heart disease, and cancers, and of course keeping you regular. The *Mind Your Body* meal plans ensure that every day is full of fiber.

the food wagon and find themselves noshing on treats they've said no to all day. At the end of the day, many people find that their willpower is weak (for solutions see "What Is Willpower?" on page 9).

8. Eat When You're Hungry

If you are not truly hungry, don't force yourself to eat. Listen to your body and skip that meal. If you get hungry before the next meal, have a small snack of eight to ten walnuts, pistachios, or almonds.

Why?

Learning to eat only when you are physiologically hungry and to stop when you have had enough (this is different from being full) is key to losing weight. Most people who struggle with weight either follow a set diet or eat out of stress, boredom, sadness, or in response to a celebration or event of some sort. Many of us have been taught to eat at set times because of work schedules, out of guilt or shame, or simply because of our family history. All of us eat occasionally when not hungry, but when it becomes a habit, it spells trouble. You lose the natural ability to listen to the quiet but very real signals your body gives when you begin to get hungry and when you have consumed an appropriate amount of food. In the next section, you will learn to use a scale of 1 to 10 to keep tabs on your hunger and to know when to start and stop eating.

Quick tip: Eat anti-inflammatory foods whenever possible, such as nuts, garlic, ginger, turmeric, sardines, and salmon. They are all rich in omega-3 fatty acids and disease-fighting antioxidants.

9. Keep Food Separate

Never let different food items touch on your plate when you serve yourself (you can mix it up after you've chosen your foods). If you are having a salad or a mixed-up meal like a stir-fry, portion out the components before you put them in the bowl to toss

The 10 Rules of the Nutritionally Fit: Recap

1. Hydrate Right
2. Always Eat Breakfast
3. Eat Fruits Solo
4. Chew Food Thoroughly
5. Eat Beverage-Free
6. Lunch Like a King
7. Don't Eat Before Bedtime
8. Eat When You're Hungry
9. Keep Food Separate
10. Eat Food That Rots

together. You've got goals, right? Portion control is what helps you stick to them and skip having seconds. In fact, seconds don't exist on *Mind Your Body* unless you're talking about exercise.

Why?

Keeping your foods from touching when you put them on your plate isn't the action of a picky eater or an OCD behavior. When you keep food separate on your plate, it helps you clearly see what you'll be eating for a meal, so you're more likely to stick to appropriate portions. This is especially helpful when you are eating out or at a buffet because you can only pile your plate so high if you are carefully keeping each part in its own place (see "The Clock Method for Proper Portions," page 160).

10. Eat Food That Rots

This is one of author Michael Pollan's twelve commandments for serious eaters, from his book *In Defense of Food: An Eater's Manifesto,* and it goes along with not eating anything your grandmother wouldn't recognize as food and avoiding ingredients you can't pronounce.

Why?

You can almost always bet that the more processed a food, the worse it is for you. Back before we had refrigerators and freezers, creating foods that had a long shelf life seemed like a good idea. Unfortunately, what makes a food last a long time usually makes it a foreign object to your human body—not a good thing. Instead, focus on eating *real* foods. In addition, eat fruits and vegetables when they are naturally abundant and in season, not shipped from across the globe. This isn't only good for your body; it helps the environment, and it's also easier on your wallet. Some experts believe that your constitution changes with the seasons of your local climate, so eating foods that are native to your habitat and in season is a natural way to incorporate the intrinsic relationship your body has with the earth.

The 10 Tools of the Nutritionally Fit

Here are 10 tools to assist you with the 10 rules for optimal nutritional fitness. The people I know who have adopted these guidelines are among the most nutritionally fit people I know. These rules make healthy eating simple, clear, and deliciously satisfying so you can quickly reach a 10 on your nutritional deserve level.

1. The 1-to-10 Hunger Scale

You may have trouble detecting your body's natural hunger signals. The first step in becoming nutritionally fit is getting back in touch with these signals. This is about learning to trust your body and mind's inner wisdom. Your body's natural hunger signals are there; you just need to learn how to reawaken them. Using a 1-to-10 scale for hunger is the perfect way to get reacquainted with your body's appetite (see chart below).

The Hunger Scale

Danger: 1 to 2
Famished: Your stomach is growling, and you have a feeling of urgency bordering on panic about eating.

3 to 4
Hungry: You need to eat, are having hunger pangs, can feel a hollow sensation in your stomach.

5 to 6
Comfortable: This is when you stop; you still feel light but know you have had enough.

7 to 8
Full: You are beginning to feel slightly too full and know you have taken a bite or a few too many.

Danger: 9 to 10
Stuffed: You are uncomfortable, feeling bloated, and possibly nauseated.

It's simple, and you can start right now. Close your eyes and take a deep breath. Now rate your hunger. Do this any time you start thinking about eating. You want to eat when you are at a 3 or 4, and to stop when you are at a 5 or 6. You never want to allow yourself to be in the danger zone at 1–2 or 9–10. Hunger and satiety signals are quiet, and it can be easy to miss them if you are rushing around and not checking in with yourself or if you are eating while doing other tasks. Begin using this tool simply to stimulate awareness—it is not about keeping tabs, shaming, or guilt-tripping.

Over time it will become second nature, and you'll enjoy eating when you are truly hungry and stopping when satisfied but not stuffed (I promise). As you'll see, the tools that follow will help you be at your most aware and awake so that "hearing" your hunger signals becomes easier. During meals, stop after a few bites and rate yourself again; halfway through, do it again; and when you decide to stop, do it again; finally, about fifteen minutes after your meal or snack, rate yourself again. You'll soon know when it's truly time to eat, and you'll be able to hear the small, quiet click that alerts you that you've had enough. As you begin doing this on a regular basis, start asking yourself how well you are doing at identifying hunger signals on a scale from 1 to 10. You'll soon see it improve.

2. Mindful Meals

Recently, I had lunch with some friends at a local gym that has a dining area. Not only was my table busy with conversation but the environment was buzzing with people and upbeat music. I was so visually and aurally stimulated that if you asked me afterward what I had for lunch or how it tasted, I would have been hard pressed to give you an answer. The sounds and sights were so overpowering that I couldn't register my meal. If I'm in an aware and centered place in my mind, sometimes I can remain mindful while eating out; other times it is more challenging. If I had asked myself how mindful that meal was on a scale of 1 to 10, my rating would have been zero. When just beginning the practice of mindful eating, it's a good idea to have at least one meal a day in complete silence (or at least without anxiety-producing interactions) and to focus on eating without distractions (this will also help you sense hunger signals). Also, eat sitting down, without music, while paying full attention to the food in front of you. Make your eating environment a screen-free zone (this includes cell phones, TV, computers, and iPads). In this way you will learn to honor, respect, and be kind to yourself and to the nourishment your body deserves. It is saying, "I am giving myself not only this food but the time and

Learning to Listen to Your Body About Food

You are unique, and you have unique likes and dislikes. Research has shown that there are three common types of taste buds that influence what different people find appealing. I am sensitive to spicy foods and find that they easily overpower dishes, while others love to have lots of heat in their foods. It's important to respect what you enjoy eating, and you are the only one who is expert on this topic. Here are some of my own personal food rules.

• Listen to signals. I listen to my body carefully and with a huge dose of respect. For example, I cannot eat desserts late at night because I break out in sweats and wake up hot and cold all night long; I can't eat too much acidy fruit or my tongue gets unpleasantly tingly and numb; and I know better than to eat fruits with a full meal because I end up feeling bloated. I've learned these things by checking in and examining what I had eaten when I ended up feeling less than best.

• Listen each day. I've also learned to review on a daily basis what I ate earlier in the day or the day before. This is especially helpful if I get a stomachache, if my energy level is off, or if I just don't feel my best. I've continually tweaked my eating to serve me better by constantly listening to my body. The other side of listening and checking in carefully is that you'll learn to eat what your body really wants.

• Listen to odd reactions. The first time I had soy milk, a food that is often pushed as ultrahealthy, I was at a friend's house and they served it with granola. I coughed about ten times immediately after the meal, and I don't usually cough. About two months later, I was at a hotel and I had some soy milk again, and again, I immediately coughed. So now I know that soy milk is not for me, something I might never have learned if I didn't listen to my body. I am sharing this story with you to illustrate how important it is for you to listen carefully to *your* body.

• Learn to let go of diets. Not listening to our bodies also comes from being raised in a diet-obsessed culture. Many of my clients who struggle with weight don't think they can trust themselves and are always looking to someone else, some other book, or some diet to tell them how to eat. I want you to do the exact opposite. I want you to strike the word *diet* from your vocabulary. I never use it because it has *die* within the word itself and feels inherently negative. By listening to your body, you will come up with an eating plan that works for you—and the weight will come off effortlessly.

attention necessary to take the best care of my body and my brain today."

3. Savvy Shopping

The grocery store can be a scary place when you are trying to follow a healthy eating plan. It's easy to go in with good intentions but come out with a cart full of unhealthy food. Here are my basic tips to help you be a confident and healthy shopper:

- Never shop when you are hungry. Whenever your stomach is growling, your perception can be easily altered. Everything starts to sound good, and you can easily find yourself buying things you know you'll regret later. Cornell researchers found that hungry shoppers buy more high-calorie foods, such as potato chips and ice cream, than those who go on a full stomach. Plus, if you have a healthy snack before your trip, you'll be less likely to partake of the unhealthy samples they hand out at the store.

- Stick to the list. Be prepared by having a thoughtful shopping list with you and only buy what you planned on buying. I've made it easy. In chapter 10, you'll find shopping lists for each week of the twenty-eight-day program. Doing a bit of planning at home and having a written list to follow will make shopping effortless and keep you on track.

- Avoid sinkholes at the store. Generally speaking, the healthier items at the grocery store are on the perimeter, while processed, highly refined, and high-sugar items tend to be in the center of the store. If you aren't feeling at your strongest, avoid areas that might be triggers for you. Also, be aware that impulse items are put at the checkout line and at eye level on shelves, so make sure to look at the top and bottom shelves for healthy items.

- Shop solo. If at all possible, it is best to go to the store without distractions or added demands. You want to be focused and fast at the store, and having kids begging for goodies or even another adult can distract you from what you are putting in your cart.

4. Strategies to Prevent Temptation

You can be entirely committed to eating healthy but still have your plans dashed in seconds when you come face-to-face with your favorite temptation if you don't have a defense in place. Temptation-prevention strategies keep you on track at high-risk times and can get you back on the wagon before you even hit the ground.

Many people who are trying to lose weight face the "what-the-hell effect." This is an actual scientific term that describes what happens when you go to a party with every intention of sticking to your eating goals but then find yourself unable to stay away from the brownies or the bread bowl. What happens is that once you find yourself halfway through your second brownie, you think you've blown the day's diet, so you exclaim, "What the hell, I might as well fill my plate!"

One of the best ways to practice prevention strategies is by using a writing strategy suggested by Julia Cameron in *The Writing Diet*. She suggests that you ask yourself four questions before you eat:

1. Am I hungry?

2. Is this what I want to eat?

3. Is this what I want to eat now?

4. Is there something else I can eat instead?

This exercise helps you move from impulsive eating to mindful eating, to action. "You might start out to graze on cold pizza, but if you ask the questions, you might end up noshing on a Granny Smith apple," says Cameron. Other methods include delaying, not denying something you desire, having if/then planning in place (see page 133), and asking yourself how well, on a scale of 1 to 10, you are doing at resisting temptations. There are specific exercises to cultivate these skills in the 4-week plan that begins just a few short pages away in chapter 7.

5. A "Clean" Kitchen

If you lost weight and your clothes were too big, would you save them for when you got fat again? Not unless you were planning an "escape route" from your weight loss plan (see rule 7 in chapter 2, Extinguish Escape Routes). If you were truly committed to the new you, you would give your big clothes to charity.

The same goes for food. Keeping junk foods or highly processed foods is a way of keeping an escape route handy. How healthy is your kitchen right now on a scale from 1 to 10? Go through and toss out anything that is not helping you with your goals: candy, chips, sodas. When you are done, rate your kitchen again. In chapter 10, you'll use shopping lists that will help you restock your kitchen with *Mind Your Body* approved foods.

6. Optimistic Dining

Your thoughts and feelings alter your chemistry—negative ones can make you crave highly refined carbs

Taming Triggered Eating

The other day a client told me how upset and guilty she felt because she'd indulged in two peppermint patties the night before. "I'd been good all day, but then I got in an argument with my husband, and the next thing I knew, I was eating, actually scarfing, those darn candies," she said.

I asked her how guilty she felt on a scale from 1 to 10. She said she was at an 8, and she went on to say that she'd been so upset with herself that she'd gone to bed instead of working on the screenplay she was writing. I pointed out that this was an awful lot of energy to carry around for 120 calories. I asked her how she'd felt while she was eating the candies.

"I love peppermint patties. They taste so good," she said.

Setbacks like having an unplanned dessert aren't that big a deal; it's the guilt, shame, and remorse you bombard yourself with that really set you up for self-sabotage and throw you off track. The reality is that slipping off your eating plan will happen from time to time. Your brain is wired so the irrational sometimes wins out.

You have a couple of options. One is to pause any time you feel triggered and address with awareness

what is going on by saying something like, "I know I'm upset right now, and I have every right to feel what I feel. Sugar will give me a temporary feeling of pleasure."

Then you have to decide on your next step. One possibility is to delay the gratification by promising yourself that you will have the treat in forty-five minutes if you still feel like it (often a craving will pass, and so will triggered emotions, in about twenty minutes). The second option is to go ahead and have the treat but be fully aware that you are making a conscious choice and that you are going to enjoy it and have no bad feelings connected to it. You can adjust the rest of your menu or do a longer workout for that day, or the next day, to compensate for the treat. Then, if you are going to have your dessert, really enjoy it. I would have told my client to put those peppermint patties on a plate and sit down without any distractions, so she could have the full experience and not just stuff them in her mouth. Finally, kiss remorse goodbye. Guilt and shame are toxic emotions. They can cause further overeating or damage your self-worth, drain your energy, waste your time, and keep you from getting back on track.

and sugars—so make sure that eating time is a comfortable, relaxing, and enjoyable experience, and that your attitude is also on board. When eating time approaches, be dedicated to having a positive outlook so you won't sabotage yourself with feelings of shame or guilt about what you are eating. Don't eat in a setting that is stressful, anxiety producing, or negative. If you are dining in the company of others, focus on positive, joyous, peaceful topics—the old no-religion-no-politics rule would apply here.

Even if you are eating alone, it's important to do so in a positive frame of mind, according to a study just released by the Women's Health Initiative, a long-standing national research project that looks at women and health behaviors. In this study, University of Arizona researchers tracked more than 43,000 women and found that those who had the most positive mindset had healthier nutritional habits and were more successful at losing weight and improving the nutritional quality of their diets when compared to women who had pessimistic attitudes. The skills identified by the researcher included using self-reflection, keeping a journal or food diary, and using coping strategies such as saying affirmations, taking a break to go for a walk, or calling a friend who supports your healthy goals. To be sure to set the right tone for your meal, before you eat, review the affirmation that was prescribed for that day in chapter 7, and repeat it silently while taking slow, deep breaths, releasing any tension in your body and mind.

7. Quick Fixes

There are times when you need a quick fix to stay on track. Life gets busy, so you have to be prepared to adjust to any obstacle or challenge that might surface. Maybe you left your lunch at home, or you suddenly found out that you have to work through your dinner hour, or maybe the kid's Little League game is going on hour three, and you have to make do with food from the Snack Shack. Having a pitfall plan in place for these times is essential to keep you from getting sidetracked. Here are the basics:

Vending machines. Look for the nuts. Try to choose ones that don't come with dried fruit or chocolate chips. If you're on a road trip, rest stop machines sometimes have fresh fruit, string cheese, boiled eggs, or even sandwiches. If you choose a sandwich, ditch the white bread and go protein style.

Convenience stores. These days we are lucky. Most quick marts and gas stations offer options like single-serve string cheese, baby carrots, boiled eggs, and nuts. Some even offer apples and bananas. If you're stuck, grab one of these as a snack, along with a big bottle of water.

When Should I Eat?

Generally speaking, I recommend eating every three hours or so. That said, I still want you to check in with your hunger signals (see chart on page 73). Here are recommendations (since everyone wakes at a different time of day, adjust the times accordingly):

7 A.M.: Breakfast (eat within thirty minutes of waking)

10 A.M.: Snack (about three hours after breakfast)

12:30 P.M.: Lunch (about two and a half hours after your first snack)

3:30 P.M.: Snack (about three hours after lunch)

6:30 P.M.: Dinner (about three hours after your last snack)

If it gets to be 8:30 or within three hours of your bedtime, it is best to skip a full dinner and have one of the Power Drinks on pages 193–98.

The airport. I can't promise that airports will be budget friendly, but you can usually find healthy salads galore.

Fast food. In the appendix, "Quick Solutions" (page 205), I've created a go-to list of healthy suggestions for specific fast food restaurants. Generally speaking, you can always order a salad, hold the dressing and croutons, chips, or Asian-style noodles. If you are going for a sandwich, aim for the grilled chicken, skip the sauce, and ask for protein style (you'll get your burger or chicken sandwich wrapped in lettuce instead of a bun.

8. Smart Eating

When it comes to losing weight or improving your health, you don't need to eat less; you need to eat smarter. What this means is making meals and snacks as high quality as possible, combining foods that boost the nutritional quality of what you are eating, and never skipping meals unless your body tells you it isn't hungry (see rule 8, page 71).

The 10 Tools of the Nutritionally Fit at a Glance

1. The 1-to-10 Hunger Scale
2. Mindful Meals
3. Savvy Shopping
4. Strategies to Prevent Temptation
5. A "Clean" Kitchen
6. Optimistic Dining
7. Quick Fixes
8. Smart Eating
9. Basic Cooking Skills
10. Reflect on Meal Quality

Smart eating means you fill your plate with nutritionally dense foods and ditch refined carbohydrates such as white rice, white bread, pasta, cookies, ice cream, and sugary drinks. The number one goal for successful weight loss is to avoid getting too hungry or thirsty, and if you eat smart, this won't happen. The foods in the *Mind Your Body* meals are jam-packed with fiber, nutrients, complex carbohydrates, healthy proteins, and healthy fats so you never feel starved or deprived. The longer you go without healthy foods, the more your body breaks down muscle and craves unhealthy foods. Plus, not eating enough or skipping meals lowers blood sugar and lessens mental sharpness. Avoiding snacks may sap your willpower. When your brain is deprived of its primary fuel (glucose), you struggle to stop eating.

9. Basic Cooking Skills

While you don't need to go to culinary school to learn to eat healthy, it does help to learn some simple cooking methods. The ones outlined in this book don't take any special brainpower. They are simple and easy, and just by following the recipes in chapter 10 you'll learn many basic techniques that will help you build your healthy cooking repertoire. If you are less than sure of your cooking skills, use this affirmation daily: "*I cook healthy meals with ease. It's a pleasure to spend time in my kitchen, and people compliment me often on my cooking.*" Here is a quick review of my favorite healthy cooking methods:

- Steaming. This is using a steaming basket inside a pot with a little boiling water to cook your food. Steaming cooks vegetables and fish, sealing in flavor so you don't need to add fat.

- Stir-frying. A technique for stove-top cooking of foods at very high heat for a very short time. This is often done in a wok but can just as easily be done in a large skillet. Since food is cooked rapidly, you'll want to be prepped ahead of time, so have all the ingredients sliced and diced before starting to cook.

- Roasting. Cooking vegetables at a moderately high heat in the oven caramelizes their natural sugars and makes them delectable. It's a wonderful method that uses very little oil.

- Poaching. To poach foods, you gently simmer ingredients in a small amount of broth or water until they are cooked. This is a great way to do fat-free cooking (see also "The Perfectly Poached Egg," page 161).

10. Reflect on Meal Quality

To find out what is right for you, take stock of how you feel after you eat as well as before you eat. Do this an hour after your meal and again a few hours later. How is your energy? How does your stomach feel? If you experience indigestion or other discomfort, take note. You may begin to see patterns. And if you are not feeling your best, I want you to think over what you ate. Not every plan is right for every person.

Final Words

You have all the tools and rules you need to think, move, and eat for success. Now you are prepared to start the twenty-eight-day program. Buckle up, it's time to take off into the 4-week plan.

PART THREE

GO!

The Action Plan

The 4-Week Plan   Week 5 and Beyond

7

The 4-Week Plan

The 4-Week Plan at a Glance

Week 1	Week 2	Week 3	Week 4
Shifting Your Energy	Motivation	Being Present	Thinking Outside the Box
pages 88–92	*pages 93–97*	*pages 98–102*	*pages 103–107*
Day 1: page 88	*Day 8: page 93*	*Day 15: page 98*	*Day 22: page 103*
Day 2: page 89	*Day 9: page 94*	*Day 16: page 99*	*Day 23: page 104*
Day 3: page 89	*Day 10: page 94*	*Day 17: page 99*	*Day 24: page 104*
Day 4: page 90	*Day 11: page 95*	*Day 18: page 100*	*Day 25: page 105*
Day 5: page 90	*Day 12: page 95*	*Day 19: page 100*	*Day 26: page 105*
Day 6: page 91	*Day 13: page 96*	*Day 20: page 101*	*Day 27: page 106*
Day 7: page 91	*Day 14: page 96*	*Day 21: page 101*	*Day 28: page 106*

It's time to get started! I've made the following plan super simple in several ways. So while it might look like a lot of information, this plan is going to save you loads of time while delivering amazing results. You'll wake up your mind with daily mindful exercises to keep you focused so you don't waste energy feeding negative feelings. You're going to eat delicious home-cooked meals, but because of how I've designed the *Mind Your Body* meals, you'll actually be saving time in the kitchen. Plus, you'll get a daily workout in fifteen minutes that will work every muscle from every angle.

Before you get started, there are just a few housekeeping items we need to handle.

Setting Goals

Believing in yourself is the first step, but nailing down your intention in writing and having a plan of action will give substance and stickiness to your goals. In one University of Pennsylvania study, women who had a clear vision of how their weight loss success would happen, the commitment it would take, and the focus and motivation they'd need lost twenty-six pounds more than women who just proclaimed that they would lose weight without thinking it through. The difference happens when you blend your positive mindset with a realistic action plan—which is what we're doing right now. I have found that success is most often gained from going after specific positive desires and taking specific, sensible steps to achieve these goals. Personally, I want to feel *stimulated*. So that drives me to change my course of action and try new things, which in turn causes me to increase my deserve levels in all ten categories from fitness to family and friends to goals.

Grab your notebook and a pen, and have a seat. Relax your body by taking a few slow, deep breaths. Now, think of something someone else is doing right now that sounds thrilling to you, and write it down.

For example, maybe you have a friend who is training for a triathlon or climbing Mount Kilimanjaro.

Next I want you to write down three specific feelings that you wished you felt more of on a regular basis—for example, passionate, carefree, and worthy.

1. _____

2. _____

3. _____

Once you've finished this exercise, it's time to write down specific goals. This is about setting yourself up to succeed, so make sure your goals are realistic and specific (for example, I want to lose twenty pounds, or I want to be able to do fifty push-ups).

1. _____

2. _____

3. _____

Write down your deserve levels.

Before you begin, copy your deserve levels below from pages 19–28. You'll repeatedly track your changes and progress on these deserve levels as you move through the next twenty-eight days.

Categories	Deserve level ratings (from pages 19–28)	What number would you realistically like your deserve level to be?
1. Fitness		
2. Nutrition		
3. Family and friends		

4. Nest

5. Spiritual
   condition

6. Work

7. Attitude

8. Finances

9. Hobbies and
   interests

10. Dreams

Your total score
(a perfect score is 10 x 10 = 100)

Now let's start to bridge the gap in these numbers!

How to Use the 4-Week Plan

Remember that the *Mind Your Body* plan is centered on incorporating a Whole-istic approach that includes your mindset, moves, and meals to create the most positive environment for unstoppable success. The more fully you implement the tools, rules, and exercises, the more you'll absorb the 10 Core Concepts for Optimal Success.

Mindset

In the mindset sections, you'll find an affirmation for each day. In addition, turn to the page prescribed for that day in chapter 9, you'll find an extended list of exercises that relate to that day. It's great to start with the affirmation in this chapter, but if you truly want to see the results that come from living by the Core Concepts for Optimal Success, it's important to incorporate the mindful exercises in chapter 9.

Moves

In the moves sections are workouts in a specific order for that particular day, with page numbers for detailed instructions and pictures. The moves are organized day by day to work different body parts in a specific sequence; for a well-balanced body, do them in order. Keep these things in mind:

Listen to your body. Only do exercises that feel comfortable. If any move bothers your knees, back, hips, or any other body part, stop immediately.

Balancing. If you have trouble balancing in any of the exercises, keep a sturdy chair nearby.

Footwear. I like working out barefoot, and most of the workouts are designed to be done shoeless, but it is best to mix it up by wearing shoes from time to time so that you work your muscles differently.

Kneeling. If you find any of the kneeling positions uncomfortable, use a folded towel to support your knees.

Meals

In the meals sections for each day, you will see the recipe name, a number or numbers in parentheses, and sometimes a page number. The number in parentheses indicates which serving you are eating of the recipe you prepared.

For example, let's take a look at what's for dinner for day 2: Ginger Lentil Soup (2 of 2) and Simple Kale Salad (1 of 3). This tells you that you are eating your second serving of the soup (you had the first serving of soup for lunch on day 1), and your first serving of the salad. You'll pack up portions 2 and 3 of the salad and store them in your refrigerator for later meals. You're going to be having kale salad as part of dinner for day 3 and as part of lunch on day 5.

What About Beverages?

Besides the power drinks, make water your favorite beverage for the next twenty-eight days, and hopefully for the rest of your life. As far as the rest . . .

Coffee
I'm not a coffee drinker. I love the smell but not the taste. That said, if you love your java, stick to one cup a day in the morning, as research shows it provides lots of antioxidants and is safe in moderation.

Tea
Feel free to drink green or black tea in the morning. Tea has been shown to be full of antioxidants, may protect against some cancers, lowers stress, improves cholesterol levels, and slightly increases metabolism.

Alcohol
I like to have a cold beer every week or so, but this program is designed to be fully alcohol-free for the next four weeks, so raise a glass with sparkling water.

Any time you see a recipe listed that has more than one serving and no other directions, you'll store the leftovers in the refrigerator.

Mind Your Body is designed for one person. If you are cooking for a family, feel free to double recipes where it makes sense. You may end up with a bit extra for leftovers, but many recipes are freezer friendly, and extra portions can be saved for future lunches.

Shopping Lists
You'll find easily printed weekly shopping lists on pages 150, 152, 154, and 156. Make a point to review your shopping list a night or two before beginning the new week to see what items you need and what you already have. You'll buy the most before starting your first week. I've designed the 4-week plan to be superior in nutrient quality but extremely budget friendly.

Friends Night
On days 7, 12, 22, and 28, I've designed dinner to be shared with a friend or family member. Not only will these dinners be an opportunity to increase your family and friends deserve level and nurture your social skills but you'll share a delicious meal and an enlightened way of life with your loved one. Plus, you'll make your friends happy, because you'll be sending them home with leftovers!

Desserts
I've included four delectable desserts (pages 202–204).

Coconut Truffles

Gooey Chocolate Power Brownies

Peanut Butter Avocado Cookies

Vegan Chocolate Mousse

Pick the treat you'll enjoy the most and prepare it for your first friends night on day 7. The remaining dessert can be stored in the refrigerator or freezer to be spread out over the three remaining weeks.

Muffins
There are two muffin recipes on pages 201 and 202. Each makes twelve muffins. Please choose the recipe you think you'll enjoy most and bake it at the beginning of week 1. Put two muffins in the refrigerator, and bag and freeze the remaining ten. Each week, take two muffins from the freezer and have them as a bonus snack on an afternoon or evening when you feel extra hungry. At the end of the first four weeks, you'll have four muffins left for two more weeks.

Substitutions

In the menus, you may find a dish that won't work for you because of dietary restrictions, allergies, or personal reasons. If so, return to the list and choose a different option. Be sure to adjust your shopping list accordingly.

Soup: Vitamin A Soup (8 servings), page 167

Salad: Quinoa Sweet Potato Salad (6 servings), page 173

Entrée: Curried Spinach and Sweet Potato Freekeh (5 servings), page 180

Sides: Spinach and Navy Beans (4 servings), page 191

Track Your Weight Loss

To change your body, it is crucial to be a realist and know where you stand. Weigh yourself first thing in the morning and write your daily weight in your journal. This will help you track your progress. A realistic goal is 1 to 2 pounds per week. Start now by numbering a page from 1 to 28, and write your goal weight next to day 28.

Day	Weight	Day	Weight
1.		15.	
2.		16.	
3.		17.	
4.		18.	
5.		19.	
6.		20.	
7.		21.	
8.		22.	
9.		23.	
10.		24.	
11.		25.	
12.		26.	
13.		27.	
14.		28.	

(Goal Weight)

WEEK 1

Shifting Your Energy

This week is about change and making an investment in yourself, who you want to be, and what you put out into the universe.

Note: The number of servings per recipe is shown in parentheses.

MINDSET

Body Language

Today's affirmation

"I move forward in life with confidence and sincerity, wanting only to do good. I love exactly who I am today. I am strong and capable."

Do the day 1 mindset exercises on page 123.

Moves

Arms Workout A, page I-17

Abs Workout A, page I-9

Meals

Breakfast: Spinach and Mushroom Omelet (1 serving), page 162

Snack: Watermelon Juice (1 serving), page 198

Lunch: Tomato, Avocado, and Hearts of Palm Salad (1 of 2), page 176; Ginger Lentil Soup (1 of 2), page 164

Snack: Handful of almonds

Dinner: Seared Salmon Steaks (1 of 2), page 185; Garlic Spinach (1 of 2), page 188

Quick tip: To make almonds more digestible and help you get maximum nutrients from them, place them in a glass of water in the fridge and let sit for one hour before consuming.

MINDSET
Simplicity

Today's affirmation

"I handle everything I encounter with clarity and patience. I let go easily."

Do the day 2 mindset exercises on page 124.

Moves

Legs Workout A, page I-60

Meals

Breakfast: Coconut Muesli (1 of 8), page 159

Snack: Watermelon Juice, page 198

Lunch: Seared Salmon Steaks (2 of 2); Tomato, Avocado, and Hearts of Palm Salad (2 of 2)

Snack: Handful of pistachios

Dinner: Ginger Lentil Soup (2 of 2); Simple Kale Salad (1 of 3), page 176

A goal is a dream with a deadline.
—NAPOLEON HILL

MINDSET
Let Go of Your Past

Today's affirmation

"My thoughts and actions are my own. I create them, and I can uncreate them."

Do the day 3 mindset exercises on pages 124–25.

Moves

Back Workout A, page I-27

Meals

Breakfast: Apple Pumpkin Salad (1 of 6), page 168

Snack: 1 celery stick with 1 spoonful of almond butter or natural peanut butter

Lunch: Roasted Beet with Freekeh (1 of 4), page 174; Garlic Spinach (2 of 2)

Snack: Watermelon Juice, page 198

Dinner: Beef and Okra Stir-Fry (1 of 2), page 178; Simple Kale Salad (2 of 3)

A true friend is the one who knows all about you and still loves you.

Day 4

MINDSET
Smile

Today's affirmation

"I am full of generosity. I know that everyone is doing the best they can, and I have an abundance of love to give. Smiling comes to me easily."

Do the day 4 mindset exercises on pages 125–26.

Moves

Chest Workout A, page I-54

Abs Workout B, page I-11

Meals

Breakfast: Collards Scramble (1), page 159

Snack: Apple Pumpkin Salad (2 of 6)

Lunch: Beef and Okra Stir-Fry (2 of 2)

Snack: Artichoke and Spinach Hummus (1 of 6), page 199, with two baby carrots and one stalk of celery

Dinner: Roasted Beet with Freekeh (2 of 4); Lemon Asparagus (1 of 2), page 189

Quick tip: Smile when it is raining or you are having a rough day. Close your eyes and think how much worse things could be and how grateful you are for your life. If we all put our problems on the table, I am sure you would choose yours over those of someone else.

Day 5

MINDSET
Energy Distribution

Today's affirmation

"I love myself, and I will always be here for me. I feel comfort and ease. I create my new reality."

Do the day 5 mindset exercises on page 126.

Moves

Buns Workout A, page I-36

Meals

Breakfast: Coconut Muesli (2 of 8)

Snack: 1 cup cottage cheese with 1 teaspoon cinnamon and 1 teaspoon sunflower seeds

Lunch: Roasted Beet with Freekeh (3 of 4); Simple Kale Salad (3 of 3)

Snack: Apple Pumpkin Salad (3 of 6)

Dinner: Ginger Shrimp (1 of 4), page 182, and Lemon Asparagus (2 of 2)

Practice is good, but perfect practice is better.

—UNKNOWN

MINDSET
Sleep

Today's affirmation

"I drift off with ease into a deep restful slumber. My dreams take me on beautiful, joyful journeys. I wake feeling well rested and energized."

Do the day 6 mindset exercises on page 127.

Moves

Cardio Workout A, page I-46

Meals

Breakfast: Apple Pumpkin Salad (4 of 6)

Snack: Edamame, ½ cup

Lunch: Ginger Shrimp (2 of 4); Parsnip Soup (1 of 4), page 166

Snack: 1 banana

Dinner: Roasted Beet with Freekeh (4 of 4); Ginger Shrimp (3 of 4)

Quick tip: Get seven to nine hours of sleep a night. If you don't get the proper sleep, you don't get the proper recovery, and then you can't do the next workout.

MINDSET
Floating

Today's affirmation

"My mind works perfectly; whenever I need an idea or inspiration, I simply relax, and it comes to me effortlessly."

Do the day 7 mindset exercises on pages 127–28.

Moves

Shoulders Workout A, page I-71

Abs Workout C, page I-13

Meals

Breakfast: Spinach and Mushroom Omelet (1), page 162

Snack: Apple Pumpkin Salad (5 of 6)

Lunch: Ginger Shrimp (4 of 4); Parsnip Soup (2 of 4)

Snack: Edamame (half cup)

Dinner: Pork Tenderloin (1–4 of 8), page 184; Roasted Turmeric Cauliflower (1–2 of 4), page 190; Rosemary Brussels Sprouts (1–2 of 4), page 190

Friends night! This meal is meant to be shared with a friend. You and your company will enjoy two portions of pork, two portions of cauliflower, and two portions of Brussels sprouts. You will give your friend two portions of pork to take home. This leaves you with four servings of pork and two servings each of the vegetables, which will be used in upcoming meals.

Week 1 Review

Congratulations! You've finished your first week of *Mind Your Body* living. Before going on to the next seven days, take a moment to write in your original deserve level results to the right (you wrote them at the beginning of this chapter on pages 84 and 85), and then go back to page 19 and retake the test to see how you are doing after your first week. Add your updated scores to the right in the second column, "Week 1 Deserve Level Ratings."

Categories	Original Deserve Level Ratings	Week 1 Deserve Level Ratings
1. Fitness		
2. Nutrition		
3. Family and friends		
4. Nest		
5. Spiritual condition		
6. Work		
7. Attitude		
8. Finances		
9. Hobbies and interests		
10. Dreams		

Plan ahead for day 15. You will be directed to schedule a massage; book it now.

WEEK 2

Motivation

To move full speed in the direction of your goals, you must first let go of everything that is weighing you down—and that's what this week is all about.

I don't believe in luck. Luck equals leaving things to chance and to the outside world. I believe in being harbingers of our fate, taking action, and creating our own path and destiny in life. Your life is yours to create—don't let others do it for you.

—CELESTINE CHUA

MINDSET
Mentor Advice

Today's affirmation

"I am my own remarkable person. People are drawn to me from every direction. I am building the life I want."

Do the day 8 mindset exercises on pages 128–29.

Moves

Legs Workout B, page I-65

Meals

Breakfast: Coconut Muesli (3 of 8)

Snack: Handful of soaked almonds

Lunch: Pork Tenderloin (5 of 8); Roasted Turmeric Cauliflower (3 of 4)

Snack: Apple Pumpkin Salad (6 of 6)

Dinner (Veggie Night): Parsnip Soup (3 of 4); Rosemary Brussels Sprouts (3 of 4); Squash Mash (1 of 2), page 192

MINDSET
Gratitude

Today's affirmation

"I appreciate all that I am and all that I see and do. I am grateful for all the universe offers me."

Do the day 9 mindset exercises on page 129.

Moves

Arms Workout B, page I-22

Abs Workout D, page I-15

Meals

Breakfast: Seitan Sausage Sandwich (1), page 161

Snack: Orange Lime drink, page 197

Lunch: Parsnip Soup (4 of 4); Pork Tenderloin (6 of 8); Rosemary Brussels Sprouts (4 of 4)

Snack: Five macadamias

Dinner: Mom's Salmon Croquettes (2 of 10 patties; freeze additional patties in four small bags of two patties each), page 183; Roasted Turmeric Cauliflower (4 of 4)

MINDSET
Public Speaking

Today's affirmation

"My thoughts flow easily; I express and share my ideas with confidence and grace."

Do the day 10 mindset exercises on pages 129–30.

Moves

Back Workout B, page I-31

Meals

Breakfast: Poached Eggs and Kale (1 of 2), page 160

Snack: Ginger Mango drink, page 195

Lunch: Mom's Salmon Croquettes (3 and 4 of 10 patties); Squash Mash (2 of 2)

Snack: Green Tea Juice, page 196

Dinner: Pork Tenderloin (7 of 8), with Bok Choy Salad (1 of 4), page 170

We all have ability. The difference is how we use it.

—STEVIE WONDER

MINDSET

Free Time

Today's affirmation

"I have an abundance of time. I am able to do everything I want whenever I want to do it."

Do the day 11 mindset exercises on pages 130–31.

Moves

Buns Workout B, page I-40

Meals

Breakfast: Poached Eggs and Kale (2 of 2)

Snack: Handful of walnuts

Lunch: Pork Tenderloin (8 of 8); Arugula Salad (1 of 2), page 169

Snack: Plum Punch, page 198

Dinner: Bok Choy Salad (2 of 4); Creole Lima Beans (1 of 8), page 187; Lemon Zucchini Soup (1 of 4), page 165

MINDSET

$$$$$$$

Today's affirmation

"Money continually flows to me from every direction. I have an abundance of riches to do exactly what I want whenever I want to do it."

Do the day 12 mindset exercises on page 131.

Moves

Chest Workout B, page I-57

Abs Workout A, page I-9

Meals

Breakfast: Coconut Muesli (4 of 8)

Snack: 1 cup cottage cheese with two slices of tomato and a dash of paprika

Lunch: Arugula Salad (2 of 2); Creole Lima Beans (2 of 8); Lemon Zucchini Soup (2 of 4)

Snack: Four figs

Dinner: Bok Choy Salad (3 and 4 of 4); Poached Halibut (1 and 2 of 4), page 184; Indian Sweet Potatoes (1–4 of 8; freeze leftovers), page 189; Creole Lima Beans (3–6 of 8)

Friends night! Share with a friend or loved one, then send your friend home with two servings each of sweet potatoes and lima beans.

Quick tip: Plan ahead to hydrate. It takes twenty minutes for 8 ounces of water to hydrate your body, according to a University of North Carolina study.

MINDSET
Forgiveness

Today's affirmation

"I accept myself and am good enough just the way I am today. I forgive myself and let go of any harm to others or myself."

Do the day 13 mindset exercises on page 132.

Moves

Cardio Workout B, page I-49

Meals

Breakfast: Collards Scramble (1), page 159

Snack: Date Shake, page 194

Lunch: Creole Lima Beans (7 of 8); Poached Halibut (3 of 4); Indian Sweet Potatoes (5 of 8)

Snack: 1 Greek yogurt with cinnamon and almonds

Dinner: Poached Halibut (4 of 4); Lemon Zucchini Soup (3 of 4); Quinoa Salad (1 of 4), page 173

MINDSET
If/Then Plans

Today's affirmation

"I handle whatever comes in my direction with simplicity and ease."

Do the day 14 mindset exercises on pages 132–33.

Moves

Shoulder Workout B, page I-49

Abs Workout B, page I-11

Meals

Breakfast: Seitan Sausage Sandwich (1), page 161

Snack: Avocado Milk Shake, page 193

Lunch: Indian Sweet Potatoes (6 of 8); Lemon Zucchini Soup (4 of 4); Quinoa Salad (2 of 4)

Snack: Four figs

Dinner: Creole Lima Beans (8 of 8); Chicken Farro Salad (1 of 2), page 171

Life is 10 percent what happens to you and 90 percent how you respond to it.

—LOU HOLTZ

Week 2 Review

Great job! You are two weeks into transforming your life. Make sure to take time to reward yourself for all your hard work. Get a massage, go see a play, or spend some time with some special friends on day 15, since that is your day to skip working out. Take a moment for self-reflection. How do you feel about your effort? Your progress? What areas can you pump up a notch, and where do you think you can put in a little more effort? Are there places you can walk rather than drive? Can you go for a hike with a friend instead of talking on the phone? This is about you and your goals. As Arnold H. Glasgow said, "In life, as in football, you won't go far unless you know where the goalposts are."

Categories	Original Deserve Level Ratings	Week 1 Results	Week 2 Results
1. Fitness			
2. Nutrition			
3. Family and friends			
4. Nest			
5. Spiritual condition			
6. Work			
7. Attitude			
8. Finances			
9. Hobbies and interests			
10. Dreams			

WEEK 3
Being Present

How much time do you spend thinking about the past or future—worrying about what could, should, or might happen tomorrow? This week focuses on keeping you living in the here and now.

Be mindful of the present moment, because the past is over and the future doesn't exist. The only moment is now.

—UNKNOWN

MINDSET
Taste

Today's affirmation

"I eat and drink only nutritious foods and beverages that replenish my body and leave me feeling energized and restored."

Do the day 15 mindset exercises on pages 134–35.

Moves

Massage. Today is your day to treat yourself if you have faithfully stuck to the *Mind Your Body* moves. Do something nice for your body. Ideally it would be best to get a whole body or foot massage. Sometimes we don't realize how much our body needs it until we feel the therapist working to soothe our muscles.

Meals

Breakfast: Oatmeal Shake (1), page 197

Snack: 1 cup cottage cheese with 1 teaspoon chia seeds, two cherry tomatoes, and four slices of cucumber (salt and pepper to taste)

Lunch: Chicken Farro Salad (2 of 2); Quinoa Salad (3 of 4); Squash Casserole (1 of 6; freeze half the recipe), page 191

Snack: Baba Ganoush (1 of 4), page 199, with two baby carrots and one stalk of celery

Dinner: Squash Casserole (2 of 6); Turkey Burgers with Spinach and Feta (1 of 6; freeze three of the burgers), page 186

Day 16

MINDSET
Monitor Your Mood

Today's affirmation

"I have control over how I feel and act. When I trust myself and monitor my impulses, I am able to help myself and others."

Do the day 16 mindset exercises on page 135.

Moves

Legs Workout A, page I-60

Meals

Breakfast: Coconut Muesli (5 of 8)

Snack: One hard-boiled egg

Lunch: Squash Casserole (3 of 6); Turkey Burgers with Spinach and Feta (2 of 6)

Snack: Baba Ganoush (2 of 4) on two slices of jicama

Dinner: My Sister Paige's Gazpacho (1 of 4), page 166; Quinoa Salad (4 of 4)

Day 17

MINDSET
Outer Appearances

Today's affirmation

"A sense of balance, serenity, and strength comes from looking my best. I give myself the time to be healthy and vibrant. Each and every one of my cells glows with illuminating energy. People always say how attractive I am."

Do the day 17 mindset exercises on page 136.

Moves

Arms Workout A, page I-17

Abs Workout C, page I-13

Meals

Breakfast: Banana Almond Shake

Snack: Four pieces of endive and half an avocado

Lunch: My Sister Paige's Gazpacho (2 of 4); Asparagus Barley "Risotto" (1 of 4), page 178

Snack: Half a grapefruit

Dinner: Turkey Burgers with Spinach and Feta (3 of 6); My Sister Paige's Gazpacho (3 of 4)

MINDSET
Honor Code

Today's affirmation

"I come from a place of love, honesty, and kindness. I say what I mean and I mean what I say. People respect me because I am trustworthy, tolerant, and loving."

Do the day 18 mindset exercises on page 137.

Moves

Back Workout A, page I-27

Meals

Breakfast: Spinach and Mushroom Omelet (1), page 162

Snack: ½ cup blueberries and ½ cup grapes

Lunch: Mom's Salmon Croquettes (5 and 6 of 10 patties); Asparagus Barley "Risotto" (2 of 4)

Snack: Five macadamias

Dinner: My Sister Paige's Gazpacho (4 of 4); Edamame Salad (1 of 4), page 172

MINDSET
Smell

Today's affirmation

"I take in all the rich aromas around me. Wherever I go, I stop and smell; it is a window into my present moment. My sense of smell draws me to healthy nutritious foods that nourish my body."

Do the day 19 mindset exercises on pages 137–38.

Moves

Buns Workout A, page I-36

Meals

Breakfast: Seitan Sausage Sandwich (1), page 161

Snack: ½ cup Brazil nuts

Lunch: Edamame Salad (2 of 4); Asparagus Barley "Risotto" (3 of 4)

Snack: Pineapple Punch, page 197

Dinner: Chicken Stir-Fry (1 of 2), page 179

MINDSET
Work

Today's affirmation

"I am creative. I am unique. I have a job that I love doing, and I get paid great money for doing it."

Do the day 20 mindset exercises on pages 138–39.

Moves

Shoulders Workout A, page I-71

Abs Workout D, page I-15

Meals

Breakfast: Coconut Muesli (6 of 8) with ½ cup almond or flax milk (6 of 8)

Snack: Green Dream, page 196

Lunch: Chicken Stir-Fry (2 of 2); Asparagus Barley "Risotto" (4 of 4)

Snack: ½ cup blueberries and ½ cup grapes

Dinner: Edamame Salad (3 of 4); Turmeric Chicken Soup (1 of 6; refrigerate two portions and freeze remaining three), page 167

MINDSET
Other People

Today's affirmation

"I enjoy being in the presence of others. We are all unique human beings, and we each have our own purpose. I surround myself and appreciate all my loving relationships."

Do the day 21 mindset exercises on pages 139–40.

Moves

Cardio Workout A, page I-46

Meals

Breakfast: Collards Scramble (1), page 159

Snack: Avocado Milk Shake, page 193

Lunch: Edamame Salad (4 of 4); Sweet Potato Chips (1 of 2), page 192

Snack: Half a grapefruit

Dinner: Turmeric Chicken Soup (2 of 6)

Quick tip: Share your goals with your friends and loved ones. It will help you remain accountable.

Week 3 Review

Well done! Tomorrow marks your twenty-second day on the *Mind Your Body* 4-week plan. For three weeks, you've practiced new thinking, moving, and eating strategies. You feel more energized from deep in your core. What are some of your best accomplishments? What compliments have you heard? How was this last week different from the first? How has your thinking changed? Take some time to reflect on your progress. Update your deserve level ratings to the right and see how you are doing.

Categories	Original Deserve Level Ratings	Week 2 Results	Week 3 Results
1. Fitness			
2. Nutrition			
3. Family and friends			
4. Nest			
5. Spiritual condition			
6. Work			
7. Attitude			
8. Finances			
9. Hobbies and interests			
10. Dreams			

WEEK 4

Thinking Outside the Box

To get different results, you have to change your actions. Doing the same thing and expecting a different outcome is a common definition of insanity. This week is about thinking bigger and better, breaking out of your comfort zone to reach greater heights.

Logic will get you from A to B. Imagination will take you everywhere.

—ALBERT EINSTEIN

MINDSET

Setting Daily Intentions

Today's affirmation

"Today I honor myself by sticking to my goals. I will eat nutritiously so I have optimal energy to be of maximum service to others and myself. I will look at life from new angles."

Do the day 22 mindset exercises on pages 140–41.

Moves

Chest Workout A, page I-54

Abs Workout A, page I-9

Meals

Breakfast: Prune Shake, page 198

Snack: Hard-boiled egg

Lunch: Turmeric Chicken Soup (3 of 6); Sweet Potato Chips (2 of 2); Avocado and Kale Salad (1 of 4), page 170

Snack: ¼ cup dried cranberries

Dinner: Mom's Salmon Croquettes (7–10 of 10 patties); Avocado and Kale Salad (2–3 of 4); Garlic Eggplant Mash (1–2 of 8), page 188

Friends night! Share with a friend and then freeze half of the Garlic Eggplant Mash, unless your friend wants to take it home.

MINDSET
Clean Out
Your Closet

Today's affirmation

"I joyously release and easily give away any excess in my life. I encourage the flow of life. New things come to me with ease."

Do the day 23 mindset exercises on pages 142–43.

Moves

Legs Workout B, page I-65

Meals

Breakfast: Coconut Muesli (7 of 8)

Snack: A quarter honeydew

Lunch: Garlic Eggplant Mash (3 of 8); Black Bean Soup (1 of 4; freeze half the recipe), page 163

Snack: One pear

Dinner: Shrimp and Spinach Salad (1 of 2), page 175

_____

Don't confuse motion and progress. A rocking horse keeps moving but doesn't make progress.

_____

MINDSET
Dreams

Today's affirmation

"Tonight I go to sleep with a clear mind; I know I'll receive answers to all my questions when I wake. I dream with clarity and peace of mind."

Do the day 24 mindset exercises on page 143.

Moves

Back Workout B, page I-31

Meals

Breakfast: Collards Scramble (1), page 159

Snack: A quarter honeydew

Lunch: Shrimp and Spinach Salad (2 of 2); Black Bean Soup (2 of 4)

Snack: Electrolyte Punch, page 195

Dinner: Garlic Eggplant Mash (4 of 8); Avocado and Kale Salad (4 of 4)

_____

If you have hit a plateau in your workouts, mix it up by going for a swim to jump-start you.

_____

Day 25

MINDSET
Ideal Job

Today's affirmation

"I appreciate my source of income. I am open to new opportunities. Each and every day, I express more and more of my talents and abilities. I chase my bliss."

Do the day 25 mindset exercises on pages 143–44.

Moves

Arms Workout B, page I-22

Abs Workout B, page I-11

Meals

Breakfast: Pomegranate Punch, page 198

Snack: Hard-boiled egg

Lunch: Sweet Turkey Loaf (1 of 6; freeze half the recipe), page 185; Mom's Zucchini Soup (1 of 6), page 165

Snack: A quarter honeydew

Dinner: Halibut and Artichokes (1 of 2), page 182; Broccoli and Black-Eyed Pea Salad (1 of 6), page 171

All children are artists. The problem is how to remain an artist once he grows up.

—PABLO PICASSO

Day 26

MINDSET
Eulogy

Today's affirmation

"I make active choices that are in line with my creative self. I know that I am in the process of changing into the butterfly I'm meant to be. I am a risk taker."

Do the day 26 mindset exercises on pages 144–45.

Moves

Buns Workout B, page I-40

Meals

Breakfast: Spinach and Mushroom Omelet (1), page 162

Snack: A quarter honeydew

Lunch: Halibut and Artichokes (2 of 2); Collard Greens (1 of 2), page 187; Mom's Zucchini Soup (2 of 6)

Snack: Artichoke and Spinach Hummus (2 of 6) with two carrots and one stalk of celery

Dinner: Sweet Turkey Loaf (2 of 6); Almond Slaw (1 of 4), page 186; Broccoli and Black-Eyed Pea Salad (2 of 6)

Man's mind, once stretched by a new idea, never regains its original dimensions.

—OLIVER WENDELL HOLMES

MINDSET
Visualize Abundance

Today's affirmation

"My body is made perfect. I have the power to correct what is wrong. I am profoundly magnetic to the abundance the universe has to offer. I shift into a place of possibility."

Do the day 27 mindset exercises on page 145.

Moves

Cardio Workout B, page I-49

Meals

Breakfast: Coconut Muesli (8 of 8) with ½ cup almond or flax milk

Snack: Orange Zing (1), page 197

Lunch: Sweet Turkey Loaf (3 of 6); Collard Greens (2 of 2); Broccoli and Black-Eyed Pea Salad (3 of 6)

Snack: Mom's Zucchini Soup (3 of 6)

Dinner: Eggplant Chili (1 of 6), page 181; Walnut Salad (1 of 4; your fridge will now have items to keep you eating healthy), page 177

Quick tip: Think abundance. There is a wealth of all that is good in the universe, and it is available for you to take when you are ready.

MINDSET
The Power of Pause

Today's affirmation

"A craving is a thought. I am not my thoughts. I don't have to react or respond to my thoughts. I have the power to choose how I will react and behave. My cravings are not me."

Do the day 28 mindset exercises on pages 145–46.

Moves

Shoulders Workout B, page I-76

Abs Workout C, page I-13

Meals

Breakfast: Zucchini Omelet (1), page 162

Snack: Green Power, page 196

Lunch: Mom's Zucchini Soup (4 of 6); Broccoli and Black-Eyed Pea Salad (4 of 6)

Snack: 1 cup fresh berries

Dinner: Eggplant Chili (2–5 of 6); Artichoke Amaranth Salad (1–4 of 4), page 168

Friends night—time to celebrate! Have your single-portion servings for dinner and fill your fridge for the next day or let your friends take the rest home.

---

*Don't allow food cravings to manipulate you
into eating what you know you shouldn't;
you are in control of your cravings.*

Week 4 Review

To truly understand how far you've come in a relatively short time, take a moment to review your progress over the last four weeks by revisiting the test on page xx, "Are You Who You Want to Be?" You may find that your choices have changed, and I want you to embrace your new self by taking a few minutes to reflect. This is about taking control of your focus and your condition. After you finish circling the words, pull out your notebook and answer the following questions:

1. Have you chosen different words?

2. Are you closer to being who you want to be? How does that make you feel?

3. What three actions can you take to bring you even closer to your desired self?

Final Words

Congratulations! It's time to celebrate. You've completed four weeks of total body- and mind-transforming techniques, strategies, and exercises. You have laid down new neural pathways and created new habits to make healthy living automatic. This is a success that must be celebrated. Keep treating yourself with a 10 on the deserve levels of respect, love, and self-worth. I've left you with items in your fridge and freezer to make it easy to continue on the path of eating quality nutrient-dense foods for the upcoming week. The following chapter will help you bring your journey to the next phase.

8

Week 5 and Beyond

Now that you've completed the first four weeks of *Mind Your Body* and have taken many wonderful steps to establish a new way of living with presence, dedication, and diligence, it's time to begin the next phase of the *Mind Your Body* way of life. Remember, the last and most important brain-boosting tool is self-reflection. That's where you'll start the next stage of change.

Retake the Test

To get started, retake the 10 × 10 Deserve Level Test (pages 19–28) and compare your scores. You don't need to do an adjusted score, because you are now able to see your true self in your personal mirror. Write down the ratings in your notebook, making a chart like the one at right. In the final column, put what you would like your deserve level to be for each category.

Set New Goals

Where will you turn your attention now? Will you continue to work on weight loss goals, further improve your fitness, or is it time to turn your attention elsewhere? Jot down any ideas that come to mind. The more specific you are, the less obstructed the path to get there.

Categories	Original Deserve Level Ratings	Present Deserve Level Ratings	Ideal Deserve Level Ratings
1. Fitness			
2. Nutrition			
3. Family and friends			
4. Nest			
5. Spiritual condition			
6. Work			
7. Attitude			
8. Finances			
9. Hobbies and interests			
10. Dreams			

Using the numbers from your retest, fill in the chart below, then answer the questions that follow in your notebook:

Questions	Category	Rating
1. Which category has the lowest deserve level?		
2. Which category showed the biggest change?		
3. Which category has the highest deserve level?		

Growth

1. What changes are you most proud of?

2. What were your biggest accomplishments?

3. What compliments did you receive?

Reflection

1. Looking back over the rules and tools in this program (see charts on pages 72 and 78), what are your greatest strengths?

2. In what areas do you still need to improve?

3. How will you celebrate your successes? Write down three ideas for rewarding yourself for your hard work.

Goals

1. As you move into the next phase of your journey, what are three specific goals?

2. What will be your first step in implementing these goals? Write down three first steps in your notebook.

Feelings

Answer these questions in your notebook:

1. What three feelings are you experiencing now?

2. What three feelings would you like to be experiencing now?

What Now?

I designed the 4-week plan to be repeated. There is so much variety that you could easily go back to week 1 and start over. You could also mix up the weeks or do a week more than once. You could substitute week 2 for week 1, or if you love week 3, repeat it a few times. Any order is fine.

To take it a step farther, you can break the program down even more.

Moves

For the exercise portion, you can mix and match by week but not by day. Remember, I designed the workouts so your muscles have optimal time to recover and repair, hence you see maximum benefits in minimal time. So you can substitute week 2 for week 1, or week 3 for week 4, but keep weeks together to work every muscle from every angle. Turn to pages I-6 and I-7 to pick exercises.

Mindset

You can rearrange mindset days in any order that works for you. I do suggest keeping a day's exercises complete, because they are made to relate to one another.

Meals

Mix and match meals from the recipes in chapter 10. Be creative. Just aim to swap breakfasts for breakfasts, lunches for lunches, and so on. Pick your favorites to do your own menu design.

Making Your Own Meals

During the past twenty-eight days, you got plenty of variety. I designed your meals to provide maximum nutrients, antioxidants, and fiber, as well as the right proportion of healthy carbohydrates, proteins, and fats. That said, if you're ready to design your own meals, use the planner on page 114 and pick from the food lists on pages 112 and 113 to design your own meals. Also see "The Clock Method for Proper Portions" (page 160).

Write What You Eat and Lose More Weight

I have done all the footwork in designing your meal program for the last four weeks, but for you to keep progressing toward your goals, consider tracking what you eat each day in a food journal, or print and use copies of the daily menu planner on page 114. Why does writing work?

When you write something down, it works as sort of a mini-rehearsal. When you write down what you plan to eat, it triggers your brain to play out this scenario. Then, when it comes time to actually eat, you'll be more likely to eat the healthy foods you wrote down. Plus, keeping a daily food diary can double the amount of weight you lose, according to a study published in the *American Journal of Preventive Medicine*. While two-thirds of the nearly 1,700 dieters in the study lost an average of nine pounds, those who kept a food diary lost up to twenty pounds, more than twice as much as those who did no record keeping. Even though you have the idea that you're going to eat healthy today, it can be easy to ignore this goal if it is just a thought in your head, whereas writing down every bite you eat keeps you on target.

How Much Should I Eat Each Day?

Aim for 30 percent protein, 30 percent fat, 40 percent healthy carbohydrates, and 30 grams of fiber per day.

But How Many Servings of Each Food Is That?

To figure out your calories and servings for the day takes a little more work. I want your body to feel satiated and your mind to feel content. Watch your mind to see whether you are being indulgent. Your nutrient needs are based on your age, height, gender, and activity level. The U.S. Department of Agriculture offers some helpful tools to portion your daily allotment of food (see http://www.choosemyplate.gov/myplate/index.aspx). Within a couple of minutes, you'll have some general guidelines for counting out portions for the day.

What About Calories?

The general rule about weight loss, exercise, and calories—eat less, move more—is misleading. Your body does not work like a simple math equation. You process calories differently based on their nutritional makeup. There is not the same nutritional value in 120-calorie portions of chocolate cookie, chicken, blueberries, broccoli, and Greek yogurt. All calories are not created equally. Some take up a large amount of space, such as the blueberries and broccoli; others take much longer to digest, such as the chicken and Greek yogurt, while the cookie is just a little jolt of energy without any real nutritional benefit. At a deeper level, when you eat different foods, your body and brain respond by triggering hormones and neurotransmitters that tell you what to do with the food. Most alarmingly, refined carbohydrates and sugars tell your body to make fat, then they make you crave more of the same.

The idea to take away is that you can't choose a given number of calories and then eat any set of nutrients and get the response you're looking for. If you want to lose weight, build muscle, get fit, boost energy,

Mind and Body Nourishing Foods

Vegetables

Portion = 2.5 cups of vegetables per day
Dark green vegetables = 1.5 cups weekly
Orange vegetables = 5.5 cups weekly

Asparagus	Carrots	Garlic	Okra	Squash, winter
Avocados	Cauliflower	Green beans	Olives	Sweet potatoes
Beets	Celery	Green peas	Onions	Swiss chard
Bell peppers	Collard greens	Kale	Potatoes	Tomatoes
Bok choy	Corn	Leeks	Romaine lettuce	Turnip greens
Broccoli	Cucumbers	Mushrooms, crimini	Sea vegetables	
Brussels sprouts	Eggplant	Mushrooms, shiitake	Spinach	
Cabbage	Fennel	Mustard greens	Squash, summer	

Fruits

Portion = 1.5 cups a day

Apples	Cantaloupe	Grapes	Papaya	Prunes
Apricots	Cranberries	Kiwifruit	Pears	Raspberries
Bananas	Figs	Lemons/limes	Pineapple	Strawberries
Blueberries	Grapefruit	Oranges	Plums	Watermelon

Nuts and Seeds

Best used as garnishes for salads and stir-fries in small amounts, or have eight to ten nuts as a snack

Almonds	Peanuts	Pine nuts	Sunflower seeds
Cashews	Pecans	Pumpkin seeds	Walnuts
Flaxseeds	Pili nuts	Sesame seeds	

Protein Foods: 5–7 ounces per day

Beans and Legumes

Black beans	Kidney beans	Navy beans	Soybeans
Dried peas	Lentils	Pinto beans	Tempeh
Garbanzo beans (chickpeas)	Lima beans	Seitan	Tofu
	Miso	Soy sauce	

Eggs and Dairy

Cheese, grass-fed	Cow's milk, grass-fed	Eggs, pasture-raised	Yogurt, grass-fed

Seafood

Cod	Sardines	Shrimp
Salmon	Scallops	Tuna

Poultry and Meats

Beef, grass-fed	Chicken, pasture-raised	Lamb, grass-fed	Turkey, pasture-raised

Herbs and Spices

Portion = unlimited use

Basil	Cilantro and coriander seeds	Cumin seeds	Oregano	Sage
Black pepper		Dill	Parsley	Thyme
Cayenne pepper	Cinnamon, ground	Ginger	Peppermint	Turmeric
Chili pepper, dried	Cloves	Mustard seeds	Rosemary	

Grains

Portion = 6 ounces a day

Barley	Buckwheat	Millet	Quinoa	Whole wheat
Brown rice	Freekeh	Oats	Rye	

Fats

Portion = 2 tablespoons max a day

Extra-virgin olive oil	Grapeseed oil	Butter	Coconut oil	Flaxseed oil

*This Mind and Body Nourishing Foods table is for you to
copy and keep handy.

balance your moods, and sleep well, then it's best for you to minimize refined carbohydrates and sugars and maximize healthy proteins, carbs (fruits and whole grains), fats, and vegetables. Consult the Department of Agriculture website to get specific recommendations about your individual nutritional needs.

The table on the two previous pages is for you to copy and keep on your desk, your refrigerator, or anywhere you will see it at least once a week. Part of eating healthy is to make sure to get plenty of variety. If you notice you haven't had something in several weeks, put it on your shopping list. Choose organic, grass-fed, and additive-free products whenever possible. Portions are included in the table, but visit http://www.choosemyplate.gov/myplate/index.aspx to get a more accurate idea of proper portions.

Whole-istic Menu Planner

Meal or Snack	Item/Amount
Breakfast (eat within thirty minutes of waking and aim for at least 7 grams of fiber)	
Snack (three hours after breakfast, at least 3 grams of fiber)	
Lunch (two to three hours after last snack, at least 7 grams of fiber)	
Snack (three hours after lunch, at least 3 grams of fiber)	
Dinner (two to three hours after last snack, and not within 3 hours of bedtime; at least 7 grams of fiber)	

Final Words

You did it! It has been a month since you started this journey, and you are now equipped with all the rules, tools, and components to be your own weight loss, fitness, and life coach, as well as so much more. In yoga there is a philosophy called Aparigraha that promotes nonpossessiveness—a deep understanding of not taking more than you need, knowing how to let things go when they no longer serve you, opening yourself up to fresh ideas and more harmonious ways of living and being. In other words, living the *Mind Your Body* way of life. With this knowledge in mind, you are ready to start designing your own Whole-istic plan composed of exercises for your mind and your body. You've learned so much about how to think, move, and eat for optimal success. What gift can you give to those you love that is better than being free of tension, positive, energized, and empowered? I'm so proud of you! I encourage you to hold on to the essential *Mind Your Body* philosophy: that the path to a richer life and to true success, happiness, and health is centered in your mind. May your journey continue to be bigger and better than you ever thought possible.

PART FOUR

YOUR TOOLBOX

Mindset:
Your 4-Week Plan

Meals:
Your 4-Week Plan

Moves:
Your 15-Minute Workouts

9

Mindset

Your 4-Week Plan

The 4-Week Mindset Plan at a Glance

Week 1	Week 2	Week 3	Week 4
Shifting Your Energy	Motivation	Being Present	Thinking Outside the Box
pages 123–28	*pages 128–33*	*pages 134–40*	*pages 140–46*

ere, in detail, are the mental tools as they are prescribed in the 4-week plan. Each day is designed to address and improve your 10 deserve level scores to create maximum success, happiness, and balance. You will find some suggestions more challenging than others—that's normal, but don't skip them. The exercises that take the most effort are often the most beneficial. Each activity serves a specific purpose, with the aim of building a mind that you want to live within. You are creating a powerful relationship with yourself, where you'll learn to fully understand that you control your thoughts and do not have to let them control you.

How It Works

Each day's mindful practice should take roughly ten minutes. Only do one day's prescribed exercises. These exercises are designed to be absorbed over a full twenty-four-hour period to deliver maximum benefit.

When to Practice

Ideally, you'll want to practice the day's exercises in the morning and then repeat them in the evening, but feel free to add a midday session. The more you keep these positive strategies in the front of your mind, the better.

Before You Retire for the Day

At the end of each day, I want you to take a couple of minutes to take a daily inventory, or a mental scan, of your 10 deserve level categories (page 17). As you bring each category to mind, pause to reflect on how you feel about your deserve level in that area. Then congratulate yourself on a job well done.

Brain-Boosting Tool How-Tos

Below is a quick review of the 10 brain-boosting tools and how to put them to best use. Here you'll find a basic description of how to use the tool most effectively.

1. Meditation Exercises

There is nothing easier. You simply sit quietly and focus on your breath. You can do this anywhere—even while eating, walking, sitting in a meeting, or walking around the grocery store. Here's a simple way to begin from researchers at the University of Wisconsin: Sit comfortably. Relax and close your eyes. Focus on the flow of your breath at the tip of your nose. If a thought arises, acknowledge the thought and then let it go by gently bringing your attention back to the flow of your breath. Part of meditation is to learn to let thoughts, feelings, and emotions float by like clouds in the sky. So view your mind as the sky, and thoughts, feelings, and emotions as the weather—rain, clouds, wind, sun, etc. The weather comes and goes; it arises, exists, and passes. You don't need to ride the clouds, get soaked in the rain, or be blown away by the wind. In other words, you don't need to feel or think a certain way to take the action you want to take toward your goals.

2. Visualization Exercises

To get the most out of imagery exercises like the ones described in this chapter, it's key to include all your senses. If you want to relax, for example, it isn't enough to just see yourself sitting on a sandy beach. You must *smell* the salt from the ocean, *feel* the warmth of the sun on your skin, and *hear* the waves crashing on the beach. By doing this, you fully immerse yourself in the mental picture you are painting, so your brain actually believes you are at the beach and you trigger a relaxation response. Your heart rate, pulse, and breathing slow down.

How to Visualize Success

Set a timer for three minutes. Close your eyes and create a mental picture of yourself having achieved all your goals and dreams. Picture yourself filled with happiness, confidence, abundance, prosperity, peace, and a sense of purpose. Allow yourself to not only see it but really feel it. See yourself at your ideal weight and feeling strong and healthy. Now, as you look inwardly at this strong, confident person, feel the energy of this ideal you flooding into the actual you. Feel your chest lift, feel yourself growing more self-assured, full of passion for your life, full of respect and love for yourself: you are graceful, capable, and strong. Imagine your successful environment. Bring an image of your ideal living space into mind. What does it look like? What is the quality of the light? How does it make you feel? Smell how fresh, soothing, and clean it smells. Imagine your family and friends. Hear them laughing and sharing loving words with you. Continue to expand this visualization into all areas by imagining your ideal workspace, career, finances, hobbies. See yourself happily doing, hearing, smell-ing, seeing, and feeling all your dreams and goals. Stay with this inner vision for as long as you can, and make it feel as genuine as possible. Throughout the rest of your day, periodically call this visualization back into your mind as you go about your normal ac-tivities. Pause and remember that you *are* this confi-dent, worthy person. Similarly, if a snag arises in your day, pause and remember the self-assured, graceful, worthy person you are. The more you repeat this exer-cise, the more your brain will rewire to make you into the person you were always meant to be.

3. Writing

In the box below you'll find basic rules for keeping a journal. For the full background on how writing can help you boost your mind power, see page 42.

see page 42

Journaling Basics

The Rules

Plan on writing for roughly ten to fifteen minutes each morning and again each evening, focusing on insights, ideas, and struggles. Write freely, forget-ting about spelling, grammar, and punctuation, and write as quickly as you can for the full time you've allotted. Don't let your hand stop moving, and don't allow your inner critic to surface. Everything you write is exactly as it should be.

In the Morning

Take a few minutes to review how yesterday went, enjoy what went right, contemplate what you could have done better, and acknowledge that this is a new day. I like to think over anything that knocked me off center, shifted my mood, or made me strug-gle with energy, feelings, or food cravings. I also like to review how I slept and jot down any dreams I re-member. Next, take a few minutes to think about your plans for the upcoming day. Write out a little to-do list, then think about how you can address your day with a good attitude and an optimistic spirit. End your writing session by writing down three intentions for the day. I often write that I will eat for optimum health, I will get in a great and en-ergetic workout, I will focus on releasing any tension and anxiety that arises, and I will make positive con-nections with everyone I encounter.

At Night

You can also use writing at the end of your day to review what and how you did. This sort of self-reflection helps me stay centered; I feel like I put the day to rest, and in the morning I can start again with a clean slate. This cultivates self-awareness about patterns of eating, feelings, and energy. I know that if I don't take good care of myself, I won't be any good to anyone else.

4. Affirmations

> "I am in Charge of How I Feel and Today I am Choosing Happiness."

Think of affirming statements as self-talk that programs you for what you want in your life. When you practice affirmations, you are choosing to focus on what you value for yourself. Just as you are influenced by the messages you receive from other people and the outside world, you are also influenced by what you say to yourself.

When you first try out an affirmation, you may experience some arguing in your head. This is a normal response when you are used to an attitude of failure and negative thinking. This is your brain creating negative mental noise; you can choose to buy into it or not. So if you say, "I am quickly reaching my healthy weight," and you find yourself thinking, "I've always failed at weight loss," you can respond, "That is the way I used to feel, but it is now an outdated and unhelpful belief. I am not my thoughts, I choose my thinking, and today I choose to love myself." You observe the negative thought without engaging it. You can also create a positive affirmation out of a negative thought, so the thought above becomes "I have learned to be successful at weight loss."

How to Practice Affirmations

When you wake and when you are getting ready for bed are ideal times to say affirmations. At the beginning of your day, an affirmation will help set the tone for your day. Before you retire, affirmations help focus your mind on the positive as you drift off to sleep, which can help your dreams send powerful positive messages to you as you slumber. You can also practice affirmations while stuck in traffic, as you stand in line at the grocery store, during a lunch break, while walking, or even as you sit in a restroom stall. It's great if you are able to speak the words out loud, but affirmations also work by thinking and feeling them in your mind. Read the affirmation for your day several times. Then close your eyes and repeat it in your mind, and say it out loud to let it resonate. You can also write out the affirmation several times.

Creating Your Own Affirmation

When creating affirmations for yourself, always make sure they are in the present tense: "I have perfect balance" instead of "I am going to have perfect balance." When you express something in the future tense, it stays just out of reach in the future. Always be specific and clear. Finally, keep it positive. Try to avoid words such as *don't, should, bad,* or anything that brings up a negative connotation. Take these steps to stay laser-focused on your goals.

5. Spirituality-Boosting Exercises

Spirituality is interwoven in the mindfulness exercises given in the 4-week plan, but I also encourage you to celebrate and foster spirituality in your own way. Write out spiritual values that speak to you, such as tolerance, love, kindness, honesty, courage, integrity, and grace, and honor these daily. You could say something as simple as this: "May I be honest, authentic, humble, true to myself, kind, loving, and compassionate to others, may I bring harmony, may I be graceful and wise, and may I be of maximum service to myself, my loved ones, and all others." If you belong to a church or other spiritual group but have let your membership or attendance lapse, make a point to revisit and see if it is helpful to you in moving toward your goals. Ask a friend to go with you to solidify your commitment and allow you to spend quality time with someone you may not have seen in a while. This might involve making a regular trip into nature, listening to spiritual music, or meditating, as well as attending church or temple services. If you are not religious, you can still turn things over or pray to a Higher Power, Higher Self, Enlightened Energy, or Nature.

6. Social-Building Strategies

Look at it this way: each chance meeting you have in a day can provide a small boost in your life. View social interactions as a chance to connect positively with those you come into contact with. This can be a smile and some small talk, lending a helping hand (holding a door open for someone), or letting someone go before you in line. If they don't thank you, don't fret. You are responsible for your karma, not theirs. Get even deeper benefits by meeting with a friend or connecting with a loved one at least a couple of times a week. If you are too busy for face-to-face dates, Skype or phone chats will do, but it is important to have physical contact at least once a week with someone you care about.

7. Sleep Strategies

If you have trouble sleeping, try the following tips to improve your snooze time:

- Don't exercise within three hours of bedtime.

- Avoid alcohol in the evenings (it might make you feel sleepy, but it actually interrupts sleep).

- Don't consume caffeine after 2 P.M.

- Check that your medications don't interfere with sleep.

- Establish a regular bedtime and wake-up time, and stick to it.

- If you nap, keep it to under an hour per day.

- Cooler bedroom temperatures promote sleep.

- Remove or cover lights, glowing screens, or lit displays.

- Use a white-noise maker or a fan if outside noises keep you up.

- Get black-out curtains if daylight or outside lights are an issue.

- Allow only sleep and intimacy in the bedroom; do all other activities in other areas of the house.

8. Making Music Work for You

Most of us know that music can elicit exhilaration, joy, sadness, and a wealth of other feelings. It can uncover long-lost memories, bring back visions of the past, help us exercise longer and harder than we thought, and ease tension at the end of a stressful day. You can use music to help rebalance your mind and body when you are feeling off kilter. Remember, you might not like the same music every day, so check in with yourself to see what you are in the mood for. I have one client who listens to Broadway show tunes on some days, but on others she chooses classical. Another client can only listen to classic rock; as soon as I turn it on, his face lights up, and he's ready to, well, *rock*. And sometimes silence is the best music. I have a client who has music piped in at work all day, so she chooses quiet and is invigorated by listening to nothing but the city sounds. Experiment and see what works best for you. Change it up from time to time. Play a few songs and see how they make you feel. Sometimes I like movie soundtracks because it helps me connect to the creativity of the movies and characters and takes me to another place.

9. Breathing Exercises

Throughout the twenty-eight days, you will do daily breathing exercises for the mental portion of *Mind Your Body*. Experiment with the different options and do what works best for you. Depending on your mood, you may find that some exercises feel more comfortable than others. Do what feels the most soothing to your body. Try fast breathing, shallow breathing, deep breathing, and slow breathing to see what feels best and gives you the result you desire. It's common for people to breathe shallowly when they feel preoccupied, and breathing exercises help you be relaxed and open.

Basic Directions

Find a quiet, comfortable place to sit or lie down. Fold your arms gently and loosely across your belly. Now, take a normal breath, then exhale. With each successive breath, begin to inhale and exhale more deeply and slowly. With each breath in, your arms should rise along with your belly. If they don't, you aren't fully using your diaphragm and are not fully relaxed. Continue to breathe in slowly through your nose, allowing your chest and lower belly to rise as you fill your lungs. Let your abdomen fully expand. Pause at the top of your breath for a second, then exhale slowly and completely through your mouth (or your nose, if that feels more natural), feeling your lungs release air. As you take these first breaths, do a scan of your body, acknowledging and releasing any noticeable areas of tension. Then check in with the quality of your mind. Is it filled with rambling, repetitive, or noisy thoughts? When your mind wanders or you follow a thought, or you get distracted by a noise or bodily discomfort, gently bring your mind back to your breath.

Quick tip: Don't leave negative feelings lying around—they'll fester. Whenever you become aware of negative feelings (sadness, jealousy, anxiety), imagine the feeling floating into the sky and evaporating into thin air. You don't want to leave toxic emotions lying around on the sofa, or on your desk at work, or even floating into traffic—they might transfer to someone else or end up as weeds in your front yard.

10. Self-Reflection

At the beginning of this chapter, I asked you to reflect daily on your deserve level categories; you will review your progress several times as you move through the 4-week plan. This is incorporated seamlessly so that self-reflection becomes a habit. This will help you increase your awareness and learn to reshape negative patterns into positive ones. A lot of times bad patterns continue for years because we are like hamsters on their wheels, going round and round with our consciousness completely asleep. I call it the treadmill of life. These habits got you where you are today. To be your own best coach, you need to get in the habit of regularly self-reflecting.

How to Self-Reflect Anytime, Anywhere

Whenever you are waiting for someone and have a few minutes to spare, think back on your moods over the past week. Were they positive or negative? Then imagine you are sitting across the room looking at yourself. What would you have to say about that person? Do you see a tired person slouching over? Do you look annoyed? Would you want to approach this person? This is not an exercise in becoming self-absorbed. This is how, by being present and responsible, you become a realist.

"Happiness Is . . .
. . . . an Inside Job."

WEEK 1

Shifting Your Energy

This week you'll find exercises that help you visualize success, shift your perspective to successful thinking, shut off mental static, and improve sleep.

Day 1

MENTAL STRATEGY
Body Language

Your body language is not an accident. Your posture, the way you walk, your facial expressions, and your physical gestures and features all make up the nonverbal vehicle that communicates your self-perception to others—and to yourself, according to Amy Cuddy, social psychologist at Harvard University. Cuddy's research shows that how you use your body influences not only how others perceive you but also how you feel and think about yourself—and it takes only two minutes to start a real change in your body and your mind!

Thought for the Day

Think about how you are standing and sitting today. Notice if you tend to make your body small by hugging yourself, tucking your legs up underneath you, or slouching. These are all ways of saying, "I am powerless in this world." Whenever you catch yourself making your body small, correct it. Use the next exercise to begin opening up your body—and, in turn, your inner power.

Body Language Exercise

Stand with your back against a flat, sturdy wall, with your heels flush or one inch from the baseboard, whichever is more natural. While looking straight ahead, imagine that a string is attached to the top of your head and is pulling up, elongating you all the way from your heels through your hips, spine, neck, and head. Roll your shoulders up, back, and down. Now, scan your body, taking a few deep breaths and letting go of unnecessary tension with each exhale. Relax your mind and focus on your breathing. After a few more breaths, imagine that there are three strangers standing behind you. How would each describe you by your body language? What messages is your body telling them? Would they see irritation, confidence, laziness, or . . . ? Now let joy, assertiveness, peace, light, and love flood into your body, and imagine that these strangers see only positive body language. Relax your arms to your sides and lift your chin. Continue to breathe away tension. Be aware of how your body shifts as you move through this exercise.

Breathing Exercise

You are going to take five breaths, inhaling slowly and deeply, then exhaling slowly and completely. Each time you inhale, allow your mind to take you to a tense part of your body. Imagine that there is a balloon in this spot, and imagine it expanding. Keep your chest lifted as you exhale. Visualize negative tension, thoughts, and feelings drifting off into the sky to disappear forever. Repeat, moving your attention to another tense area for a full five breaths. Throughout your day, each time you check the time, take ten seconds to check in with any points of tension or negative thoughts and breathe them away.

Affirmation

"I move forward in life with confidence and sincerity, wanting only to do good." "I love exactly who I am; I am strong and capable."

MENTAL STRATEGY
Simplicity

Cluttered homes equal cluttered minds.

Simplifying Exercise

Pick a drawer or stack of papers in your home that needs to be organized. Take it to a different room. For example, if you want to clean a desk drawer that is in your office, take it to the kitchen table. Take everything out, or if it is a stack of papers, put it on a table. Put an empty trash can and a recycling container nearby. Imagine someone is watching you. This creates a feeling of validation and responsibility. Go through each item one by one and toss it, take action, or save (only if you will use the item within the coming six months). If the paper or item calls for an immediate action, stop and do it. Whenever you come across areas in your nest that represent unfinished projects or business, it creates anxiety. The goal, when you have finished your stack or drawer, is to be left feeling able to find anything you need quickly and easily.

Thought for the Day

Whenever a circumstance, event, or situation arises, pause and take time to think of the most direct path to resolve the issue, make the decision, or deal with the event.

Breathing Exercise

Inhale slowly to a count of four, and exhale slowly to a count of four. Repeat this four times. Then read the next meditation, close your eyes, and repeat the breathing exercise while focusing on the meditation.

Meditation

While practicing the breathing exercise, begin to incorporate this thought: "Everything inside and around me is perfectly organized. I release all confusion and conflict. I appreciate, value, and am drawn toward simplicity."

Affirmation

"I handle everything I encounter with clarity and patience. I let go easily."

Feel good, live simply, and laugh more.

—UNKNOWN

MENTAL STRATEGY
Let Go of Your Past

The family you grew up with may have taught you good or bad things—or, most likely, some of both. Often people continue to think, feel, and act out based on coping strategies they learned as children, but you don't have to live in your childhood anymore. It's time to let go of the past and learn new and empowering feelings, thoughts, and actions. How you feel, think, and behave today is what defines you, not who you were in the past.

Changing Childhood Patterns

Think back over this last week. What thoughts did you have or what did you say or do that didn't really come from who you are? This could be something you were taught in your youth or a habit or expression you developed during your childhood that doesn't match who you are or who you want to be today. Don't criticize or judge; simply allow the awareness of how the past still affects your present and realize that you can let go of whatever doesn't work for you today. Your thoughts are your choice.

Affirmation

"I don't respond or react immediately. I pause and listen to my thoughts before I speak. My thoughts and actions are my own. I create them, and I can uncreate them."

Breathing Exercise

Throughout your day today, practice taking a slow, deep inhale and a slow, full exhale before you speak, respond, or react to anything, even yourself.

Meditation

After reading the following statement a few times, close your eyes and repeat it several times while taking slow deep breaths: "I say what I mean and mean what I say. I have transparent beliefs."

Day 4

MENTAL STRATEGY

Smile

Smile as big and bright as you can while you read the following exercises. Smiling triggers activity in the areas of your brain that register happiness, so do it even when you don't feel happy, and you'll instantly improve your mood. Plus, smiling is contagious, according to recent research from Wayne State University in Detroit. Your smile triggers happiness in the brains of those around you as well as in yourself.

Thought for the Day

Today I want you to think about spreading your smile. All day today, smile at every person you see. Don't expect a response or return smile. Just give your smile away, pass it on, even if it feels awkward at first. Don't think about it. Just do it.

Meditation

After reading the following statement a few times, close your eyes and think it while taking slow deep breaths: "I see only loving people around me. Even if their outsides don't show it, I know that we are all the same at our center—loving, kind, and caring."

Breathing Exercise

Any time you run into an unpleasant situation, experience, or person today, pause and then inhale deeply, breathing in all negativity, and then exhaling fully and releasing positive energy back into the universe. You have the power and abundance to transform energy from negative to positive. It just takes a breath to clear away undesirable energy. You can use this whenever you run into an undesirable situation. Try combining this breathing exercise with the visualization below.

Visualization

Close your eyes and visualize negativity flying at you in the form of negative signs from every direction. Imagine that you are breathing in this negative energy, and as you exhale, see them come out as positive energy in the form of plus signs (+ + + +). Imagine that you are releasing positivity out into the universe. Feel your body relax each time you transform a "– – –" into a "+ + +."

Affirmation

"I am full of generosity. I know that everyone is doing the best they can, and I have an abundance of love to give. Smiling comes to me easily."

Sometimes your joy is the source of your smile, but sometimes your smile can be the source of your joy.

—THICH NHAT HANH

Day 5

MENTAL STRATEGY
Energy Distribution

Today is about doing an energy makeover. Paying attention to what saps your energy during the day and making conscious choices about where to devote your energy will help you get more out of your day.

Thought for the Day

Use lights as triggers to check in with your energy today. Whenever you see a light fixture (table lamp, chandelier, wall sconce, or candle), let it remind you of energy. Pause for a moment to take stock of how you are feeling. Be aware of your energy; imagine what someone would see if your energy and emotions expressed themselves as light and color. For example, if you are hot with anger, your light might be bright red. If you are exhausted, maybe it is just a dim yellow light.

Affirmation

"I love myself, and I will always be here for me. I feel comfort and ease. I create my new reality."

Energy Distribution Exercise

Do a quick scan of the areas you feel are draining you of energy. What areas in your body or places in your life drain you of power? Write down the top three that come to mind. Inhale deeply and slowly, and as you exhale fully, let them go. You will feel immediately lighter.

What energizing, uplifting, joyful feelings do you want to feel? Write three of them down on sticky notes and put them where you can see them. Now inhale deeply, breathing in energizing feelings, and exhale a radiating light.

Visualization

Close your eyes and imagine what is draining you of energy. See these things visually. If work is one of these, imagine your desk, your boss, or a meeting that you dread. Hear the sounds of phones ringing, smell the office, see the bright lights. Imagine whatever is overwhelming in your life with all your senses. When you can clearly visualize an image and hold it, begin to shrink it down. Next, picture a big trash can or dumpster and imagine yourself throwing your draining images into it. In goes the boss, the office, the meeting. Finally, see the trash men coming, and watch as they haul off the waste that you no longer have room for in your life.

Meditation

Sit in silence for one minute and focus on taking full breaths of love. With each inhale and exhale, imagine a golden light radiating out from every one of your pores. You are glowing with energy and light.

Day 6

MENTAL STRATEGY
Sleep

Quality and quantity go hand in hand when it comes to sleep. If you sleep deeply (quality), but for just a few hours a night (lack of quantity), your brain and body don't get what they need to rejuvenate. If, on the other hand, you spend plenty of time in bed at night, but the quality of sleep is poor—you'll have the same problems. You deserve to be well rested and to sleep in peace for the appropriate amount of time.

Thought for the Day

Fake it till you make it. Whenever someone asks you how you sleep, respond that you sleep like a baby. You'll create a new story about yourself, and that will make it into a reality.

Affirmation

"I drift off into a deep restful slumber with ease. My dreams take me on beautiful, joyful journeys. I wake feeling well rested and energized."

Bedtime Practice

While you are lying in bed tonight, take a moment to examine the quality of your thoughts. Sometimes, when I'm going to bed I realize that I have to get up early and I won't get all the sleep I know I need. I start thinking about how sleepy I'm going to be in the morning, and I have to catch myself, because I know this sort of thinking can disrupt the quality of sleep that I do have available. Instead, I say an affirmation: "I am going to wake up easily, feeling awake and alive. I am going to have a perfect night of sleep."

Bedtime Writing Exercise

Keep a notebook and a pen by your bed, and use it as a safe holding place for your thoughts. If you find your mind racing at bedtime, write down any to-dos, worries, ideas, or goals. Trust that they'll be waiting right there for you tomorrow. For now, you can rest easy.

Day 7

MENTAL STRATEGY
Floating

Today is about unplugging and allowing your mind to let go and float.

Free-Your-Mind Meditation

Take a pen and paper and sit in a comfortable chair. Let your mind drift off for around ten minutes. Allow your thoughts to wander freely. Imagine that your mind is a river; see your thoughts floating along with the current. If a thought arises that feels pressing, urgent, or persistent, simply jot it down, then come back to the river. Listen to the sounds of the water lapping against the shore. See the sun shining and feel its warmth on your skin. Feel your body melt, releasing all tension. When you notice that you are following a thought or have been hooked into an emotion, take a deep breath, jot it down, and let it go.

Thought for the Day

Fire your autopilot and hire your creative mind. We often limit ourselves when it comes to creating ideas, because we feel hindered by fear of judgment. You can change this pattern by freeing your mind. When it's time to come up with an idea, allow your mind to wander for a few minutes (as in the "Free-Your-Mind

Meditation" on page 127). The process of disconnecting and letting your thoughts flow freely will engage your creative side to produce more effective, intuitive, and inspired ideas.

Affirmation

"My mind works perfectly, and whenever I need an idea or inspiration, I simply relax, and it comes to me effortlessly."

Floating Visualization

Sit comfortably and close your eyes. Imagine that you are drifting up into the sky. Feel how light your body feels, how your arms and legs just float out to your sides and feel weightless. See yourself among the clouds in the blue sky. Feel how comfortable and secure you feel. Continue this exercise for about three minutes, making the visual world as real as possible. See and hear birds flying by; see the houses and the tops of trees down below. Then gently feel your body floating down onto a warm, sandy beach. Feel the sand between your toes and the sun on your skin.

WEEK 2

Motivation

This week is all about creating confidence and drive, cultivating grit, empowering yourself, and learning to be a doer. You're going to learn how to eliminate roadblocks and escape routes.

Day 8

MENTAL STRATEGY

Mentor Advice

Today is about remembering the wisdom that your parents, a teacher, or a mentor instilled in you. I want you to take a few minutes and think back to what sayings or advice you have been given that still floats around in your brain. For example, my mom always told me, "It is nice to be nice" and "Make a decision or someone else will make it for you." It's time for you to consciously decide if these messages from the past are still helpful to you today. Are they positive, negative, or just plain useless? Take a piece of paper and fold it in half lengthwise and write down the old messages as fast as you can. Then take the ones that are negative, and on the other side of the paper rewrite them so they are positive. An old message one client of mine shared with me was "If you do that, they are going to think you are nuts," which she rewrote as "I accept and love myself just as I am, and people are drawn to me from every direction. My mind is unique and creative."

Affirmation

"I am my own remarkable person. People are drawn to me from every direction. I am building the life I want."

Visualization

Close your eyes and see your parents on a stage in front of an enormous audience. Hear them saying how incredibly talented you are and how proud of you they are. Visualize old defeating messages and thoughts drifting away. Let yourself feel your parents' loving presence, unconditional love, and overflowing pride in you.

Breathing Exercise

Take five deep breaths; with each exhale, feel your body relax as you settle into who you are in this very moment. As you breathe, repeat to yourself, "I am enough just the way I am today."

Day 9

MENTAL STRATEGY

Gratitude

When we are grateful, we sleep better, have lower blood pressure, and stay healthier. Practicing gratitude is taking a moment to consciously acknowledge a benefit that is already in your life or coming your way. Unfortunately, we tend to live extremely busy lives, and it is easy to overlook what is going right in our lives, which can lead to negativity. Today is about practicing the art of giving thanks for what is good in our lives. Everyone I know likes to be thanked; I've never met anyone who liked being taken for granted or overlooked. Most people like to do things for people

who appreciate it. Our true selves are accustomed to being generous and gracious.

Thought for the Day

Keep the following thought as a running theme for your day: I am sensitive and aware of all that goes on around me. I see the positive, and I say "thank you" easily. It slips off my lips with ease.

Affirmation

"I appreciate all that I am, and feel gratitude for all that I see and do. I am grateful for all the universe offers me."

Visualization

Close your eyes. Scan the past week and see all the things you have to be thankful for. Maybe there was a day that was particularly beautiful. See the sunshine, feel the warmth, and hear the birds singing. Take a moment to create an image of what brought the feeling of gratitude into your being. Inhale each grateful moment and smile.

Day 10

MENTAL STRATEGY

Public Speaking

The more confidence we have, the easier it is to propel ourselves forward. Everyone I know who has taken a class in public speaking or acting, including myself, has said that it was one of the best things they ever did for themselves. Some people say they were terrified to get up in front of a crowd, but once they went through it, they felt rejuvenated and empowered. Why? Because it allows you to get in front of others and express yourself confidently. You do this in your daily life. You have to convey your thoughts to others to communicate your needs, wants, and desires.

Thought for the Day

Think about where you could communicate more effectively in your life. Think of an idea or concept you wanted to share, and share it today with a trusted friend or co-worker. After you've expressed yourself, ask for feedback. One of my clients, Serina, told me that she wanted to take voice lessons when she was growing up, but her parents couldn't afford them. Today she is very successful and could easily pay the price. Serina passed my next client, a famous singer, as she was leaving our appointment. At our next appointment, she asked me if I'd ask the singer about a voice teacher. I told her I would, but that I thought it would be better for her to do it. After a few weeks, she finally got up the courage. And after a year of voice lessons, she's so good that she's now performing in a big show in the city. Taking risks pays big.

Affirmation

"My thoughts flow easily; I express and share my ideas with confidence and grace."

Visualization

Close your eyes and imagine that you are standing in front of a huge crowd of people. You have just completed an amazing lecture, lost weight, finished a marathon, or achieved another enormous success. Feel people patting you on the back and hear them shouting words of praise and congratulations on a job well done.

Stress is not driven by the things that happen in life; stress is driven by your perception of what happened.

MENTAL STRATEGY
Free Time

We all have the same twenty-four hours in a day. Most of us have work obligations and other commitments, but ultimately, how you use your time, especially your free time, is up to you. If you say "time zips by," it will. If you think, "I never have enough time," then you never will. Negative affirmations are self-defeating and must be eliminated if you want to empower yourself to make healthy changes. Take control! Think about how you typically spend your leisure time. Are you watching TV, surfing the web, or on your phone? The average American spends about 8.5 hours a day in front of screens of one sort or another—that's an entire day not spent on your goals. Pay attention to what is sucking up your unscheduled time, and make sure it matches your goals.

Thought for the Day

Today I want you to think about being responsible for yourself. Being self-responsible is dynamically liberating and endlessly energizing. Before you can support others, you have to learn how to nurture yourself.

Writing Exercise

Grab a pen and paper and spend a few minutes brainstorming on what you could do to take care of yourself. Pick three things, and take the first step on one project today. Learn to knit, speak Spanish, or play tennis. Find a local class and schedule an appointment today.

Affirmation

"I have an abundance of time. I am able to do everything I want whenever I want to do it."

Visualization

Sit comfortably and close your eyes. Think of your hobbies and the activities you fantasize about doing. Let's say you want to go on a hike. Feel the rocky path under your feet and the sun on your shoulders. Breathe in the fresh mountain air. Hear the birds chirping in the trees around you. See yourself smiling and losing track of time because you are having such a good time.

Day 12

MENTAL STRATEGY

$$$$$

Money is a great motivator, but does it have power over you? Is lack of money causing you to feel trapped? What are your inner thoughts about money? Get clear on them. When one client first started coming to me, he would say, "I'm never going to make great money; my parents will always have to pay for me." Negative thinking like this creates a negative reality. Instead of freeing you to do what you want, does money trigger insecurity, anxiety, or low self-worth? If it does, then it has control over your moods and your life. To be truly powerful, you have to face your fears about money, cleaning up any debts you created, and doing the work to bring in money.

Thought for the Day

Today, consider redefining your relationship to money. Understand that while there are limits that come with financial difficulties, there are also opportunities and possibilities that you are missing. If you are in this state, think about how you can make a game of reducing your spending as much as possible, paying off debt if you have it, while raising your quality of life.

Affirmation

"Money continually flows to me from every direction. I have an abundance of riches to do exactly what I want whenever I want to do it."

Visualization

Sit quietly and close your eyes. Bring to mind the image of a hundred-dollar bill. Feel the bill with your hands. Imagine that you are looking up and you begin to see hundred-dollar bills falling rapidly from every direction. It's as if you are caught in a storm of hundred-dollar bills. See yourself walk to your mailbox and open it; as you do, see hundred-dollar bills pouring out. Imagine looking at your windows and your door and seeing hundred-dollar bills coming in through every crack. See all this prosperity coming to you. Feel how you deserve to have this financial abundance in your life.

Breathing Exercise

You can start feeling successful right now with your breath. As you take in a slow, deep inhale, imagine that you are breathing in success, abundance, and prosperity. As you exhale, release negative feelings and stress about money. As you inhale again, feel your chest lift and your body center itself in the endless abundance you deserve.

No one can make you feel inferior without your consent.

—ELEANOR ROOSEVELT

MENTAL STRATEGY
Forgiveness

Do you have past actions that you don't feel good about? What do you need to forgive yourself for? Do you feel you have been wronged? Do you hold grudges? Forgiving others and yourself is the path to true serenity. It is time to accept responsibility and move into peace and acceptance. To truly forgive yourself, it is of paramount importance that you free yourself and make amends where appropriate.

Thought for the Day

Holding on to resentment attaches you to anger and bitterness, paralyzing your growth. Today, aim to let go of resentment and embrace forgiveness wherever possible.

Amends Exercise

Make a list of all wrongs, big or small, that you feel you owe an apology for or need to make restitution on—anything that makes you squirm or cringe. Quickly jot down desired amends without worrying about grammar, punctuation, or spelling. When you are done, go over your list and brainstorm what action you need to take. You might need to write a letter, make a phone call, or go in person to say you are sorry. Now go stand in front of a mirror and say "I'm sorry" several times. Say it until it feels easy. Let go of how the other person might react or any wrongs they may have done to you. This is about cleaning up your side of the street. Forgiveness is freedom.

Affirmation

"I accept myself and am good enough just the way I am today. I forgive myself and let go of any harm to others or myself."

Visualization

Sit comfortably and close your eyes. See the people on your list. Imagine that you have made amends and see your loved ones, friends, and acquaintances smiling and looking at you with warmth. Hear them say you are forgiven. See yourself laughing with them. See everyone at peace.

Meditation

Sit quietly and focus on your breath, paying attention to each inhale and exhale. After a few minutes, turn your attention to your heart. Feel your heart opening. Feel the hurt you've carried around for years. Feel love and goodwill flow in with your in-breath and out with your out-breath. Feel the hurt and pain flowing out. Be patient and give your body some time to adjust. Feel any bitterness or resentment lifting from your heart and body, flowing out through every pore. Feel how light and open you feel. See the particles of pain as they drift off into the sky and evaporate like mist in the sunshine. There can be no darkness where you shine light.

A loving heart is the beginning of all knowledge.
—THOMAS CARLYLE

MENTAL STRATEGY
If/Then Plans

I find that a lot of people stay stuck and don't move forward with their dreams because of fear, so that's often where I start my work with people. If you want to move forward, it's important to identify what is holding you back. The simplest and most effective way to do this is by making an if/then list. When a challenge surfaces in my life, I focus on how to fix the problem instead of worrying about it happening. Worry is a useless emotion that just fuels anxiety.

Thought for the Day

Think about the day in front of you. What plans do you have? What obstacles or challenges might you encounter? How can you apply the "if this happens, then I will do this" way of thinking throughout your day today?

If/Then List

Grab a piece of paper and fold it vertically in half. On the left side, list your worries and what you fear will happen. On the right side, brainstorm solutions. For example, Suzy, a client of mine who was trying to lose weight, wrote down that she was worried about going to happy hour with her friends because having a few drinks added unnecessary calories and made it harder to skip appetizers. Her solution was to tell her friends that she wasn't in the mood for alcohol and she would order sparkling water instead. Having a plan in place, Suzy smoothly made it through the evening, stuck to her goals, and had fun. You can, and should, use if/then planning any time you are heading into a potentially challenging situation.

Affirmation

"I handle whatever comes in my direction with simplicity and ease."

Visualization

You can do if/then planning as a visualization exercise anytime you are feeling worried, concerned, or fearful about something. In the example above, I would have told Suzy to sit quietly with her eyes closed and see herself at happy hour ordering the alternative drink, socializing with her friends, and having fun. I'd ask her to hear ice clinking in the glasses, to see the appetizers being passed around and being so focused on scintillating conversation that she doesn't even notice the food. Now it's your turn: If you have something on your mind and you're not sure how you're going to get through it, think it through carefully. Be creative and flesh it out completely. Visualize everything that could go wrong and all the solutions you can come up with. Make sure to see yourself successfully getting through the situation.

If/Then Planning

This is a technique you can employ any time you want to prepare for a potentially challenging event. The strategy is extremely useful for bolstering your resolve in times of temptation and helping you stick to your goals. So, if you are committed to following the *Mind Your Body* plan but have an upcoming party where you know temptations will be flying in your face all evening, grab pen and paper and fill in the statement "*If* X happens, *then* I will do Y." You might write something like this: "If I have a party to go to where there may be cupcakes or other tempting treats, then I will eat a healthy snack ahead of time and take a healthy food item to the party." Surprisingly, this simple exercise can radically improve your success rate in losing weight and changing just about any other habit, according to a New York University review of ninety-four studies that investigated the technique.

WEEK 3

Being Present

Do you easily find your mind slipping into an auto-pilot mode of ruminating about past occurrences or future possibilities? This week is about acting with an intention to live in the present moment, encouraging self-trust, and helping you follow through when times are challenging.

Day 15

MENTAL STRATEGY
Taste

Are you ever in such a hurry that you inhale your food so fast you don't taste a single bite? Eating is supposed to be an enjoyable process where you savor each mouthful. Mealtimes are meant to be a time to celebrate nourishing your body with delicious healthy foods. I want you to experience pleasure in the taste that food brings to your palate. This isn't a practice in decadence or overindulging. When you are fully conscious and present for your food, overeating is much less likely.

Thought for the Day
Today, take time to register the flavors, textures, temperatures, and aromas of the food you are eating. Your hunger is appeased faster when you pay attention.

Taste Meditation
Right now, take a moment to wake up your mouth. Close your eyes and notice the tastes in your mouth. Take your tongue and circle it around the perimeter of your teeth. Start at the top and then move to the bottom. Then massage the roof of your mouth with your tongue. When you eat your next meal, take a mouthful of food and then set your food and utensils down. Chew this first mouthful slowly, focusing intently on the flavors, texture, and temperature of the food. Chew this mouthful until it is the consistency of baby food, then swallow. Take your next bite. Repeat, noticing the flavors and chewing carefully. Continue like this, pausing between bites, focusing intently, and chewing carefully. Notice how it feels to eat like this. Do you get full faster? Try to do this at one meal a day for the next week, and get in the habit of checking in. You'll increase awareness of hunger and satiety signals and avoid mindless eating.

Affirmation
"I eat and drink only nutritious foods and beverages that replenish my body and leave me feeling energized and restored."

Visualization
Close your eyes and bring to mind an image of the inside of your refrigerator. Visualize each shelf and drawer overflowing with a wide variety and abundance of healthy fresh foods. Imagine that you pick up various items and smell them, see the vividness of the different colors, and feel a great desire to eat these wonderfully nutritious foods.

Breathing Meditation
Allow yourself time to relax today while you are eating. As you enjoy the meal, be aware of your breathing. As you pause between bites, take a few deep breaths. Sit back as you chew your food so you can breathe easily. If you are eating with others, try to be

the slowest eater at your table. Notice your posture. If you are slouching or hunched forward, sit up and lift your chest so you can breathe easily.

Day 16

MENTAL STRATEGY
Monitor Your Mood

It is easy to get caught up in the emotions around us or to get swept away by another person's mood. However, you are accountable for your own feelings, and you don't have to let someone else's emotions blow you about. To maintain a healthy emotional balance, I find that it is best to stay in a neutral place, ask questions, and refrain from jumping to conclusions. This can be difficult when dealing with someone who is acting irritable, but if you can avoid taking it personally, instead staying impartial and asking questions, you'll understand the situation better. You'll be much more likely to resolve the problem without being knocked off balance.

Thought for the Day

Let the following statement be your theme for the day: "I don't have to dominate or control others. I create my own moods, and I take responsibility for my mental state."

Self-Reflection Meditation

Sit quietly and reflect on the past week. What was your overriding mood? How did you feel today? How do you want to feel? Take a moment to monitor what you are feeling right now, and then imagine a positive emotion. Examine what it feels like—and then acknowledge that you are feeling what you are practicing. Let yourself be conscious and fully aware of this moment.

For example, if you are feeling a sense of urgency, take a moment to visualize what patience and tolerance feel like. Settle into those feelings of patience and tolerance. Allow your body to relax, and acknowledge to yourself, "Yes, this is how I am feeling now." Sometimes it takes multiple repetitions to release negative emotions; practice releases and frees you from the reactivity of negative thoughts. The more I practice a positive emotion, the more it becomes a healthy habitual reaction.

Affirmation

"I have control over how I feel and act. When I trust myself and monitor my impulses, I am able to help myself and others."

Visualization

Find a comfortable and quiet place to sit. Close your eyes. Imagine that you are seeing yourself from far away. Imagine there is an aura of light around you that represents your current attitude. What do you see? Is the energy around you positive or negative? What does it feel like? Now imagine that the negative vibrations and colors are fading, and the positive colors and vibrations are growing more and more vivid. See the people around you, your home, your pets, and your work as having the same positive colors and vibrations surrounding them. Everything your energy touches is enhanced with a positive, upbeat energy.

Breathing Meditation

As you take five deep breaths, repeat, "Inside each of us are all the good traits the universe has to offer. I breathe in the white light of universal energy, and I breathe out universal peace."

MENTAL STRATEGY

Outer Appearances

We all want to feel and look our best, but many people don't realize that this involves more than just eating right and exercising. Your perception, feelings, and attitude all play an important part in how you look to the outside world. All the cells that make up your body have a direct relationship to your feelings and thoughts. My most successful clients always look amazing because they work to feel their best from the inside out. These people know that to look stunning, they must also feel their best. When you groom and dress yourself in the morning, do you take the time to look your best? If not, why not? How can you change that?

Thought for the Day

Consider this: the better you feel about yourself, the higher your self-worth, the more you love yourself—all this will translate into outer beauty, and you'll worry less about how you look to the outside world.

Tension Release Exercise

Feeling overly tense shows up as lines on your face. Tension can start from your feet (which ground you and propel you forward) and spread all the way up your body. Foot massages have been shown to relieve headaches, back pain, and overall tension. Try the following foot treatment to release tension and make you look beautiful all over. While seated in a comfortable chair, sit barefoot and bring your left foot up onto your right leg. Take both hands and massage your foot. Use your fingers to knead every crevice and gently pull each toe. Allow yourself to relax and let go of tension. Then switch sides and massage the other foot. While you are doing this, think of actions you can take to look your best.

Affirmation

"A sense of balance, serenity, and strength comes from looking my best. I give myself time to be healthy and vibrant. Each and every one of my cells glows with illuminating energy. People always say how attractive I am."

Visualization

Sitting comfortably, close your eyes and take a few slow, deep breaths. Then bring your attention to your feet. Imagine that your feet look beautiful, fully manicured, and smooth. Move your attention up to your ankles, calves, and thighs, visualizing them as the picture of perfection. Move on to your bottom and belly. Be very specific. If you want to lose your stomach, see and feel it flat and firm. See these areas exactly as you've always dreamed. Now do the same for your back, chest, shoulders, and neck. Let go of any excess weight until you are perfect. See your beautiful face and hair. Pretend you are making a sculpture of yourself the way you want to be. The more you crystallize your vision of yourself as pure beauty, the clearer your attractiveness in your mind's eye, the faster it will become your reality.

Breathing Exercise

Take a slow, deep inhale and feel what it feels like to have an amazing body. Then exhale fully, slowly, and completely, letting imperfections go out with your breath. Repeat, inhaling beauty into your bones, muscles, and cells and exhaling insecurity and self-doubt. Repeat for a total of five breaths, settling into the beautiful person you truly are.

Day 18

MENTAL STRATEGY
Your Honor Code

Having a set of moral principles can help you stay anchored in the present moment. An honor code is a set of qualities or principles you have deemed important enough to uphold even under duress. These are core values you believe in that you can return to whenever you begin to feel off balance. Other people learn that they can expect certain things from you based on the values you hold dear. For example, if you live by a code of honesty, love, and kindness, you'll be more likely to have genuine, loving, kind relationships. The more you value an attitude of appreciation, patience, and understanding, the more you will be surrounded by these qualities. Spending time defining the values you want to live by will help you decide what you must change in your behavior to align your life with who you want to be. In this way, having an honor code helps you define your sense of self, and knowing who you are is paramount in eliminating noise (see rule 1 on page 6).

Thought for the Day

Today I want you to consider what makes up your honor code. What virtues did you learn as a child? What still holds true? What are the values of the people you spend the most time around? What are they doing with their lives? How successful, optimistic, spiritual, or loving are they? Do your principles match? What do you believe in, but don't behave in accordance with? What values from your childhood or friends will you keep? What will you abandon?

Affirmation

"I come from a place of love, honesty, and kindness. I say what I mean and I mean what I say. People respect me because I am trustworthy, tolerant, and loving."

Visualization

Sit quietly and imagine yourself attracting loving relationships. Visualize what it feels like to be in healthy relationships with each of your family members, friends, co-workers, and anyone you surround yourself with. Pick five people who are closest to you, and bring them into your imagination. See yourself having a pleasant conversation. Feel their enthusiasm and how it energizes you. See yourself being fully nourished and nourishing.

You are the average of the five people you spend the most time with.

—JIM ROHN

Day 19

MENTAL STRATEGY
Smell

Of all your senses, which is your strongest? Your nose is the main sensor for smelling and tasting. That's why you have trouble tasting food when you are congested. Aromas and scents trigger memories, lift your spirits, and often cause cravings. Ever been at the airport or mall and been hit by the intoxicating aroma of cinnamon buns? It makes you want to drop your bags, rush to the front of the line, and bite into one immediately. Smell can increase or decrease appetite, so it is imperative to be aware of what you're smelling and what it might trigger. Your sense of smell deteriorates with age, but you can keep it alive and kicking by stimulating your sense of smell in healthy ways.

Thought for the Day

Pay close attention to the smells in your environment as you move through the day. What is your favorite smell? The smell of a lemon, lavender, or fresh muffins? As you go about your day, be aware of smells and how they make you feel. Do they trigger snacking? Do they make you want to eat unhealthy snacks? What makes your stomach grumble? What wakes you up? Pause several times to smell your surroundings. Be conscious of the perfume of flowers wafting by if you are outside. How does the cafeteria, dining room, or restaurant smell at lunchtime? Notice how your home smells when you return home. Light a special candle or burn some incense and enjoy the aroma today.

Practice Scent Sense

While standing, reach your arms straight above your head with palms facing forward and fingertips pointing to the ceiling. Inhale deeply through your nose, and as you exhale, bring your arms to your sides with the tempo of your breath. Relax your hands at your sides. Take another breath in through your nose, and this time notice what aromas are in your environment. Are they pleasant or unpleasant? How do they make you feel? Do they bring up memories? Repeat this a couple of times. Next, cup your hand around your mouth and inhale, smelling your breath. Is it good or bad? Most people never take the time to smell their own breath. If it doesn't smell good, fix it. You want to attract people to you; bad breath is a sure way not to.

Affirmation

"I take in all the rich aromas around me. Wherever I go, I stop and smell; it is a window into my present moment. My sense of smell draws me to healthy nutritious foods that nourish my body."

Breathing Exercise

While sitting quietly, take a deep inhale through your nose and exhale fully through your mouth. Close your eyes. As you continue to breathe, feel the sensation of air passing in and out of your nostrils. Allow this to set the stage for awakening your sense of smell.

Day 20

MENTAL STRATEGY

Work

Most of us spend most of our waking hours in a place of business. Is your occupation fulfilling? Are your thoughts about your career limited by your beliefs? If something doesn't feel right, it might be time for a change. Maybe you just need to adjust your attitude, or perhaps your future is calling you to a new adventure. Even if your work is challenging or tough, remember that all experiences are opportunities to grow, cultivate grit, and become more talented.

Thought for the Day

Spend some time today thinking about your current work situation and how your attitude might be influencing your perception of your career. Nathan, a client of mine, used to complain about his job through entire training sessions. After listening a few times, I asked him how he would feel about himself if he were the employer. Did he see himself as a valuable employee? He laughed and told me he wouldn't think much of himself as an employee—not when he knew what sort of attitude he was carrying around. I told him that he had just explained why he was so unhappy with work. His face went flat, and he looked confused.

"If you wouldn't want you working for yourself, why would anyone else?" I asked.

He tried to explain that his boss was annoying, but I cut him off with a "so?" And I suggested he try giving the boss what he had been hired for, do the work, and stop taking advantage of his boss, and then see if he still found the boss irritating. I told him that I thought he was irritated with himself and projecting it onto his boss. At our next session, Nathan came in looking sheepish.

"Well?" I asked.

"Well, I did what you suggested, and the boss is off my back, and he actually complimented me on a project I proposed this past week," he said.

Affirmation

"I am creative. I am unique. I have a position that I love doing, and I get paid great money doing it."

Visualization

Close your eyes and conjure up an image of your workplace. See yourself going to your office or workspace at the start of the day. What does it look like? What sounds do you hear? What smells do you smell? What feelings and thoughts come up? Really go deep into the feeling. Now imagine that you are having a fabulous day. Co-workers are complimenting you. Your supervisor is praising your work. See yourself leaving at the end of the day, tired but feeling fantastic. You have done well today. You were helpful and useful to your co-workers, to the mission your job stands for, and you have provided for yourself and your family.

Breathing Exercise

Take five deep breaths, inhaling deeply and fully, and exhaling slowly and completely, and imagine you are being praised for a job well done. Sense what it feels like to be commended on your talents and abilities.

MENTAL STRATEGY
Other People

We all have to deal with other people, some of us more than others. I see the world get a wee bit more self-absorbed day by day and it saddens me, but it is within our power to reverse the wave. I need your help. It's easy to forget that we are all part of one universe. It's easy to separate yourself from others, but it doesn't have to be that way. Your mind is the universal mind, and the way you access the collective mind we all share is by tapping the present moment and connecting with those around you.

Thought for the Day

Think about the other people in your life—not just friends and family, but people you see often, such as the doorman, the mail carrier, your barista. Consider that each person you cross, drive next to, or see on the street has good days and bad, triumphs and defeats, loves and rejections. We are all one. We share many of the same experiences, but some of us have harder lives than others.

Writing Exercise

Write thank-you notes. Think back over the past few months and list five people who did something nice for you. It doesn't have to be a big gesture. Maybe a food server was particularly attentive. Maybe a friend called to see how you were doing. Grab a note card or head to the store and pick out five cards, and write each person a thank-you note. Make the notes all about them and how much their gestures meant to you. If you don't know someone's address, personally hand it to that person.

Affirmation

"I enjoy being in the presence of others. We are all unique human beings and each of us has a purpose. I appreciate the loving relationships I am surrounded with."

Meditation

Allow yourself a few minutes to sit quietly and focus on yourself. Thank yourself for taking care of yourself. You go to work, you are eating heathy, you are exercising and making healthy changes. You are reading this book and attempting to take part in a total transformation. Be grateful for yourself. Write a thank-you note to yourself. Sense what it feels like to be appreciated and noticed for what you say and do.

WEEK 4

Thinking Outside the Box

It's time to get creative, tap your imagination, and open your mind. Remember, you deserve better than the best, and being willing to try new ideas and solutions is the first step. Plus, anytime you are open to learning something new, you literally wake up your brain. It doesn't matter if you decide to take up knitting, sign up for guitar lessons, or learn to play chess—your brain will respond whenever you try something new by rebuilding neurons and creating new pathways. This mental stimulation in turn stimulates and energizes your body.

It's your road, and yours alone. Others may walk it with you, but no one can walk it for you.

—RUMI

Day 22

MENTAL STRATEGY
Setting Daily Intentions

On page 84, you identified goals you wanted to achieve. Congratulations! You are now on day 22 and have actively set a positive intention for change by following these daily prescriptions. Now it is time to start thinking about how you can design your own daily intentions to continue to carry you toward your dreams. Do you still have the same dreams you did at the beginning? Are they true to the real you who is emerging? It's okay—in fact it's great—if you want to tweak or shift your goals. That's part of growth. Now is the time to upgrade them.

Each and every day counts, even if some days it feels like you take two steps back for every step forward. Missteps and slip-ups are just as valuable as accomplishments if you are awake to see the lessons that can be learned. If you went to a party and got caught by the chocolate fountain, it might make you want to throw in your workout towel, but it can actually be a fantastic opportunity to examine what happens to you at social gatherings. You can go back to day 14 (page 132) and practice some if/then brainstorming so you will hit the next event prepared. As long as you continue to walk in the same direction, you will get to your destination. Most roads aren't smooth, and life doesn't come with an "undo" button. Our lives twist and turn, with potholes and detours, but if you keep the faith and continue with persistence in the direction of your goals, you will make it. Never underestimate the power of taking consistent small steps.

Thought for the Day

Are you headed in the right direction? Take a moment to review the 10 categories in the test on pages 19–28. Scan these critical areas of your life and review the goals you have set for yourself. Are you on your path? It is not necessary to beat yourself up. Just check in with yourself and think through where you want to go. It's never too late to start over. It's okay if you've had a shift since you started *Mind Your Body*; just adjust your intention to match today's goals. If you have the thought, you have the ability to make it happen. Adjusting goals doesn't create stress; it releases tension. By staying current with daily intentions, you will make sure that your goals have maximum meaning and purpose. Decide what is most important to you today. What action will you take to move toward your goal? That is your day's intention.

Mind Game

Today is about mixing it up. Take the items in your right pocket and put them in your left, or if you have a purse, carry it on your opposite side. Use your nondominant hand when you need to get something out of your pocket or purse. Do this for daily tasks, too: brush your teeth and use your computer mouse or TV remote with the "other" hand. You'll tap into unused areas of your brain and wake up your creative mind. It's a great way to shift your perspective, see things in a new light, and open yourself to creative thinking.

Affirmation

"Today, I honor myself by sticking to my goals. I know that I will eat nutritiously so I have optimal energy to be of maximum service to others and myself. I will look at life from new angles."

Breathing Meditation

Sit quietly with your eyes open. Let your gaze rest softly a few feet in front of you, not focusing on anything specific. Let sounds and sights float around you while you focus on your breath. Feel the air flow into your nostrils as you inhale, pause, and then feel your belly deflate as you completely exhale. Accept outside sounds as they occur, rise, and then fall into silence. Let the silence between the sounds settle you. Think of your dreams and imagine what it feels like to have your dreams come true in the present moment. Repeat this five times, feeling the payoff for your many days of setting intentions.

MENTAL STRATEGY
Clean Out Your Closet

The way you dress is an expression of who you are. Most of us fall into patterns of dressing. We create "uniforms," even if we have no dress code for work. Does the way you dress reflect the true you, or is it the product of old patterns?

Thought for the Day

When you go to your closet, do you pull out items that you can't wait to wear because they help you feel alive, inspired, and empowered? It's time to think outside your closet. Today, watch other people on the street, flip through some magazines, or look up some fashion ideas on Pinterest. What styles inspire you? Think about putting yourself in one of these outfits.

Affirmation

"I joyously release and easily give away any excess in my life. I encourage the flow of life. New things come to me with ease."

Create Closet Space

Grab some bags and head to your closet. Close your eyes, then take a deep inhale and a full exhale. Repeat a few times, allowing your mind to clear, your body to relax, and your thoughts to settle. Now open your eyes. Starting on one side of the closet, go through each item. If you are unsure of whether something fits, try it on. If it is too big, put it in the bag. If it is something you haven't worn in the last year, put it in the bag. If it is too tight, put it on the other side of your closet; you will wear it soon. Any piece of clothing that doesn't feel right doesn't belong in your wardrobe. You are opening yourself up to the new. Organize your closet as you

go. Pants with pants, skirts with skirts, tops with tops, and so on. You can also organize by color—blacks, browns, blues, pinks, and so on. When you are done, take the filled bags and put them by your front door to be taken out the next time you leave the house.

Visualization

After you finish your closet, stand in your underwear in front of a full-length mirror and look at yourself. Remember that this week is about committing to breaking out of old thinking and tapping into a new mindset. With this intention in mind, smile and say out loud to yourself, "I am full of joy and beauty. I love and express my true self today." Scan your body and visualize exactly how you want to look and feel. Refuse to criticize yourself. If you are having a hard time, act as if you are encouraging a dear friend. When you do this, you draw the law of attraction into your world. You create an energetic field that will help you manifest the body you desire faster than you think.

When Writing Brings Up Difficult Feelings

Sometimes writing can bring up emotional or traumatic memories. While this can make you feel depressed and increase stress in the short term, research shows that over the long haul your mood will be improved, and you'll relieve stress. When you write about a difficult memory, it can cause you to relive the event and might provoke distressing emotions. If you do find that journaling leaves you with mood swings you are not comfortable with, talk to a close friend. If your depressed mood is not alleviated within a week, consider talking with a therapist. I'm a big believer in therapists. I think it is like going to a personal trainer for your mind.

Breathing Exercise

Take a deep inhale and, as you exhale, allow your mind to relax. Release negative thoughts and feelings. Inhale again, allowing the positive energy of the universe to flow into you. Recognize that you are a perfect expression of love and health. As you continue to focus on your breath, invite in love and appreciation for who you are today.

Day 24

MENTAL STRATEGY

Dreams

You can tap into the abundance offered by your subconscious mind as you sleep at night. By tapping into your dreams, you can gain insight from hidden fears, wishes, and desires, which are often expressed in dreams. This can help you gain insight into internal feelings and give you the power to make healthy changes.

Thought for the Day

As you go about your day today, think about unresolved questions or problems in your life. Consider the possibility that tonight when you go to bed, your dream world may help you solve these issues.

Writing Exercise

This evening before you go to bed, sit with a pen and paper and make a list of the problems you thought about during the day. Put this list by your bed, and before you fall asleep, add any recurring thoughts to your list, even small things such as remembering to pick up the dry cleaning or to return a library book. Clear your mind of all mental static—your paper is your holding place for these thoughts. When you have cleared your mind, reread your list. Choose one item

to focus on and think of a question you wish to have answered. Focus intently on this question, then release it as you drift off to sleep. Trust that when you wake up you will have your answer. Give it a try. It may take more than one night, but it works.

Affirmation

"Tonight, I go to sleep with a clear mind, and I know I'll receive answers to all my questions when I wake. I dream with clarity and peace of mind."

Breathing Meditation

Sit quietly in a comfortable position and say to yourself, "May I experience true happiness. Please allow all my dreams to come true." Remind yourself that you deserve to be happy. The happier you are, the more happiness you can spread and share with others on their journey.

Day 25

MENTAL STRATEGY

Ideal Job

Most of us spend many hours at our jobs, and work can, if you allow it, take up a huge amount of mental space. Even if you are fully satisfied with your work, it's important to know how to let it go during your off hours. Your work doesn't need to be the exact reflection of who you are. The goal is to love it while you are doing it—to feel useful and of service, to be inspired and happy, and to earn a good living for yourself. Aim for a balance between work and home; that is an ideal job.

Thought for the Day

As the hours in your day go by, consider how you are using your time. Think about yourself from the perspective of an outsider. What would another person see if they saw you at work? How would you want to be perceived? Passionate? Fulfilled? Creative? If that's not the picture you're seeing, it doesn't mean you should storm out of the office. Instead, think of small steps you can take to adjust your attitude, environment, and responsibilities so that they are more in line with the work you want to do. If you feel stuck in this area, make a date with a friend to brainstorm about this. If you are toying with the idea of another career, reach out and connect with someone who already has that job and offer to take him or her to lunch. The more you investigate the job, the clearer your path will become.

Affirmation

"I appreciate my source of income. I am open to new opportunities. Each and every day I express more and more of my talents and abilities. I chase my bliss."

Visualization

Sit comfortably in a quiet place with your eyes closed. Conjure up a vision of your office. Imagine that you are sitting in your workplace. Hear the office sounds surrounding you. Smell your work's smell. What feelings come up? Is your energy drained or expanding? Visualize yourself as inspired and fulfilled. See yourself in control of the energy you carry with you at work. See yourself having great power over your work environment. See how you are helpful to others, how you serve a purpose at work.

Breathing Exercise

Sit comfortably with your eyes closed. As you take a deep, slow inhale, allow gratitude to grow. Be thankful and blessed that you have a job. As you exhale, send out feelings of gratitude to those you work with. On your next inhale, feel yourself open to new prosperity, abundance, and an increase in salary. As you exhale, sense what it feels like to be appreciated and to be open to prosperity.

MENTAL STRATEGY
Eulogy

What will be your legacy? Have you ever wondered what others will remember about you? Rather than a morbid exercise, imagining what it would be like to attend your own memorial is an enlightening way to get clear on your life, just as Ebenezer Scrooge did in *A Christmas Carol*—we all know what a transformative experience that was. Writing your eulogy allows you to reflect on your past and helps guide you to create the future that you want.

Thought for the Day

Today, reflect on your mortality. Acknowledge that this blessed life is limited, and think carefully about how you can live your life with purpose. What do you think your friends and family would say about you today? If there are things you don't like, what will you do to change how you are remembered?

Writing Exercise

Grab a pen and paper and describe what you imagine will be said about you at your funeral. Do this for five minutes. Keep your hand moving, with no thought of spelling, punctuation, or grammar. Think of all the things you have already done. After five minutes, turn your paper over and write down how this makes you feel. What are you uncomfortable about? What do you most want to change? Now think outside the box. What do you want said about you? How would you like to be remembered? How will you take actions to make these wishes a reality?

Visualization

Close your eyes and see yourself doing everything on the list you just created. Imagine it as if it had happened. Hear your friends and family remembering you with great honor, respect, and love. Imagine that you have lived the life of your dreams and accomplished everything you desired.

Affirmation

"I make active choices that are in line with my creative self. I know that I am in the process of changing into the butterfly I'm meant to be. I am a risk taker."

Breathing Exercise

As you sit quietly, inhale deeply, feeling the air go deep into your navel. Pause at the top of your breath, then begin to exhale slowly and fully, and as you do, say out loud, "Z." Inhale again, and as you exhale, say, "Y." Continue breathing and saying the alphabet in reverse until you get to A. This simple exercise will keep you going step by step toward the true you.

Day 27

MENTAL STRATEGY

Visualize Abundance

How open are you? Do you say "no" more often than "yes," or "yes" more often than "no"? Today is about being receptive to all the universe has to offer you. Yes, *you*. It is about opening up all your 10 categories and allowing the sun to shine in. Too many people live below their potential. You have many gifts and you may have achieved some success, but there is always more room in your life for growth and richness.

Thought for the Day

You can manifest everything you desire if and only if you are truly coming from a place of love, open-mindedness, and honesty. As you step forward into your day, commit to being completely receptive to all the universe has to offer. Allow yourself to listen and

be open to what is going on around you. Be awake. Look for stepping-stones, not roadblocks. Allow yourself to be open to new paths. Expect the unexpected.

Affirmation

"My body is made perfect. I have the power to correct what is wrong. I am profoundly magnetic to the abundance the universe has to offer. I shift into a place of possibility."

Visualization

Sit quietly and close your eyes. Think back to the last time you heard or saw someone doing something stimulating and thrilling. Take time to fully visualize this scene. See it clearly in your mind's eye. Hear the sounds that are happening in this vision, smell the smells, and see all the details. Now imagine you are the person doing this thrilling act. Feel how it feels to take a risk and succeed. Hear the applause and take a bow.

Meditation

Sit quietly with eyes closed and take some calming, soothing breaths. After you've taken a few slow, full inhales and slow, complete exhales, open your mind to the mindset of abundance. Experience being open to new opportunities. Feel the enthusiasm and joy that comes with learning something new. Let yourself settle into this feeling of abundance and success. Let it sink in, so when the next opportunity comes your way, you'll be ready to say, "Yes, I'd love to."

Day 28

MENTAL STRATEGY

The Power of Pause

Waiting is a positive and powerful action, and taking a breather in silence is a good thing, but learning these skills takes practice. All too often we react to people, situations, and experiences without taking even one conscious moment to consider what is happening. Our biological wiring is largely responsible for this, according to scientific studies from the Massachusetts Institute of Technology. When you react instantly, your brain actually shuts down conscious evaluating circuits and puts you on autopilot. There is no ability to consider the wide variety of choices available to you when you are in the middle of a reactive habit. Take cravings, for instance. Have you ever headed to a party with the best intentions, only to find yourself gobbling down homemade chocolate chip cookies and wondering how you went astray? The answer is that your brain shuts off in these circumstances and only turns back on when you are neck deep in sugar overload. The good news, according to a fresh study from McGill University, is that you can wake up your brain by using the power of mindful pausing. Researchers had 196 men and women use various mindful meditation techniques to reduce cravings, and after just two weeks, those who were able to pause and be conscious about what was happening reduced powerful cravings for chocolate compared to those who didn't wake up their brains.

Thought for the Day

Awareness is the word of the day. Your goal is to notice and identify as many reactive habits as you can. Think about common pitfalls you encounter on a regular basis. Maybe you hit the vending machine during your afternoon slump, or possibly you have a sugary coffee drink despite promising yourself each morning that today will be different. You might feed dollars to the candy machine or order at the coffee bar before you even realize what you are doing. Think ahead to your personal challenges, and when you come across these triggers, *pause* and recite today's affirmation. You can say it out loud or to yourself. Repeat it many times.

Affirmation

"A craving is a thought. I am not my thoughts. I don't have to react or respond to my thoughts. I have the power to choose how I will react and behave. My cravings are not me."

Feeling Visualization

Pause when you feel triggered by a craving, a person, or a situation. Go to a quiet place and close your eyes. What are you feeling inside? Notice the quality of your breath. Is it fast and shallow? Slow your breath until it is even and relaxing. What is the quality of your gut? Is it tight, nauseated, clutching, or calm? What is the quality of your head, neck, and shoulders? Are they tense, sore, or aching? Breathe into these areas and let them relax. What is the quality of your mind? Is it racing? Breathe into your mind and let all the tension flow away. See yourself sitting serenely and relaxing. See yourself waiting and not struggling. See yourself trusting that the answers will come; there is no rush. All is as it should be. All reality is what it is.

Spiritual Meditation

Sit quietly and bring your attention to your breath. Let your mind soften, allowing feelings and thoughts to flow by like clouds in the sky. Scan your body and release any areas of tension. When you feel settled, turn your attention toward your conception of a higher power. Even if you don't consider yourself religious, you can still tap the divine that flows all around you in the universe. You can turn things over or pray to a Higher Power, a Higher Self, an Enlightened Energy, Nature, or simply to the interdependent web of all existence. Say a prayer or wish of your choice. A nonreligious prayer might go like this: "Please let me always be divinely guided toward the highest good. Let the light of my best self shine from my core to all beings. May I feel the divine connection to all beings. I commit to my highest self and act from the most enlightened perspective."

Final Words

This concludes four weeks of detailed activity for a healthy mind. I encourage you to refer here often as you move forward on your journey.

10

Meals

Your 4-Week Plan

This chapter has all the simple, healthy, and delicious recipes you'll need for the *Mind Your Body* meal plan. You'll also find weekly shopping lists to print that correspond to the 4-week program. As my grandfather always told me, "If you don't take care of your body, your body won't take care of you." Your body knows what to do; the kidneys filter out toxins, the liver flushes out waste, the lungs breathe out pollutants, and our digestive system absorbs the nutrients that keep us alive. That's why I created a whole program filled with a variety of color, with totally accessible recipes that are bursting with rich flavors while being highly nutrient dense. Healthy eating doesn't have to be bland. If what you are eating doesn't taste good, you won't enjoy your food, and that takes the fun out of eating. That's why I've created a lifestyle plan, not just a quick-fix regime.

Recipe Code Key

The following codes indicate recipes that are vegetarian, vegan, dairy-free, gluten-free, nut-free, and freezer-friendly.

Dairy-free	DF
Freezer-friendly	FF
Gluten-free	GF
Nut-free	NF
Vegetarian	VEG
Vegan	VGN

Recipes at a Glance

Cooking Made Easy

These four kitchen gadgets don't take up much space, and they'll save you considerable time when preparing the recipes in *Mind Your Body*. Consider adding them to your kitchen tools.

Nutribullet

This high-powered mixer takes multiple tough ingredients such as carrots and ice, and blends them silky smooth without you having to jab even once with a wooden spoon.

Four-Piece Minimeasuring Beaker Set

Measuring spoons and cups are fine, but they do spill easily, which can be frustrating. I found that these beakers made measuring even the smallest amount a breeze, without making a mess.

Nut Chopper

These little handheld crank gadgets chop up any sort of nut and keep the pieces all neatly contained, so you can pour it directly into the recipe.

Vegetable Chopper

I used this for many of the recipes I prepared for this book, and it really saved a lot of time and made dealing with carrots, onions, and potatoes simple and quick.

Shopping Lists

On the following pages you'll find weekly shopping lists and weekly menus. You will be making more than one trip to the store each week. At times you may be able to consolidate some of your shopping, but the list is organized this way so you can purchase the highest-quality, freshest ingredients available. Make sure to go shopping a day or two before day 1 in order to be prepared for your next twenty-eight days. Then you'll return to the store on day 5, day 7, day 12, day 14, day 16, day 19, day 21, day 23, and day 25.

Week 1 Shopping Lists

This will be the biggest shopping trip of the four weeks because you'll stock your pantry with items that will last the entire month.

Produce

1 container mushrooms
1 bag spinach
1 bunch asparagus
1 carton cherry tomatoes
1 orange bell pepper
1 red pepper
1 bunch celery
1 avocado
1 bunch kale
3 medium white onions
3 red tomatoes (enough for 2 diced cups)
7 medium-size beets
12 ounces frozen or fresh okra
1 bunch collard leaves
1 bunch asparagus
1 carton edamame
1 large carrot
2 large parsnips
4 lemons
2 limes
1 banana
2 oranges
1 small watermelon
2 red apples
1 two-inch stalk ginger
1 bunch mint
1 bunch cilantro
1 bunch basil (optional)
1 bunch parsley
2 garlic bulbs

Dairy

1 dozen eggs
1 small block cheddar cheese
1 small block parmesan cheese
1 small container nonfat feta cheese
1 cup cottage cheese
1 carton unsweetened flax milk
1 carton almond milk

Seeds

1 cup pumpkin seeds
1 cup sunflower seeds
1 bag chia seeds
1 container ground flaxseed
1 container hemp seeds

Nuts

5 cups walnuts
5 cups almonds
2 cups pecans
1 large bag pistachios
1 small bag pine nuts
1 small bag cashews
1 small bag pili or pine nuts
1 small bag macadamias
1 cup Brazil nuts

Protein

2 fresh salmon steaks
½ pound flank steak

Spices

cinnamon
nutmeg
cumin
turmeric
paprika
curry powder
sea salt
pepper
dried or fresh rosemary
tarragon
garam masala
thyme
chili powder
parsley flakes
dill weed

Pantry

1 cup lentils
4 cans chickpeas
1 can artichoke hearts
1 small jar tahini
1 can or jar hearts of palm
1 cup dried tomatoes
1 container rolled oats (4 cups minimum)
1 bag unsweetened coconut flakes
1 jar honey
1 bag dried fruit (your choice)
1 bag raisins
1 box beef bouillon cubes
1 box chicken bouillon cubes
1 large box veggie broth (enough for 4 cups)
1 small bag date sugar
1 small bag spelt flour
1 small can green chilies
1 small jar dijon mustard
1 bottle coconut water
1 can pumpkin puree
1 container natural almond butter
1 bag freekeh
1 can navy beans
1 jar apple cider vinegar
1 bottle light soy sauce
1 bottle extra-virgin olive oil
1 bottle avocado oil
1 small jar red palm oil
1 small jar coconut oil
1 jar light mayo made with olive oil
psyllium husk

Day 5 Shopping Trip

1 pound shrimp, peeled and deveined
2 pounds pork tenderloin
1 cup fresh snow peas
1 medium head of cauliflower
15 Brussels sprouts

Week 1 Meals

Day 1

Breakfast: Spinach and Mushroom Omelet, page 162

Snack: Watermelon Juice, page 198

Lunch: Tomato, Avocado, and Hearts of Palm Salad (1 of 2), page 176; Ginger Lentil Soup (1 of 2), page 164

Snack: Handful of walnuts

Dinner: Seared Salmon Steaks (1 of 2), page 185; Garlic Spinach (1 of 2), page 188

Day 2

Breakfast: Coconut Muesli (1 of 8), page 159

Snack: Watermelon Juice, page 198

Lunch: Seared Salmon Steaks (2 of 2); Tomato, Avocado, and Hearts of Palm Salad (2 of 2)

Snack: Handful of pistachios

Dinner: Ginger Lentil Soup (2 of 2); Simple Kale Salad (1 of 3), page 176

Day 3

Breakfast: Apple Pumpkin Salad (1 of 6), page 168

Snack: Celery stick with a spoonful of almond butter or natural peanut butter

Lunch: Roasted Beet with Freekeh (1 of 4), page 174; Garlic Spinach (2 of 2)

Snack: Watermelon Juice, page 198

Dinner: Beef and Okra Stir-Fry (1 of 2), page 178; Simple Kale Salad (2 of 3)

Day 4

Breakfast: Collards Scramble, page 159

Snack: Apple Pumpkin Salad (2 of 6)

Lunch: Beef and Okra Stir-Fry (2 of 2)

Snack: Spinach and Artichoke Hummus (1 of 6), page 199; with two baby carrots and stalk of celery

Dinner: Roasted Beet with Freekeh (2 of 4); Lemon Asparagus (1 of 2), page 189

Day 5

Breakfast: Coconut Muesli (2 of 8)

Snack: 1 cup cottage cheese, 1 teaspoon cinnamon, 1 teaspoon sunflower seeds

Lunch: Roasted Beet with Freekeh (3 of 4); Simple Kale Salad (3 of 3)

Snack: Apple Pumpkin Salad (3 of 6)

Dinner: Ginger Shrimp (1 of 4), page 182; Lemon Asparagus (2 of 2)

Day 6

Breakfast: Apple Pumpkin Salad (4 of 6)

Snack: ½ cup edamame

Lunch: Ginger Shrimp (2 of 4); Parsnip Soup (1 of 4), page 166

Snack: Banana

Dinner: Roasted Beet with Freekeh (4 of 4); Ginger Shrimp (3 of 4)

Day 7

Breakfast: Spinach and Mushroom Omelet (1)

Snack: Apple Pumpkin Salad (5 of 6)

Lunch: Ginger Shrimp (4 of 4); Parsnip Soup (2 of 4)

Snack: ½ cup edamame

Dinner: Pork Tenderloin (1–4 of 8), page 184; Roasted Turmeric Cauliflower (1–2 of 4), page 190; Rosemary Brussels Sprouts (1–2 of 4)

*Friends night

Week 2 Shopping Lists

Produce

1 large spaghetti squash
1 red tomato
1 bag spinach
3 small onions
1 bunch kale
2 cups bok choy
1 large carrot
6 cups arugula
1 carton cherry tomatoes
3 mushrooms
1 green pepper
3 medium zucchini
1 bulb garlic
1 red onion
2 limes
3 lemons
1 banana
1 cup strawberries
1 pineapple
3 oranges
1 mango
1 papaya
4 figs
1 plum
1 kiwi
1 carton blueberries

Dairy

1 dozen eggs
2 small plain 2% Greek yogurts
1 cup cottage cheese

Protein

1 seitan sausage patty
2 cups salmon from salmon fillets or canned
1 package turkey bacon

Pantry

1 loaf of Ezekiel Bread (store in freezer)
1 container horseradish
1 cup bread crumbs/ panko crumbs
1 jar coconut water
1 box green tea
1 bottle tamari sauce
1 bottle balsamic vinegar
1 can (15 ounces) chopped tomatoes
2 cups fresh or canned lima beans
1 small bag of jasmine rice
1 container (8 ounces) veggie broth
1 small container cacao powder
1 cup quinoa
1 cup spelt berries
1 cup farro

Day 12 Shopping Trip

Produce

1 container cherry tomatoes
3 large sweet potatoes
2 medium white onions
2 bunches collard greens
1 red pepper
1 avocado
1 bunch asparagus
3 scallions
1 shallot
1 bulb garlic
fresh thyme
1 orange
4 figs
3 dates

Protein

4 halibut fillets (4 ounces each)
2 boneless, skinless chicken breasts

We are indeed much more than what we eat, but what we eat can nevertheless help us to be much more than what we are.

—ADELE DAVIS

Week 2 Meals

Day 8
Breakfast: Coconut Muesli (3 of 8)
Snack: Handful of almonds
Lunch: Pork Tenderloin (5 of 8); Roasted Turmeric Cauliflower (3 of 4)
Snack: Apple Pumpkin Salad (6 of 6)
Dinner: Veggie Night: Parsnip Soup (3 of 4); Rosemary Brussels Sprouts (3 of 4); Squash Mash (1 of 2), page 192

Day 9
Breakfast: Seitan Sausage Sandwich, page 161
Snack: Orange Lime drink, page 197
Lunch: Parsnip Soup (4 of 4); Pork Tenderloin (6 of 8); Rosemary Brussels Sprouts (4 of 4)
Snack: 5 macadamias
Dinner: Mom's Salmon Croquettes (2 of 10 patties), page 183; Roasted Turmeric Cauliflower (4 of 4)

Day 10
Breakfast: Poached Eggs and Kale (1 of 2), page 160
Snack: Ginger Mango drink, page 195
Lunch: Mom's Salmon Croquettes (3–4 of 10 patties); Squash Mash (2 of 2)
Snack: Green Tea Juice, page 196
Dinner: Pork Tenderloin (7 of 8); Bok Choy Salad (1 of 4), page 170

Day 11
Breakfast: Poached Eggs and Kale (2 of 2)
Snack: Handful of walnuts
Lunch: Pork Tenderloin (8 of 8); Arugula Salad (1 of 2), page 169
Snack: Plum Punch, page 198
Dinner: Bok Choy Salad (2 of 4); Creole Lima Beans (1 of 8), page 187; Lemon Zucchini Soup (1 of 4), page 165

Day 12
Breakfast: Coconut Muesli (4 of 8)
Snack: 1 cup cottage cheese, 2 slices tomato, paprika
Lunch: Arugula Salad (2 of 2); Creole Lima Beans (2 of 8); Lemon Zucchini Soup (2 of 4)
Snack: 4 figs
Dinner: Bok Choy Salad (3–4 of 4); Poached Halibut (1–2 of 4), page 184; Indian Sweet Potatoes (1–4 of 8), page 189; Creole Lima Beans (3–6 of 8) *Friends night!

Day 13
Breakfast: Collards Scramble, page 159
Snack: Date Shake, page 194
Lunch: Creole Lima Beans (7 of 8); Poached Halibut (3 of 4); Indian Sweet Potatoes (5 of 8)
Snack: 1 Greek yogurt with cinnamon and almonds
Dinner: Poached Halibut (4 of 4); Lemon Zucchini Soup (3 of 4); Quinoa Salad (1 of 4), page 173

Day 14
Breakfast: Seitan Sausage Sandwich, page 161
Snack: Avocado Milk Shake, page 193
Lunch: Indian Sweet Potatoes (6 of 8); Lemon Zucchini Soup (4 of 4); Quinoa Salad (2 of 4)
Snack: 4 figs
Dinner: Creole Lima Beans (8 of 8); Chicken Farro Salad (1 of 2), page 171

Week 3 Shopping Lists

Produce

1 peach
1 carton strawberries
1 cucumber
1 bag baby carrots
1 bunch celery
1 eggplant
1 lemon
1 garlic bulb
1 bunch fresh mint
3 yellow squash
 (2 pounds)
2 medium tomatoes
1 onion

Dairy

1 small 2% Greek yogurt
1 cup cottage cheese
1 small container feta
 cheese

Pantry

1 jar tahini
1 large carton veggie
 broth
rice vinegar
whey protein
1 small bag barley

Day 16

Produce

1 bag spinach
2 red tomatoes
1 jicama
1 carton cherry tomatoes
1 green pepper
1 bunch endive
1 avocado
2 onions
1 bunch asparagus
1 cup mushrooms
1½ cups cooked shelled
 edamame beans
2 large carrots
3 scallions (⅓ cup)
1 bunch cilantro
1 lemon
1 banana
½ fresh pineapple
1 carton blueberries
1 cup grapes
1 grapefruit

Dairy

1 carton almond milk
1 dozen eggs

Protein

1 pound ground turkey

Day 19

Produce

2 cups broccoli
1 yellow squash
1 bunch kale
1 bag spinach
1 white onion
1 large sweet potato
2 large carrots
2 parsnips
2 cups green cabbage
1 bunch parsley
1 lemon

Protein

2 cups diced rotisserie
 chicken meat
2 chicken breasts

Pantry

8 cups chicken broth
1 jar coconut water

---

*Win your personal battles and your
life becomes clearer and easier.*

Week 3 Meals

Day 15

Breakfast: Oatmeal Shake, page 197

Snack: 1 cup cottage cheese, 1 teaspoon chia seeds, 2 cherry tomatoes, and 4 slices cucumber

Lunch: Chicken Farro Salad (2 of 2); Quinoa Salad (3 of 4); Squash Casserole (1 of 6), page 191

Snack: Baba Ganoush (1 of 4), page 199; 2 baby carrots; stalk of celery

Dinner: Squash Casserole (2 of 6); Turkey Burgers with Spinach and Feta (1 of 6), page 186

Day 16

Breakfast: Coconut Muesli (5 of 8)

Snack: Hard-boiled egg

Lunch: Squash Casserole (3 of 6); Turkey Burgers with Spinach and Feta (2 of 6)

Snack: Baba Ganoush (2 of 4) and 2 slices jicama

Dinner: My Sister Paige's Gazpacho (1 of 4), page 166; Quinoa Salad (4 of 4)

Day 17

Breakfast: Banana Almond Shake, page 178

Snack: 4 pieces endive, half an avocado

Lunch: My Sister Paige's Gazpacho (2 of 4); Asparagus Barley "Risotto" (1 of 4), page 178

Snack: Half a grapefruit

Dinner: Turkey Burgers with Spinach and Feta (3 of 6); My Sister Paige's Gazpacho (3 of 4)

Day 18

Breakfast: Spinach and Mushroom Omelet, page 162

Snack: ½ cup blueberries and ½ cup grapes

Lunch: Mom's Salmon Croquettes (5–6 of 10 patties); Asparagus Barley "Risotto" (2 of 4)

Snack: 5 macadamias

Dinner: My Sister Paige's Gazpacho (4 of 4); Edamame Salad (1 of 4), page 172

Day 19

Breakfast: Seitan Sausage Sandwich, page 161

Snack: ½ cup Brazil nuts

Lunch: Edamame Salad (2 of 4); Asparagus Barley "Risotto" (3 of 4)

Snack: Pineapple Punch, page 197

Dinner: Chicken Stir-Fry (1 of 2), page 179

Day 20

Breakfast: Coconut Muesli (6 of 8)

Snack: Green Dream drink, page 196

Lunch: Chicken Stir-Fry (2 of 2); Asparagus Barley "Risotto" (4 of 4)

Snack: ½ cup blueberries and ½ cup grapes

Dinner: Edamame Salad (3 of 4); Turmeric Chicken Soup (1 of 6), page 167

Day 21

Breakfast: Collards Scramble, page 199

Snack: Avocado Milk Shake, page 193

Lunch: Edamame Salad (4 of 4); Sweet Potato Chips (1 of 2), page 192

Snack: ½ grapefruit

Dinner: Turmeric Chicken Soup (2 of 6)

Week 4 Shopping Lists

Produce

2 avocados
3 sweet potatoes
4 cups kale
1 bunch celery
1 bag carrots
1 red pepper
3 small white onions
1 red onion
1 cup raw shelled edamame
1 eggplant
6 new potatoes (golf-ball size)
3 fingerling potatoes
1 garlic bulb
1 bunch cilantro
1 cup mushrooms
3 lemons
1 grapefruit
1 banana
1 pear
1 honeydew melon

Dairy

2 small 2% Greek yogurts
1 dozen eggs

Protein

1 package turkey bacon

Pantry

4 prunes
½ cup dried cranberries
2 cups dried black beans
3 cups vegetable broth
1 can (15 ounces) crushed tomatoes
2 8-ounce jars artichoke hearts in water
10 cups vegetable broth
1 tube tomato paste
¼ cup ketchup
1 cup 100% pomegranate juice
1 bag Almond Accents
1 cup wheat berries
1 cup barley
1 cup amaranth
8 green olives
1 (15 ounces) kidney beans
1 can (15 ounces) navy beans

Day 23

Produce

1 jicama
10 ounces baby spinach
1 bunch (5 cups) collard greens
3 white onions
3 medium zucchini
1 yellow onion
1 tomato
1 cup watermelon
1 carton raspberries
1 papaya
1 banana

Dairy

1 package (8 ounces) fat-free cream cheese

Protein

16 medium shrimp
1 pound ground turkey breast

Pantry

2 cups coconut water

Day 25

Produce

1 pound new red or finger potatoes
1 red pepper
2 cups broccoli florets
½ cup mushrooms
2 shallots
5 radishes

2 cups red cabbage
2 cups green cabbage
3 large eggplants
1 white onion
1 bunch fresh parsley
1 bunch cilantro
2 large tomatoes
1 yellow onion
¼ cup dried tomatoes
1 avocado
8–10 cups seasonal greens
1 cup watercress
½ cup zucchini
1 bag spinach
1 avocado
1 lime
1 lemon
1 cup fresh berries of your choice
1 cup pineapple
1 banana
2 oranges or 1 cup fresh orange juice
¼ cup fresh cranberries

Dairy

½ cup goat cheese
¾ cup mozzarella cheese

Protein

2 halibut fillets

Week 4 Meals

Day 22

Breakfast: Prune Shake, page 198

Snack: Hard-boiled egg

Lunch: Turmeric Chicken Soup (3 of 6); Sweet Potato Chips (2 of 2); Avocado and Kale Salad (1 of 4), page 170

Snack: ½ cup dried cranberries

Dinner: Mom's Salmon Croquettes (7–10 of 10 patties); Avocado and Kale Salad (2–3 of 4); Garlic Eggplant Mash (1–2 of 8), page 188
*Friends night

Day 23

Breakfast: Coconut Muesli (7 of 8)

Snack: ¼ honeydew

Lunch: Garlic Eggplant Mash (3 of 8); Black Bean Soup (1 of 4), page 163

Snack: 1 pear

Dinner: Shrimp and Spinach Salad (1 of 2), page 175

Day 24

Breakfast: Collards Scramble, page 159

Snack: ¼ honeydew

Lunch: Shrimp and Spinach Salad (2 of 2); Black Bean Soup (2 of 4)

Snack: Electrolyte Punch, page 195

Dinner: Garlic Eggplant Mash (4 of 8); Avocado and Kale Salad (4 of 4)

Day 25

Breakfast: Pomegranate Punch, page 198

Snack: Hard-boiled egg

Lunch: Sweet Turkey Loaf (1 of 6), page 185; Mom's Zucchini Soup (1 of 6), page 165

Snack: ¼ honeydew

Dinner: Halibut and Artichokes (1 of 2), page 182; Broccoli and Black-Eyed Pea Salad (1 of 6), page 171

Day 26

Breakfast: Spinach and Mushroom Omelet, page 162

Snack: ¼ honeydew

Lunch: Halibut and Artichokes (2 of 2); Collard Greens (1 of 2), page 187; Mom's Zucchini Soup (2 of 6)

Snack: Spinach and Artichoke Hummus (2 of 6), 2 carrots, stalk of celery

Dinner: Sweet Turkey Loaf (2 of 6); Almond Slaw (1 of 4), page 186; Broccoli and Black-Eyed Pea Salad (2 of 6)

Day 27

Breakfast: Coconut Muesli (8 of 8)

Snack: Orange Zing drink, page 197

Lunch: Sweet Turkey Loaf (3 of 6); Collard Greens (2 of 2); Broccoli and Black-Eyed Pea Salad (3 of 6)

Snack: Mom's Zucchini Soup (3 of 6)

Dinner: Eggplant Chili (1 of 6), page 181; Walnut Salad (1 of 4), page 177

Day 28

Breakfast: Zucchini Omelet, page 162

Snack: Green Power drink, page 196

Lunch: Mom's Zucchini Soup (4 of 6); Black-Eyed Pea Salad (4 of 6)

Snack: 1 cup fresh berries

Dinner: Eggplant Chili (2–5 of 6); Artichoke Amaranth Salad (4 of 4), page 168
*Friends night

The Health Benefits of Seeds

I love seeds. They are a great way to add a burst of fiber, healthy fats, and protein to any meal, making these little nuggets a perfect tool in helping you stay satisfied so you see more weight loss. You'll find these seeds in many of the recipes in this chapter.

Hemp

Even though these are grown on the cannabis plant, they won't alter your mind in any adverse ways. These little guys are rich in heart-healthy, stroke-reducing omega-3 fatty acids, and 2 tablespoons provide 5 grams of nearly complete protein, which is unusual for plant proteins. Hemp seeds have also been linked to reducing ADHD symptoms and alleviating skin issues such as eczema.

Flaxseed

This seed's benefits come from the fact that they are high in fiber and omega–3 fatty acids. One tablespoon gives you 150 mg of antioxidants, 2 grams of fiber, and 2 grams of healthy fats (including omega-3s). I always recommend ground flaxseed, because it's easier for your body to digest than whole seeds.

Chia

The good news is that you don't have to buy a chia pet to reap the benefits. These seeds were the original energy food, consumed by the Aztecs to boost stamina. They provide 5 grams of fiber per tablespoon and are also high in omega-3 fatty acids.

Sunflower

This seed is rich in vitamin E, an antioxidant that protects you from asthma, osteoarthritis, hot flashes, diabetes, heart disease, and some forms of cancer. A quarter cup of sunflower seeds supplies more than 80 percent of your recommended daily allotment of vitamin E.

Pumpkin

Also called pepitas, pumpkin seeds are rich in zinc (10.5 mg in 3.5 ounces) when you buy the unshelled form, which is what I recommend in all my recipes. A quarter cup provides nearly half your daily magnesium, and this seed is also rich in antioxidants that protect you from cancer.

You don't have to cook fancy or complicated masterpieces—just good food from fresh ingredients.

—JULIA CHILD

Coconut Muesli

10 SERVINGS • DF, GF, VEG, VGN

This cereal can be stored dry for several weeks and is a great source of fiber, protein, whole grains, and nearly a quarter of your day's quota of iron.

For a quick morning meal, scoop out ½ cup cereal and add ½ cup almond or flax milk and 1 teaspoon honey. Let soak overnight in fridge.

4 cups old-fashioned rolled oats
1 cup raw almonds, sliced
1 cup unsweetened coconut flakes
¼ cup pumpkin or sunflower seeds
1 cup dried fruit, any variety
¼ cup ground flaxseed
¼ cup hemp seeds
¼ cup chia seeds
½ teaspoon cinnamon
½ teaspoon nutmeg
2 tablespoons orange zest
dash of salt

1 Preheat oven to 350°.

2 Scatter oats and almonds on one baking sheet and coconut flakes on another, and place in oven for 5 minutes. Watch closely and remove as soon as they begin to brown. Let cool.

3 In a large mixing bowl, thoroughly mix all dry ingredients.

4 Store in a zip-lock bag or sealed container.

Per serving: **404 calories, 18.5 g fat, 47.8 g carbs, 10.5 g fiber, 13.8 g sugar, 12.2 g protein**

Collards Scramble

1 SERVING • DF, GF, VEG

3 eggs
1½ teaspoons red palm oil
1 garlic clove, minced
½ white onion, diced small
½ teaspoon turmeric
2 collard green leaves, stems removed and leaves finely chopped
salt and pepper
2 tablespoons pili nuts or pine nuts, chopped

1 Whisk eggs in a bowl.

2 Heat oil in a skillet on medium high and add garlic and onion. Sauté for 1–2 minutes or until soft. Turn heat to medium. Add turmeric, greens, and 2 tablespoons water and sauté until tender, about 3 minutes. Season with salt and pepper to taste.

3 Add eggs and scramble until eggs are ready. Sprinkle with nuts and serve.

Per serving: **408 calories, 32.2 g fat, 11.4 g carbs, 2.9 g fiber, 4.1 g sugars, 20.1 g protein**

Pili Nuts

This incredibly delicious product of Asia is now turning up in stores all over the United States. The pili nut is a good source of magnesium, phosphorous, and vitamin E, and is also rich in heart-healthy fats.

The Clock Method for Proper Portions

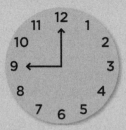

When serving your meal, pretend your plate is a clock for portion control.

12 to 6: Fill this half of your plate with vegetables.

6 to 9: This quarter is for protein.

9 to 12: Here is where you'll put healthy carbs.

Poached Eggs and Kale

2 SERVINGS • GF, NF

1 teaspoon sea salt
4 cups kale, stems removed, chopped
2 slices turkey bacon, cooked according to
    package directions
4 tablespoons vegetable broth
1 white onion, chopped
2 garlic cloves, minced
1 teaspoon rosemary
salt and pepper
2 eggs
Parmesan cheese

1 Bring a large pot of salted water to boil. Add kale and cook for 2 minutes, then drain and cool.

2 Add 2 tablespoons broth to the empty pot and put on medium heat. Add the onion and garlic, and stir until they begin to brown. Add the rosemary, the remaining 2 tablespoons of broth, and kale. Reduce heat to a simmer and cook until the kale is dark and wilted, about 20 minutes. Stir occasionally. Season with salt and pepper.

3 While the kale is cooking, poach 1 egg (save the second egg for tomorrow). See "The Perfectly Poached Egg," page 161.

4 Once kale and egg are done, crumble turkey bacon into the kale and mix. Split kale mixture into two dishes, and serve with egg and a sprinkle of parmesan on top.

Per serving: 227 calories, 8.1 g fat, 21.1 g carbs, 3.2 g fiber, 2.8 g sugars, 18.3 g protein

The Perfectly Poached Egg

Bring three inches of water in a small pan to a gentle boil. Crack the egg into a small bowl so you can easily add it to the water. (Poach eggs one at a time.) Just before you add your egg, use a wooden spoon to swirl the water, making a gentle whirlpool; this will help keep the egg white together. Lower the rim of the bowl that is holding your egg into the water and slide the egg into the bowl. If you want a runny egg, let it poach for 2 minutes. For medium, 3 minutes, and firm takes 4 minutes. Remove the egg with a slotted spoon and let it sit for a moment to allow the excess water to drain off.

Seitan Sausage Sandwich

1 SERVING • GF, VEG

This yummy breakfast provides more than a third of your iron quota for the day.

- 1 poached egg
- 1 slice Ezekiel bread
- 1 seitan sausage patty
- 1 thin slice of cheese
- 2 small spinach leaves
- 1 slice of tomato

1 While your egg is poaching, toast the bread in a toaster and heat the sausage in a skillet over medium heat for 30 seconds on each side. Put the slice of cheese on top and let it melt.

2 Build your sandwich: place sausage and cheese on the toasted bread and top with spinach, tomato, and finally egg.

Per serving: 284 calories, 12.6 g fat, 18.3 g carbs, 4.3 g fiber, 1.8 g sugars, 23.3 g protein

What Is Seitan?

Seitan is a high-protein vegetarian food made from cooked wheat gluten. It is made by washing wheat flour dough with water until all the starch has been removed, then cooking it. Seitan is often used for mock duck or chicken in Asian restaurants, but many stores also carry seitan products, including these mock meats as well as sausage, bacon, and barbecued ribs. It's high in protein but virtually free of fat, unless added to the product.

Spinach and Mushroom Omelet

1 SERVING · GF, NF, VEG

2 eggs
1 tablespoon flax milk, unsweetened
1 teaspoon chia seeds
1 teaspoon olive oil
½ cup mushrooms, chopped
⅛ cup shredded cheddar cheese
½ cup baby spinach, chopped
salt and pepper

1 Whisk the eggs, milk, and chia seeds in a bowl. Set aside to let the seeds soften.

2 Heat the oil in a nonstick skillet. Add the mushrooms and sauté until softened (2–3 minutes), then add the egg mixture and rotate pan around so the eggs cover the inside of the pan, using medium heat until almost cooked. Carefully flip omelet over, sprinkle cheese and spinach inside, season with salt and pepper, fold, and allow cheese to melt and spinach to wilt.

Per serving: 256 calories, 19.3 g fat, 4.3 g carbs, 2.4 g fiber, 1.4 g sugars, 17.1 g protein

Zucchini Omelet

1 SERVING · DF, GF, NF, VEG

3 eggs
1 teaspoon olive oil
1 clove garlic, minced
2 tablespoons onion, diced fine
½ cup zucchini, chopped fine
salt and pepper
1 teaspoon chopped fresh cilantro

1 Whisk eggs in a small bowl and set aside.

2 Heat olive oil in a nonstick skillet on medium, tilting pan to coat. Add garlic and onion and sauté for 30 seconds. Add zucchini and cook for another 30 seconds. Pour eggs on top and gently stir and cook until nearly set. Season to taste with salt and pepper. Add chopped cilantro, fold, and serve.

Per serving: 255 calories, 17.9 g fat, 5.8 g carbs, 1.2 g fiber, 2.9 g sugars, 17.6 g protein

Black Bean Soup

4 SERVINGS • FF, GF, NF, VEG, VGN

This soup freezes beautifully. Just leave out the yogurt and cilantro until you are ready to eat.

> 2 cups dried black beans, soaked overnight
> 3 fingerling potatoes, about the size of a hotel-size shampoo
> ½ teaspoon salt
> 3 cups vegetable broth
> 1 can (15 ounces) crushed tomatoes
> 1 white onion, chopped
> 2 garlic cloves, minced
> ½ cup celery, diced
> ½ cup carrots, diced
> ¼ teaspoon ground cumin
> 1 cup plain 2% Greek yogurt
> ¼ cup cilantro, chopped
> salt and pepper

1 Soak beans in water overnight in a covered soup pot. In the morning, rinse the beans and return to the pot with enough water to cover by an inch. Bring the beans to a boil on high, then turn heat to low, cover, and simmer for about 45 minutes or until soft. Cool.

2 In a small pot, add potatoes, ½ teaspoon salt, and enough water to cover the potatoes by an inch. Bring to a boil and cook 20 minutes or until soft. Drain and let cool.

3 Place beans and potatoes in a blender with 1 cup water and puree.

4 Put pureed beans, vegetable broth, tomatoes, and onion in a soup pot, and bring to a boil over high heat. Turn heat to low, add remaining ingredients (except yogurt and cilantro), season to taste with salt and pepper, and simmer for 10 minutes.

5 Put a generous spoonful of yogurt in the bottom of the bowl, pour soup on top, stir, garnish with cilantro, and serve.

Per serving: 266 calories, 1.3 g fat, 65.8 g carbs, 33.8 g fiber, 10.4 g sugars, 26.1 g protein

Ginger Lentil Soup

2 SERVINGS • DF, FF, GF, NF, VEG, VGN

This dish is a powerhouse; it provides an entire day's worth of fiber and more than half your quota of iron in one bowl.

1 cup lentils, uncooked
1 cup vegetable broth
1 cup water
1 onion, chopped
1 small can green chilies
4 cloves garlic, minced
2 ½-inch cubes fresh ginger, minced
2 cups tomatoes, diced
½ teaspoon cumin
½ teaspoon mustard
½ teaspoon turmeric
½ teaspoon paprika
salt and pepper
parsley, chopped

1 In a pot, combine lentils, vegetable broth, water, onion, green chilies, garlic, ginger, and tomatoes. Bring to a boil over medium heat. Cover pot and simmer over low heat for 30 minutes, stirring occasionally.

2 Stir in the dry spices and salt and pepper to taste. Cover and simmer for 10 more minutes. Garnish with fresh parsley.

Per serving: 208 calories, 0.7 g fat, 35.6 g carbs, 7.2 g fiber, 3.9 g sugars, 13.4 g protein

Ginger

This herb is well known for its power to soothe stomachs, but did you know that it has also been shown to be a powerful anti-inflammatory that can reduce the pain of migraine headaches and some forms of arthritis? Ginger has also been shown to reduce symptoms of menstrual pain, as well as general dizziness, morning sickness, and nausea. And that's not all! This herb seems to have a protective effect against colon cancer, diabetes, and heart disease.

Lemon Zucchini Soup

4 SERVINGS • FF, GF, NF, VEG

¼ cup vegetable broth
2 cloves garlic, minced
1 medium onion, chopped
3 medium zucchini, shredded
6 cups water
½ cup jasmine rice
4 eggs
juice from 1 lemon
½ cup fresh parsley, finely chopped
salt and pepper
2 tablespoons parmesan cheese

1 Heat vegetable broth and garlic in a soup pot over medium heat. Add onion and cook until translucent, about 3 minutes. Add shredded zucchini and stir until soft, about 3 minutes.

2 Add 6 cups water and rice. Bring to a boil, then reduce heat, cover, and simmer for 30 minutes.

3 Beat eggs and lemon juice in a metal bowl, then very slowly stir 1 cup of hot broth from the soup into the eggs. Doing it slowly will keep the eggs from curdling. Then slowly add this mixture to the soup. Sprinkle in parsley and cook 5 more minutes. Serve garnished with salt and pepper and ½ tablespoon each of Parmesan cheese.

Per serving: 144 calories, 5.7 g fat, 13.9 g carbs, 1.4 g fiber, 2.7 g sugar, 9.6 g protein

Mom's Zucchini Soup

6 SERVINGS • FF, GF, NF, VEG

3 medium zucchini
5 cups vegetable broth
1 yellow onion, chopped
1 package (8 ounces) fat-free cream cheese
1 tablespoon curry powder
salt and pepper

1 Cut off the ends of the zucchini and slice into ¼-inch rounds.

2 Put the broth in a soup pot and bring to a boil. Add cut zucchini and chopped onion. Turn heat to low and simmer for 45 minutes.

3 Cut cream cheese into dice-size squares. Drop along with curry powder and salt and pepper into hot mixture and stir until fully melted. Turn stove off and let completely cool.

4 Put into blender and blend until smooth. Can be served hot or cold.

Per serving: 66 calories, 0.6 g fat, 8.8 g carbs, 2.9 g fiber, 4.4 g sugars, 6.4 g protein

My Sister Paige's Gazpacho

4 SERVINGS • DF, FF, GF, NF, VEG, VGN

1 vegetable bouillon cube
1 cup water
1 pint red cherry tomatoes
2 stalks celery, chopped
2 carrots, chopped
1 green bell pepper, chopped
¼ teaspoon sea salt
¼ teaspoon pepper

1 Dissolve bouillon cube in 1 cup hot water, then set aside to cool.

2 When broth is cool, blend all ingredients in a blender. Chill in fridge before serving.

Per serving: **39 calories, 0.5 g fat, 7.9 g carbs, 2.7 g fiber, 5.2 g sugars, 1.8 g protein**

Parsnip Soup

4 SERVINGS • DF, FF, GF, NF, VEG, VGN

1 white onion, chopped
3 cups vegetable broth
1 large carrot, chopped
2 cups parsnips, chopped
1 tablespoon avocado oil
1 teaspoon curry powder
¼ teaspoon sea salt
¼ teaspoon pepper
1 cup almond milk

1 In a soup pot, cook onion in 3 tablespoons vegetable broth until translucent.

2 Add remaining ingredients except milk and bring to a boil. Lower heat, cover, and simmer for 15–25 minutes. Stirring occasionally.

3 Once carrots and parsnips are soft, let cool. Then process in blender in four batches. Return soup to pot, add milk, and reheat.

Per serving: **112 calories, 2.3 g fat, 17.8 g carbs, 4.9 g fiber, 5.8 g sugars, 5.1 g protein**

Turmeric Chicken Soup

6 SERVINGS • DF, FF, GF, NF

2 tablespoons olive oil
1 white onion, chopped
8 cups chicken broth
1 large sweet potato, cut in bite-size cubes
2 carrots, cut in bite-size cubes
2 parsnips, cut in bite-size cubes
2 cooked chicken breasts, about 2 cups, diced
2 cups green cabbage, shredded
1 teaspoon turmeric
2 tablespoons chia seeds
¼ cup shredded unsweetened coconut
salt and pepper
1 small parsley spray

❶ Heat olive oil on medium high in soup pot. Add onion and sauté for 5 minutes.

❷ Add remaining ingredients, except salt, pepper, and parsley, and bring to a boil. Cover and simmer for 30 minutes, stirring every 10 minutes. Season with salt and pepper, and garnish with parsley.

Per serving: 327 calories, 14.5 g fat, 24.7 g carbs, 8.5 g fiber, 7.8 g sugars, 23.9 g protein

Turmeric

This spice is a powerful anti-inflammatory that has been shown to have disease-protecting benefits. Numerous studies have shown that turmeric helps prevent the brain from developing Alzheimer's-related plaque, while other studies show that it helps reduce arthritis-related symptoms and protects against some forms of cancer.

Vitamin A Soup

8 SERVINGS • DF, FF, GF, NF, VEG, VGN

A serving of this soup provides 123 percent of your quota of vitamin A.

6 shiitake mushrooms
4 carrots
4 celery stalks
1 medium onion
1 bell pepper
1 zucchini
1 cup parsley
1 teaspoon cayenne pepper
1 teaspoon dried basil
1 tube or small can (4.5 ounces) tomato paste
10 cups water

Chop the vegetables. Place everything in a soup pot and bring to a boil. Simmer, covered, for 2 hours. Strain vegetables if you want a broth or serve as is.

Per serving, unstrained: 49 calories, 0.3 g fat, 11 g carbs, 2.9 g fiber, 5.6 g sugars, 2 g protein

Apple Pumpkin Salad

6 SERVINGS • DF, GF, VEG, VGN

This makes a great breakfast, and leftovers can be portioned for snacks and future breakfasts.

- 2 tablespoons coconut oil
- 2 red apples, cored and diced
- zest from 1 orange
- zest from 1 lime
- ¼ cup fresh mint, chopped
- ¼ cashews, chopped
- 1 cup coconut water
- 2 tablespoons unsweetened coconut flakes
- 2 teaspoons chia seeds
- 1 tablespoon honey
- 1 cup raisins
- 1 can (15 ounces) pumpkin puree
- 1 teaspoon ginger or cinnamon

Melt coconut oil. Place in a large bowl with all remaining ingredients and mix well. Eat immediately, or cover and store in the refrigerator.

Per serving: 230 calories, 9.1 g fat, 37.2 g carbs, 4.9 g fiber, 26.8 g sugars, 2.7 g protein

Artichoke Amaranth Salad

4 SERVINGS • DF, GF, NF, VEG, VGN

This salad is delicious warm or chilled.

- 1 cup amaranth
- 2 tablespoons olive oil
- 1 yellow onion, chopped fine
- 2 garlic cloves, minced
- 1½ cups vegetable broth
- ½ teaspoon curry powder
- 1 celery stalk, diced
- ¼ cup dried tomatoes, snipped with kitchen scissors into small pieces
- 1 can (15 ounces) artichokes in water, drained
- 1 cup baby spinach, chopped
- 8 green olives (optional)

1 Cook amaranth according to package directions, then cool.

2 Heat oil in saucepan over medium heat. Add onion and garlic and sauté until soft and translucent, about 5 minutes.

3 Add vegetable broth and bring to a boil. Add curry powder, amaranth, celery, tomatoes, and artichokes. Reduce heat to low and simmer covered 20 minutes, until all water is absorbed.

4 Turn off heat. Add spinach and olives.

Dressing for Artichoke Amaranth Salad

2 tablespoons olive oil
1 tablespoon balsamic vinegar
1 small shallot, minced
1 teaspoon mustard

Whisk together and drizzle over salad.

Per serving: **365 calories, 19.4 g fat, 42.2 g carbs, 8.5 g fiber, 2.8 g sugars, 9.3 g protein**

Amaranth

Amaranth is a whole grain that can be used in place of white rice, polenta, or other grains. It's got a tasty, chewy texture with a bit of crunch. It provides 7 grams protein and 7 grams fiber in a quarter cup dry grains, while white rice only has 1 gram protein and zero fiber for the same amount, and brown rice has 4 grams protein and 2 grams fiber. Amaranth also contains lysine, important for muscle growth, and oils that may lower cholesterol.

Arugula Salad

2 SERVINGS • GF, VEG

This dish is high in energy-revving iron and a good source of fiber and protein.

2 eggs, hard-boiled and sliced
6 cups arugula
5 cherry tomatoes, halved
3 mushrooms, chopped
1 tablespoon red palm oil
juice from 1 lemon
2 tablespoons balsamic vinegar
salt and pepper
1 tablespoon Parmesan cheese
2 tablespoons walnuts, chopped

1 Gently toss together the eggs, arugula, tomatoes, and mushrooms.

2 In a small bowl, whisk together the oil, lemon juice, and vinegar, and drizzle over the salad. Season to taste with salt and pepper.

3 Top with Parmesan and walnuts.

Per serving: **287 calories, 18.8 g fat, 19.3 g carbs, 6.3 g fiber, 10.9 g sugars, 15.2 g protein**

Avocado and Kale Salad

5 SERVINGS • DF, GF, VEG, VGN

This dish is high in fiber, a good source of protein, and very high in vitamins A, B$_6$, and C.

4 cups kale, stems removed and chopped
juice from 1 lemon
¼ teaspoon sea salt
1 cup celery, diced
1 cup carrots, grated
1 cup red bell pepper, diced
1 avocado, diced
1 small onion, diced
8 walnuts, chopped
1 cup edamame, shelled
1 tablespoon ground flaxseed
¼ cup olive oil
2 tablespoons apple cider vinegar
salt and pepper

1 Put the kale in a mixing bowl with juice from the lemon and the sea salt. Massage thoroughly with hands. Set aside.

2 Add the celery, carrots, red bell pepper, avocado, onion, and walnuts to the kale. Add edamame, flaxseed, olive oil, and vinegar, and mix all ingredients. Season to taste with salt and pepper.

Per serving: 324 calories, 23.6 g fat, 21.8 g carbs, 8.1 g fiber, 3.5 g sugars, 10.7 g protein

Bok Choy Salad

4 SERVINGS • DF, GF, VEG, VGN

Make sure when cleaning bok choy that you separate the stalks and rinse clean. They can have dirt hidden between the stalks.

2 cloves garlic
2 tablespoons tamari
⅓ cup apple cider vinegar
2 tablespoons honey
2 cups bok choy, chopped
1 cup celery, diced
1 cup carrots, diced
1 tablespoon raw sunflower seeds
1 tablespoon chia seeds
1 tablespoon flaxseeds
salt and pepper

1 Place garlic, tamari, cider vinegar, and honey in a large zip-lock bag and shake until well combined.

2 Add the bok choy, celery, carrots, and seeds to the bag and shake well. Season to taste with salt and pepper, and put in the refrigerator to chill and marinate for about an hour.

Per serving: 117 calories, 3.5 g fat, 17.5 g carbs, 4.7 g fiber, 4.1 g protein

Broccoli and Black-Eyed Pea Salad

6 SERVINGS • FF, GF, VEG, VGN

This salad is a great source of fiber and is high in vitamins A, B$_6$, and C.

3 pounds new red or fingerling potatoes
1 cup canned black-eyed peas, rinsed and drained
1 cup celery, diced
1 cup carrots, diced
1 cup red bell pepper, diced
½ cup white onion, diced
2 cups broccoli florets, cut into bite-size pieces
¼ cup walnuts, chopped
2 tablespoons red palm oil
1 tablespoon fresh dill, minced
4 cloves garlic, minced
2 tablespoons red wine vinegar
1 tablespoon dijon mustard
½ teaspoon sea salt
salt and pepper

1 Bring a large pot of salted water to a boil. Add potatoes and cook for 15 minutes or until tender. Drain and set aside. When cool to the touch, dice into bite-size pieces and place in a large bowl with the black-eyed peas.

2 Add celery, carrots, red bell pepper, onion, broccoli, and walnuts.

3 Melt red palm oil and combine in a separate bowl with the dill, garlic, red wine vinegar, mustard, and salt. Whisk together. Pour over the other ingredients and toss gently. Season to taste with salt and pepper. Eat at room temperature.

Per serving: 286 calories, 8.4 g fat, 47.7 g carbs, 8.1 g fiber, 5.4 g sugars, 8.8 g protein

Chicken Farro Salad

2 SERVINGS • FF, GF

Make this delicious salad for a refreshing evening meal, and have lunch all ready to go for the next day. This recipe provides 52 percent of your daily iron needs and is high in protein.

1 cup farro
6 stalks asparagus
4 cups spinach
2 boneless, skinless chicken breasts, cooked and diced
3 scallions, sliced fine
2 tablespoons cilantro, minced
5 cherry tomatoes, halved
salt and pepper
Parmesan cheese

1 Rinse the farro and put in a medium pan with 3 cups lightly salted water. Bring to a boil. Reduce heat to medium low and simmer, covered, for 30 minutes, until water is absorbed. Set aside to cool.

2 Place water in the bottom of a medium pan that you can fit with a vegetable steamer, and put on high heat. While waiting for water to boil, peel the asparagus and remove white ends, then cut into one-inch pieces. When the water is boiling, add asparagus and steam for 5 minutes, then remove from steamer and add to large bowl. Mix in the spinach with hot asparagus and farro so it will wilt.

❸ Add chicken, scallions, cilantro, and tomatoes and gently toss.

❹ Make dressing (recipe follows) and drizzle over the salad, seasoning to taste with salt, pepper, and Parmesan.

Dressing for Chicken Farro Salad

2 tablespoons olive oil
1 tablespoon shallot, minced
1 tablespoon apple cider vinegar
1 teaspoon honey
zest of 1 orange
1 tablespoon lemon juice
salt and pepper

Put all ingredients in a mason jar and shake, or whisk in a small bowl.

Per serving with dressing: 456 calories, 19.3 g fat, 21.7 g carbs, 6.7 g fiber, 12.8 g sugars, 46.7 g protein

---

If you can't say something nice, don't say anything at all.

—TRADITIONAL

Edamame Salad

4 SERVINGS • DF, GF, NF, VEG, VGN

It's fine to prepare this dish the night before. The flavors meld beautifully.

1½ cups cooked shelled edamame beans
2 large carrots, grated
⅓ cup scallions, finely sliced
2 tablespoons cilantro, chopped
2 tablespoons rice vinegar
2 tablespoons lemon juice
1 tablespoon olive oil
1 teaspoon minced garlic
salt and pepper

❶ Toss the edamame, carrots, scallions, and cilantro in a bowl.

❷ Whisk the vinegar, lemon juice, oil, and garlic in a small bowl.

❸ Toss all ingredients gently together and season to taste with salt and pepper.

❹ Cover and place in fridge to chill until serving time.

Per serving: 125 calories, 6.6 g fat, 10 g carbs, 4.2 g fiber, 2.1 g sugars, 6.9 g protein

Per ½ salad: 250 calories, fat 13.2 grams, carbs 19.9 grams, fiber 8.4 grams, protein 13.8 grams

Quinoa Salad

4 SERVINGS · DF, GF, NF, VEG, VGN

This salad is a great source of fiber.

 1 cup quinoa, cooked
 ¾ cup spelt berries, cooked
 2 tablespoons olive oil
 1 red onion, finely chopped
 4 cloves garlic, minced
 1 cup chickpeas, rinsed and drained
 ¼ teaspoon cumin
 salt and pepper
 1 red bell pepper, diced
 juice of 1 lemon

1 Cook quinoa and spelt berries according to package directions.

2 Heat olive oil over medium heat, add onion, and cook until translucent, about 5 minutes. Add garlic, chickpeas, and cumin. Stir and heat for 1 minute. Season to taste with salt and pepper. Transfer to a large glass bowl.

3 Add bell pepper and lemon juice and gently toss.

Per serving: 256 calories, 9.1 g fat, 40.2 g carbs, 7.6 g fiber, 2.8 g sugars, 7.3 g protein

Quinoa Sweet Potato Salad

6 SERVINGS · DF, FF, GF, VEG, VGN

This dish provides nearly half the daily recommended value of iron and is a good source of fiber and protein.

 1 cup quinoa
 2 large sweet potatoes, peeled and cubed
 1 package (6 ounces) baby spinach, chopped
 2 tablespoons balsamic vinegar
 ¼ cup unsweetened coconut flakes
 3 tablespoons sunflower seeds
 1 tablespoon hemp seeds
 ¼ teaspoon salt
 ¾ cup chopped almonds
 salt and pepper

1 Cook the quinoa according to package directions.

2 While the quinoa is cooking, prepare the sweet potatoes: Bring a medium pot of salted water to a boil, then add potatoes and cook until tender, about 15 minutes. Remove from heat and drain.

3 Combine hot quinoa, sweet potatoes, and spinach in a bowl. Stir, then cover for 5 minutes to let spinach wilt.

4 Add the remaining ingredients and gently toss. Season to taste with salt and pepper.

Per serving: 281 calories, 12 g fat, 36.1 g carbs, 6.9 g fiber, 1.3 g sugars, 9 g protein

Roasted Beet Salad with Freekeh

4 SERVINGS • VEG

This is even better the next day, so package extra for a delicious on-the-go meal.

Freekeh is wheat that is harvested green and then dried and roasted. It can be found in many health food stores. You can substitute barley or even brown rice for this recipe, but I encourage you to try freekeh—not only is it super rich in fiber and protein but it's delicious. You'll fall in love with its chewy, rich texture.

6 to 8 medium-size beets, scrubbed with greens removed
4 tablespoons olive oil
2½ cups vegetable broth
½ cup freekeh
7½ ounces (half a 15-ounce can) navy beans, rinsed and drained
2 teaspoons apple cider vinegar
¼ cup pistachio nuts
salt and pepper
½ cup crumbled nonfat feta cheese

❶ Preheat oven to 375°. On a baking sheet, drizzle whole beets with 2 tablespoons olive oil and bake in the middle of the oven for 30 minutes. Remove and let cool, then peel and dice.

❷ Put broth and freekeh in a pot and bring to a boil. Cover and simmer for 25 minutes, until freekeh is tender and the water is absorbed. Remove from heat and let cool.

❸ Gently mix beets, freekeh mixture, 2 tablespoons olive oil, navy beans, vinegar, and pistachios in a bowl. Season to taste with salt and pepper. Sprinkle feta on top and serve (you can also chill the salad before serving).

Per serving: 380 calories, 19.3 g fat, 39.1 g carbs, 11.2 g fiber, 18.5 g sugars, 16.9 g protein

Shrimp and Spinach Salad

4 SERVINGS • DF, GF

This dish is a great source of fiber, protein, vitamin A, vitamin B$_6$, iron, and vitamin C. Try putting extra servings into individual containers for easy grab-and-go lunches.

6 strips turkey bacon
1 red onion, sliced into rounds
1 small carton mushrooms, sliced
16 medium shrimp
2 tablespoons pine nuts or roasted pumpkin
    seeds, or a mixture
3 tablespoons red wine vinegar
1 tablespoon dijon mustard
salt and pepper
1 tablespoon olive oil
6 ounces baby spinach
1 avocado, diced
1 small jicama, diced
2 hard-boiled eggs, sliced

1 Cook bacon in a large skillet on medium until it is slightly crispy, flipping as needed, about 5 minutes. Transfer to paper-toweled plate to drain.

2 Sauté onion and mushrooms in the same skillet until onion begins to brown, about 3 minutes. Add shrimp and cook until bright pink, 3–5 minutes. Add pine nuts to pan and heat through, about 2 minutes.

3 Stir in vinegar and mustard and season to taste with salt and pepper. If the pan looks dry, you can add a dash of olive oil.

4 Divide spinach, avocado, jicama, and eggs onto four plates and top each salad with the hot shrimp mixture (each serving gets 4 shrimp). Serve.

Per serving: 339 calories, 20.2 g fat, 18.1 g carbs, 9.8 g fiber, 3.9 g sugars, 23.3 g protein

Simple Kale Salad

3 SERVINGS • GF, VEG

4 cups kale, stems removed and chopped
½ red bell pepper, diced
¼ cup pine nuts
½ cup dried tomatoes, finely chopped
1 ounce Parmesan cheese, grated
2 tablespoons olive oil
2 tablespoons lemon juice
1 tablespoon ground flaxseed
salt and pepper

Place all ingredients in a large bowl and massage with clean hands. Place in the refrigerator and allow flavors to meld for about an hour.

Per serving: 223 calories, 21 g fat, 5.9 g carbs, 1 g fiber, 2.1 g sugars, 6 g protein

Tomato, Avocado, and Hearts of Palm Salad

2 SERVINGS • DF, GF, NF, VEG, VGN

A fantastic iron- and fiber-filled salad!

4 stalks asparagus, washed, stems removed, and peeled
1 avocado, diced
juice from 1 lime
1 (8-ounce) can hearts of palm, drained and sliced
10 cherry tomatoes, halved
1 orange bell pepper, chopped
1 stalk celery, diced
¼ cup chopped cilantro or basil
salt and pepper

1 Bring a medium pot of water to boil. When boiling, drop in asparagus for 2 minutes and then remove and place in a bowl of ice water. When cool, drain and cut asparagus into 1-inch pieces.

2 Mix avocado and lime juice in a bowl.

3 Put all ingredients in a bowl. Season with salt and pepper, and gently toss the salad.

Per serving: 364 calories, 21.2 g fat, 43.4 g carbs, 18.6 g fiber, 21.1 g sugars, 10.4 g protein

Walnut Salad

4 SERVINGS • GF, VEG

8–10 cups seasonal salad greens
1 cup watercress, stems removed and coarsely chopped
Yogurt Chive Dressing or Mustard Vinaigrette (recipes follow)
½ cup walnuts, toasted and coarsely chopped
½ cup goat cheese, crumbled

1 Toss together the greens, watercress, and dressing of your choice.

2 Divide the salad into 4 servings and top each with 2 tablespoons goat cheese and 2 tablespoons walnuts.

Per serving without dressing: 156 calories, 12.6 g fat, 4 g carbs, 1.9 g fiber, 2 g sugars, 8.3 g protein

With yogurt dressing: 202 calories, 15.4 g fat, 7.5 g carbs, 1.9 g fiber, 5.1 g sugars, 10.4 g protein

With vinaigrette: 274 calories, 26.1 g fat, 4.3 g carbs, 1.9 g fiber, 2 g sugars, 10.5 g protein

Yogurt Chive Dressing

4 SERVINGS • GF, VEG

3½ tablespoons snipped fresh chives
3 tablespoons plain 2% Greek yogurt
1 teaspoon fresh lemon juice
½ teaspoon salt
⅛ teaspoon cayenne pepper

Whisk all ingredients together, then toss with salad.

Per serving: 46 calories, 2.8 g fat, 3.5 g carbs, 3.1 g sugars, 2.1 g protein

Mustard Vinaigrette

4 SERVINGS • GF, VEG

2 tablespoons red wine vinegar or white wine vinegar
1 teaspoon dijon mustard
1 garlic clove, minced
⅓ cup olive oil
salt and pepper

1 Whisk together the vinegar, dijon mustard, and garlic in a bowl. Add the olive oil gradually, whisking constantly until combined. Season with salt and pepper.

2 Toss ¼ salad greens with ¼ of the vinaigrette, saving the rest for later.

Per serving: 118 calories, 13.5 g fat, 0.3 g carbs, 0.1 g protein

Asparagus Barley "Risotto"

4 SERVINGS • FF, NF, VEG

2 tablespoons olive oil

1 large white onion, chopped

2 garlic cloves, minced

1 cup uncooked barley

4 cups vegetable broth

10 stalks asparagus, trimmed and cut into 1-inch pieces

2 tablespoons apple cider vinegar

2 tablespoons lemon juice

dash of sea salt

2 tablespoons Parmesan cheese, grated

❶ Heat olive oil in a large saucepan over medium heat. Add onion and cook, stirring until onion is translucent, about 5 minutes. Add garlic and barley and cook, stirring for 1 minute.

❷ Add broth, cover, and simmer for 8 minutes, and then add asparagus and simmer until broth is absorbed.

❸ Remove from heat, stir in vinegar, lemon juice, and salt.

❹ Serve garnished with Parmesan cheese.

Per serving: 345 calories, 13.7 g fat, 43.9 g carbs, 6.7 g fiber, 3.3 g sugars, 14.7 g protein

Barley and Oatmeal

Both these grains contain betaglucans, soluble fibers that help lower your LDL cholesterol by preventing it from being absorbed into your bloodstream.

Beef and Okra Stir-Fry

2 SERVINGS • DF, FF, GF, NF

This meal is a fantastic source of protein, fiber, magnesium, zinc, and vitamins A, B_6, and C.

You can also serve this dish over ½ cup brown rice, quinoa, or other cooked whole grain.

½ cup beef broth

1 tablespoon date sugar

2 tablespoons light soy sauce

1 tablespoon fresh lime juice

1 tablespoon spelt flour

1 tablespoon avocado oil

½ pound flank steak, cut into 2 ½-inch-thick strips

12 ounces frozen or fresh okra

1 tablespoon garlic, minced

1 tablespoon ginger, minced

¼ cup fresh mint

¼ cup cilantro

salt and pepper

1 Whisk together beef broth, date sugar, soy sauce, lime juice, and spelt flour.

2 Heat oil in a large skillet or wok and stir-fry steak over high heat until meat is brown and no pink can be detected, 4–5 minutes.

3 Heat 1 tablespoon water in a medium skillet. Add okra, garlic, and ginger and stir-fry for 2–3 minutes or until soft. Pour beef broth mixture over okra, and cook, stirring often, for 3–4 minutes.

4 Pour okra and broth mixture over beef, add mint, cilantro, and stir for 2 minutes. Season with salt and pepper, and serve and enjoy.

Per serving: 346 calories, 11.3 g fat, 24.4 g carbs, 7.9 g fiber, 2.9 g sugars, 37.7 g protein

The Magic of Magnesium

Magnesium supports normal muscle and nerve function, regulates blood sugar levels, and promotes healthy blood pressure. Magnesium has been shown to help with asthma, depression, diabetes, fibromyalgia, hearing loss, headaches, osteoporosis, premenstrual syndrome, and heart disease. This mineral is also intimately related to serotonin, the neurotransmitter known for boosting a happy disposition. When magnesium is low, so is serotonin. Getting enough magnesium in your diet ensures that serotonin levels stay high and you stay happy. The best sources of magnesium are nuts, dark green vegetables, soy products, and whole grains. Adult women should get around 320 milligrams, and adult men should aim for about 420 milligrams.

Chicken Stir-Fry

2 SERVINGS • DF, GF

This dish is very high in protein and vitamins B_6 and C.

   2 tablespoons avocado oil
   ½ onion, chopped
   1 stalk celery, chopped
   2 cups broccoli, cut into bite-size pieces
   ½ cup mushrooms, chopped
   1 yellow squash, sliced
   1 tablespoon spelt flour
   1 cup chicken broth
   1 teaspoon chili powder
   salt and pepper
   2 cups diced rotisserie chicken meat, skin removed
   1 cup cooked jasmine rice

1 Heat oil in a large skillet or wok on high heat. Add onion and celery and stir-fry for 2–3 minutes. Add broccoli and mushrooms and stir-fry for another 3 minutes. Add squash and stir-fry for 3 minutes.

2 Whisk flour into broth and add to the skillet with chili powder, adding salt and pepper to taste. Reduce heat to medium and stir until sauce thickens slightly. Add chicken, season with salt and pepper, and heat through.

3 Split into 2 portions and serve each over ½ cup steamed jasmine rice.

Per serving: 324 calories, 7.3 g fat, 16.4 g carbs, 5.4 g fiber, 5.2 g sugar, 48.2 g protein

Curried Spinach and Sweet Potato Freekeh

5 SERVINGS • DF, VEG, VGN

This is a great dish served warm, at room temperature, or chilled. Makes a great on-the-go lunch.

This dish is a great source of fiber and very high in vitamins A, B$_6$, and C. It also provides 30 percent of daily iron needs for women.

2 cups diced sweet potatoes

2 tablespoons red palm oil

½ cup tamari freekeh, cooked (See headnote about freekeh on page 174. If you can't find the tamari flavor, add 4 tablespoons tamari to regular freekeh.)

2½ cups chicken or vegetable broth

1 large green bell pepper, chopped

½ onion, chopped

2 tablespoons garlic, minced

5 tablespoons mild curry powder

¼ cup parsley, chopped

2 cups baby spinach, chopped

1 cup frozen peas, thawed

salt and pepper

½ cup sliced almonds

❶ Preheat oven to 375°. Put sweet potatoes on a nonstick baking sheet and drizzle 1 tablespoon palm oil on them. Bake for 25 minutes. Remove from oven and set aside.

❷ While the sweet potatoes are in the oven, cook the freekeh according to package directions, using the chicken broth in place of water.

❸ Heat the remaining 1 tablespoon palm oil in a large skillet over medium heat, and add the green pepper, onion, and garlic. Cook for 4–5 minutes, then toss in curry powder, parsley, spinach, and peas. Continue cooking until onion is translucent. Pour into large mixing bowl with freekeh and sweet potatoes. Season to taste with salt and pepper and add almonds. Gently toss and serve.

Per serving: 280 calories, 10.5 g fat, 38.4 g carbs, 10.3 g fiber, 11.4 g sugars, 9.2 g protein

Eggplant Chili

6 SERVINGS • FF, NF, VEG

This is a great dish to double and take to a potluck (just leave out the cheese). You can keep it warm in a crockpot.

Not only delicious, it is filled with fiber and very high in potassium!

3 large eggplants
2 tablespoons avocado oil
1 large white onion, chopped
1 tablespoon garlic, minced
3 cups vegetable broth
½ cup wheat berries
½ cup barley
1 tablespoon garam masala
2 large tomatoes, chopped
juice of 1 lime
1 can (15 ounces) kidney beans
1 can (15 ounces) navy beans
salt and pepper
¾ cup mozzarella cheese, cut into 12 dice-size cubes
1 avocado, diced and tossed in lime juice

1. Preheat oven to 400°.

2. Fork eggplant a few times and place on a baking sheet. Bake 30 minutes, then set aside to cool. (You can also do this step the night before, refrigerating the baked eggplant until you are ready to continue.)

3. Heat oil in a large pot on medium-high. Add onion and garlic, and cook until soft, about 5 minutes.

4. Add broth, wheat berries, barley, and garam masala and bring to a boil. Reduce heat and simmer for 30 minutes, covered. Stir occasionally.

5. Scoop out flesh from eggplant and cut into pieces.

6. Add eggplant, chopped tomatoes, lime juice, and drained kidney and navy beans to the pot. Season to taste with salt and pepper, and simmer, stirring, for 10 more minutes.

7. To serve, place 2 cubes of mozzarella in the bottom of a bowl and top with ⅙ portion of chili. Garnish with avocado.

Per serving: 310 calories, 11 g fat, 45.6 g carbs, 18 g fiber, 9.8 g sugars, 12.9 g protein

Ginger Shrimp

4 SERVINGS • FF, GF

1 cup vegetable broth
1 large yellow onion, chopped
2 cloves garlic, minced
½ inch ginger, minced
1 pound shrimp, peeled and deveined
1 cup snow peas, quartered
½ cup fresh cilantro, chopped
½ teaspoon sea salt
10 cashews
2 cups couscous, cooked according to package
   directions

1 Heat 2 tablespoons vegetable broth in a skillet over medium heat. Add the onion and cook until golden brown, about 10 minutes. Stir in garlic and ginger, and cook for 2 minutes.

2 Add the rest of the veggie broth, turn heat to high, and bring to a boil. Add the shrimp and cook for 2 minutes. Stir in the snow peas and continue cooking until shrimp are bright pink.

3 Stir in cilantro, dash of salt, and cashews. Serve over couscous.

Per serving: **293 calories, 4.5 g fat, 28.2 g carbs, 3.7 g fiber, 4.3 g sugars, 32.7 g protein**

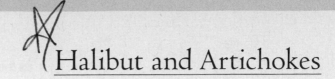

Halibut and Artichokes

2 SERVINGS • DF, GF, NF

This dish is a good source of protein.

1 jar (8 ounces) artichoke hearts in water
2 halibut fillets
1 tomato, chopped
½ lemon
½ medium onion, chopped
1 clove garlic, minced
1 teaspoon dried parsley flakes
½ tablespoon olive oil

1 Preheat oven to 375°.

2 Put 2 tablespoons artichoke water in a glass baking dish. Add fish, artichoke hearts, and tomato. Top with lemon juice, onion, garlic, parsley, and olive oil.

3 Cover with aluminum foil and bake for 25–30 minutes until flaky.

Per serving: **270 calories, 7.7 g fat, 11 g carbs, 4.5 g fiber, 2.6 g sugars, 38.7 g protein**

Mom's Salmon Croquettes

10 PATTIES, 2 PER SERVING • DF, FF, GF, NF

This dish is high in magnesium.

> 2 eggs
> 1 cup bread crumbs or panko
> 1 small onion, chopped
> 2 tablespoons fresh parsley, chopped
> 1 tablespoon dijon mustard
> 1 teaspoon lemon juice
> 1 teaspoon curry powder
> 1 tablespoon horseradish
> 2 cups salmon from leftover cooked salmon fillets, or canned
> salt and pepper
> 2 tablespoons olive oil

1. Whisk 1 egg in a mixing bowl. Add half the bread crumbs, onion, parsley, mustard, lemon juice, curry powder, horseradish, and salmon and massage well with clean hands. Season with salt and pepper. Place in refrigerator until well chilled, about an hour. While the salmon mixture is chilling, make Simple Aioli Sauce (recipe follows).

2. Remove salmon mixture from refrigerator and form into 10 patties, about 4 ounces each.

3. Whisk second egg in a bowl. Put ½ cup reserved bread crumbs in another bowl. Coat each patty first in the egg, then in the bread crumbs. Place the patties on a lightly greased baking sheet and return to the refrigerator to chill for about 30 minutes (this ensures they will hold their form when cooking).

4. Preheat oven to 350°.

5. Heat oil in a large skillet on medium-high. When hot, add the patties and brown them on each side (you may have to do this in batches). Return the browned patties to the baking sheet and bake for 10–12 minutes. Serve with Simple Aioli Sauce.

Per serving: 268 calories, 13.3 g fat, 17.9 g carbs, 1.6 g fiber, 2.5 g sugars, 19.6 g protein

Simple Aioli Sauce

10 SERVINGS OF 1 TABLESPOON • NF, VEG

> ½ cup light mayonnaise
> juice from 1 lemon
> 1 teaspoon dijon mustard
> 1 tablespoon olive oil
> 1 garlic clove, minced
> salt and pepper

Place all ingredients in small bowl, whisk thoroughly, cover, and chill in fridge for at least 1 hour for flavors to meld.

Per serving: 43 calories, 4.2 g fat, 0.7 g carbs, 0.1 g protein

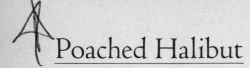

Poached Halibut

4 SERVINGS • DF, FF, GF, NF

This dish is high in protein, meets 35 percent of daily iron requirements, and is high in magnesium.

4 halibut fillets, 4 ounces each
salt and pepper
2 garlic cloves, minced
1 lemon, thinly sliced in rounds
10 cherry tomatoes, halved
¼ cup olive oil

1 Preheat oven to 300°.

2 Place fillets 1 inch apart in glass baking dish that has been wiped with a bit of olive oil.

3 Sprinkle with salt, pepper, and garlic. Top with lemon slices and tomatoes. Pour olive oil over fish and bake for 25 minutes or until fish is opaque.

Per serving: 328 calories, 16.6 g fat, 13.8 g carbs, 4.2 g fiber, 8.4 g sugars, 33.3 g protein

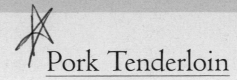

Pork Tenderloin

8 SERVINGS • DF, FF, GF, NF

2 pounds pork tenderloin
2 cloves garlic, minced
3 tablespoons red palm oil
1 tablespoon dried rosemary
salt and pepper

1 Preheat oven to 350°.

2 Put pork in a roasting pan. Mix together garlic, oil, rosemary, and salt and pepper. Brush all over pork, using about half the oil mixture.

3 Roast the pork in the oven. After 30 minutes, carefully turn the roast over. Spread with remaining oil mixture and cook another 30 minutes, until the center is no longer pink. A thermometer in the center should read 145°.

4 Serve 2 slices (about 4 ounces) with Bok Choy Salad (page 184).

Per serving: 164 calories, 4 g fat, 0.2 g carbs, 0 fiber, 0 sugars, 29.7 g protein

Seared Salmon Steaks

2 SERVINGS • DF, GF, NF

1 tablespoon olive oil
2 salmon steaks
salt and pepper

1 Heat oil in cast-iron skillet over medium heat until you see wisps of smoke.

2 Place steaks skin side down and sear without moving for 3–4 minutes, until nicely brown. When you are sure the fish won't stick, turn it carefully, add salt and pepper to taste, and sear on the other side for about 3 minutes, until fish is opaque.

Per serving: 210 calories, 14 g fat, 0 carbs, 0 fiber, 0 sugars, 22 g protein

Sweet Turkey Loaves

6 SERVINGS • DF, FF, N

2 cups mashed sweet potato
1 pound ground turkey breast
2 large eggs
1 white onion, chopped fine
2 cloves garlic, minced
¼ cup ketchup
2 tablespoons dijon mustard
¼ cup bread crumbs
1 teaspoon ground pepper
1 teaspoon salt
1 tablespoon chopped parsley
¼ cup tomato paste

1 Preheat oven to 350°.

2 Place all ingredients in a bowl and massage with clean hands until well mixed.

3 Lightly grease a muffin tray. Use a spoon to place equal amounts of the turkey mixture in six of the cups (fill the other six halfway with water to keep them from burning).

4 Bake for 30–40 minutes. After 30 minutes, check temperature with a food thermometer. The loaves are done when the internal temperature reaches 165°.

Per serving: 276 calories, 7.9 g fat, 24.1 g carbs, 3.5 g fiber, 9.2 g sugars, 26.8 g protein

Turkey Burgers with Spinach and Feta

6 SERVINGS • FF, GF, NF

- 1 cup spinach, chopped fine
- 1 medium carrot, finely grated
- 1 pound ground turkey
- 2 cloves garlic, minced
- 1 teaspoon thyme
- ½ teaspoon sea salt
- ¼ teaspoon pepper
- 1 egg
- 1 tablespoon olive oil
- 1 teaspoon lemon juice
- ½ cup crumbled feta
- 10 tomato slices

1 Place all ingredients except tomato slices in a large bowl. Thoroughly massage with clean hands and shape into 6 patties.

2 Heat oil in a large skillet on medium heat. Add patties and cook each side 4–6 minutes, until patties have no trace of pink. Serve with a slice of tomato on top.

Per serving: 180 calories, 10.6 g fat, 3.9 g carbs, 1 g fiber, 2.2 g sugars, 18.2 g protein

Almond Slaw

4 SERVINGS • DF, GF, VEG, VGN

- 2 cups finely chopped red cabbage
- 2 cups finely chopped green cabbage
- ½ cup fresh parsley, chopped
- 3 tablespoons lemon juice
- 1 teaspoon dijon mustard
- 1 teaspoon honey
- 1 tablespoon apple cider vinegar
- 1 garlic clove, minced
- ⅓ cup sliced almonds
- ⅓ cup sunflower seeds
- salt and pepper

1 Put cabbages and parsley in a large container with a lid that will seal.

2 Add lemon juice, mustard, honey, vinegar, and garlic. Seal container and shake until well mixed. Then add almonds and sunflower seeds, season to taste with salt and pepper, shake again, and serve.

Per serving: 88 calories, 4.2 g fat, 10.3 g carbs, 3.4 g fiber, 6.1 g sugars, 3.1 g protein

Collard Greens

2 SERVINGS • DF, GF, VEG, VGN

4 cups collard greens
1 tablespoon red palm oil
1 shallot, minced
¼ teaspoon sea salt
¼ cup fresh cranberries
1 teaspoon apple cider vinegar
5 radishes, chopped
5 walnuts, chopped

1. Remove and discard the thick stems from each collard leaf and chop remaining leaves.

2. Heat oil in a large skillet on medium. Add shallot and sauté for 30 seconds. Add salt.

3. Add greens and cranberries, and cook until soft, about 6 minutes.

4. Stir in vinegar and garnish with radishes and walnuts.

Per serving: 125 calories, 10 g fat, 8.1 g carbs, 4 g fiber, 0.7 g sugars, 3.2 g protein

Creole Lima Beans

8 SERVINGS • DF, FF, GF, NF

1 slice turkey bacon
½ medium onion, chopped
¼ cup celery, diced
¼ cup green bell pepper, chopped
½ can (15 ounces) chopped tomatoes
½ teaspoon honey
2 cups canned lima beans, drained
salt and pepper

1. Cook bacon in a large, deep skillet on medium high until crisp. Set aside.

2. Put onion, celery, and green pepper in pan and cook until tender, about 5 minutes, then add tomatoes and honey. Turn heat to low and cook for 15 minutes, stirring occasionally. Add a little water (if needed).

3. Add drained beans and simmer for a few minutes until heated through. Season to taste with salt and pepper. Put in dish and crumble bacon on top.

Per serving: 60 calories, 0.6 g fat, 10.5 g carbs, 2.3 g fiber, 1.2 g sugars, 2.8 g protein

Garlic Eggplant Mash

8 SERVINGS • DF, FF, GF, NF

1 eggplant
2 tablespoons olive oil
1 teaspoon fresh rosemary
6 new potatoes, golf-ball size
2 slices turkey bacon
1 small onion, chopped
2 garlic cloves, minced
1 teaspoon garam masala
salt and pepper

❶ Preheat oven to 400°.

❷ Cut eggplant in half lengthwise and rub
2 teaspoons olive oil and rosemary on cut half.
Place cut side up on a baking sheet and bake for
30 minutes, until soft.

❸ While eggplant is baking, put potatoes in a pot
and cover with water, salting lightly. Boil for about
10 minutes, or until tender when pricked with a
fork. Drain and set aside.

❹ Heat skillet on medium high and cook bacon until
brown, then set aside on a paper towel to drain.
Add onion and garlic in skillet with 1 teaspoon
olive oil, and sauté until translucent, about
5 minutes, then add to potato pot.

❺ When eggplant is cool enough to handle, remove
the skin. Place in potato pot with the garlic and
onion sauté. Add the remaining 1 tablespoon oil,
crumbled bacon, and garam masala, and season to
taste with salt and pepper.

Per serving: **164 calories, 3.9 g fat, 29.4 g carbs, 6 g fiber,
3.6 g sugars, 4.1 g protein**

Garlic Spinach

2 SERVINGS • DF, GF, NF, VEG, VGN

1 teaspoon red palm oil
3 garlic cloves, minced
1 (1-pound) bag spinach
salt and pepper

In a large skillet, heat oil on medium. Add garlic and
spinach. Toss carefully with tongs, until bright green
and just wilted. Season to taste with salt and pepper
and serve.

Per serving: **63 calories, 2.9 g fat, 6.9 g carbs, 3.4 g fiber,
0.7 g sugars, 4.6 g protein**

Indian Sweet Potatoes

8 SERVINGS • DF, FF, GF, VEG, VGN

3 large sweet potatoes
4 tablespoons olive oil
1 medium white onion, chopped
3 garlic cloves, minced
1 cup canned chickpeas, drained
1 tablespoon garam masala
2 tablespoons honey
1 tablespoon fresh ginger, minced
juice of 1 lime
1 cup vegetable broth
3 tablespoons fresh thyme
½ cup walnuts
salt and pepper

1 Bring pot of water to a boil. Add potatoes and boil for 20 minutes, or until slightly soft. Drain and set aside. When cool enough to handle, cut potatoes into bite-size pieces.

2 Wipe out pot and add olive oil, onion, and garlic. Sauté until soft, about 5 minutes.

3 Return sweet potatoes to pot, and add remaining ingredients, except walnuts, and simmer covered for 20–25 minutes. Season to taste with salt and pepper. Stir every few minutes, adding a little more broth or water if vegetables start to stick.

4 Sprinkle walnuts on top.

Per serving: **234 calories, 12.3 g fat, 27.7 g carbs, 5.2 g fiber, 10.2 g sugars, 5.9 g protein**

Lemon Asparagus

2 SERVINGS • GF, NF, VEG

1 bunch (12 spears) asparagus
juice of 1 lemon
2 tablespoons olive oil
1 tablespoon apple cider vinegar
1 tablespoon Parmesan cheese

1 Rinse asparagus with cold water, paying special attention to tips. Snap off woody base of each spear, usually the bottom quarter of the spear. If you have thick asparagus, use a vegetable peeler to lightly peel the spears. Cut into 1-inch pieces.

2 Bring a medium pot of lightly salted water to a boil. Add asparagus and continue to boil for 2 minutes. Drain.

3 While the asparagus is cooking, put remaining ingredients, except cheese, in a bowl. Whisk to blend, and add drained asparagus.

4 To serve, split into two portions and sprinkle Parmesan on each.

Per serving: **170 calories, 14.9 g fat, 9.4 g carbs, 3.8 g fiber, 3.4 g sugars, 4.4 g protein**

Roasted Turmeric Cauliflower

4 SERVINGS • GF, VEG

1 medium head cauliflower (5–6 inches in diameter)
3 garlic cloves, minced
juice of 1 lemon
2 tablespoons red palm oil
1 teaspoon turmeric
sea salt and pepper
2 tablespoons cilantro, chopped
5 cashews, chopped
2 tablespoons Parmesan cheese

1. Preheat oven to 400°.

2. Cut cauliflower into bite-size pieces, put in zip-lock bag, and add garlic, juice from lemon, oil, turmeric, and salt and pepper to taste. Shake bag until thoroughly mixed.

3. Spread in one layer in a roasting pan and bake for 25 minutes.

4. Put cauliflower, cilantro, cashews, and Parmesan cheese in a bowl and gently toss.

Per serving: 124 calories, 9.6 g fat, 6.6 g carbs, 2.2 g fiber, 2.1 g sugars, 4.2 g protein

Rosemary Brussels Sprouts

4 SERVINGS • DF, GF, VEG, VGN

15 Brussels sprouts, ends trimmed and yellow leaves removed
2 tablespoons olive oil
1 tablespoon dijon mustard
1 tablespoon rosemary
1 teaspoon sea salt
pepper
10 pecans, chopped

1. Preheat oven to 400°.

2. Put all ingredients in a bowl and massage with clean hands.

3. Spread on a baking sheet and bake for 35 minutes. Carefully stir or shake the pan a couple of times to evenly brown.

Per serving: 121 calories, 10 g fat, 7.7 g carbs, 3.5 g fiber, 1.7 g sugars, 3 g protein

Spinach and Navy Beans

4 SERVINGS • DF, GF, NF, VEG, VGN

2 tablespoons olive oil
2 pounds (10 cups) fresh spinach
1 can (15 ounces) navy or white beans
salt and pepper
garlic powder

1 Heat oil in a large nonstick skillet on medium high. Add spinach slowly, tossing carefully so the first spinach leaves will wilt and make room for the next handful. Continue until entirely wilted, just a minute or two.

2 Turn heat to low and add drained beans. Season with salt and pepper and garlic powder and heat for 4 minutes, stirring occasionally.

Per serving: 196 calories, 7.7 g fat, 24.2 g carbs, 7 g fiber, 0.6 g sugars, 10.1 g protein

Why Red Palm Oil?

Thanks to its dark red color, this oil is packed full of carotenes, which include heart-protecting and cancer-fighting lycopene and the antioxidant beta-carotene. Red palm oil was prized as a sacred food by the pharaohs of ancient Egypt. The oil was so highly valued that it was put in tombs so the dead would have access to it in the afterlife. It contains even more health boosters than tomatoes and carrots, plus the oil is packed with vitamin E.

Squash Casserole

6 SERVINGS • GF, NF, VEG

¼ cup red palm oil, melted
3 yellow squash (about 2 pounds), sliced in ½-inch rounds
2 medium tomatoes, sliced
1 medium onion, sliced
½ cup Parmesan cheese
salt and pepper

1 Preheat oven to 350°.

2 Use a small amount of the oil (reserve the rest) to grease the bottom of an 8 × 8 glass casserole dish.

3 Layer in this order: ⅓ of the squash in the bottom of the dish, ⅓ of the tomatoes, ⅓ of the onion, ⅓ of the Parmesan, ¼ of the oil, salt and pepper. Repeat until all ingredients are used.

4 Cover the casserole lightly with foil and bake for 30 minutes. Remove foil, sprinkle a little more Parmesan on top, and bake for 10 additional minutes, until beginning to brown.

Per serving: 61 calories, 2.3 g fat, 6.9 g carbs, 2 g fiber, 3.6 g sugars, 4.7 g protein

Squash Mash

2 SERVINGS • DF, GF, VEG, VGN

1 large spaghetti squash
1 tablespoon minced garlic
1 teaspoon tarragon
1 teaspoon honey
salt and pepper
2 tablespoons chopped pecans or walnuts

1 Preheat oven to 325°.

2 Cut squash in half and put it upside down in a glass baking pan, adding enough water to just cover the bottom of the dish. Bake for 30 minutes, or until soft when pricked with a fork.

3 Remove and set aside till just cool enough to handle. Scoop out the seeds and discard. Using a fork, scrape out the stringy insides and mix with remaining ingredients in a bowl. Season to taste with salt and pepper. Garnish each serving with nuts.

Per serving: 146 calories, 10.6 g fat, 13.2 g carbs, 3.2 g sugars, 2.4 g protein

Sweet Potato Chips

2 SERVINGS • DF, GF, NF, VEG, VGN

1 sweet potato
1 tablespoon olive oil
1 lime
sea salt

1 Preheat oven to 375°.

2 Wash potato thoroughly and slice as thin as possible to make thin, round chips.

3 Toss slices with oil and arrange on a baking sheet. Bake for 8 minutes, flip, and bake another 8 minutes.

4 Turn potatoes again, and reduce heat to 200°. Bake an additional 20 minutes.

5 Remove from oven, drizzle with lime juice, and sprinkle with sea salt.

Per serving: 160 calories, 7.2 g fat, 24.2 g carbs, 4.2 g fiber, 7.1 g sugars, 2.2 g protein

You will notice a small amount of fruit in some of these drinks. I've taken care to blend with ingredients that won't upset your stomach, so you don't have to worry about the rule on eating fruits solo (page 69). You can also freeze your bananas (peeled) if you prefer your drinks colder.

Coconut Water

Coconut water is a clear liquid from inside young, green coconuts. It has fewer calories, less sodium and sugar, and more potassium than sports drinks. Since it is not a heavy dairy liquid, it works perfectly in my power drinks. It does have some sugar and calories, so you don't want to guzzle it. Instead, use it prudently in these drinks. When shopping, look for raw coconut water.

Put coconut water in your ice tray and freeze to add to drinks.

Avocado Milk Shake

1 SERVING • DF, GF, VEG, VGN

Stay alert with cinnamon: the smell of this strong spice increases alertness by 25 percent, according to researchers at Wheeling Jesuit University.

½ avocado
1 cup unsweetened almond milk
1 teaspoon honey
2 teaspoons hemp seeds
1 teaspoon cinnamon

Place everything in a blender and mix until smooth.

Per serving: 294 calories, 25.2 g fat, 15.8 g carbs, 8 g fiber, 6.2 g sugars, 5.2 g protein

Banana Almond Shake

1 SERVING • DF, GF, VEG, VGN

This drink is a fully packed powerful protein breakfast, with plenty of fiber, protein, and calcium (84 percent of daily needs) to get you started off right in the morning.

  1 banana
  1½ cups unsweetened almond milk
  1 scoop whey protein powder
  1 teaspoon coconut oil
  1 teaspoon cinnamon
  1 teaspoon chia seeds
  4 ice cubes

Place all ingredients in a blender and blend until smooth. Add water for desired consistency.

Per serving: **335 calories, 11.3 g fat, 35.9 g carbs, 7.9 g fiber, 17.1 g sugars, 24.8 g protein**

Date Shake

1 SERVING • DF, GF, VEG, VGN

  1½ cups unsweetened flax milk
  5 almonds
  3 dates, pitted
  2 tablespoons cacao powder
  4 ice cubes
  2 teaspoons hemp seeds

Place everything in a blender and mix until smooth.

Per serving: **205 calories, 8.2 g fat, 6 g fiber, 16 g sugars, 6.1 g protein**

Electrolyte Punch

1 SERVING • DF, GF, NF, VEG, VGN

Eat watermelon—it's a great thirst quencher, and even though it is 92 percent water, it gives you a giant dose of glutathione, an antioxidant that has been shown to boost your immune system.

- 1 cup watermelon chunks
- 8 raspberries (fresh or frozen)
- 1 cup coconut water
- ½ tablespoon ground flaxseed
- 1 tablespoon lime or lemon juice

Place everything in a blender and mix until smooth.

Per serving: 200 calories, 2.8 g fat, 43.2 g carbs, 14.3 g fiber, 23.2 g sugars, 5.3 g protein

Ginger Mango

1 SERVING • DF, GF, NF, VEG, VGN

- 1 mango (½ cup)
- 1 dime-size slice of ginger
- ½ cup plain 2% Greek yogurt
- 1 cup coconut water
- 1 teaspoon chia seeds

Place everything in a blender and mix until smooth.

Per serving: 232 calories, 4.1 g fat, 34.7 g carbs, 6.4 g fiber, 28.1 g sugars, 14.8 g protein

Green Dream

1 SERVING • DF, GF, NF, VEG, VGN

This drink is packed with magnesium, potassium, iron, calcium, fiber, and vitamins A, B$_6$, and C.

- 1 handful kale, stems removed
- 1 handful spinach
- juice from 1 lemon
- ½ cucumber
- ½ inch ginger, peeled
- 1 cup coconut water
- 5 almonds
- 1 teaspoon ground flaxseed

Place all ingredients in a blender and mix, adding water to achieve consistency desired.

Per serving: 176 calories, 5 g fat, 28.6 g carbs, 7.3 g fiber, 7.2 g sugars, 7.8 g protein

Green Power

1 SERVING • DF, GF, VEG, VGN

- 1 cup fresh spinach
- ½ avocado
- 2 tablespoons lemon juice
- 4 cashews
- 1 cup unsweetened almond milk
- 1 scoop psyllium fiber

Place everything in a blender and mix until smooth.

Per serving: 290 calories, 24.6 g fat, 18.8 g carbs, 13.7 g fiber, 1.5 g sugars, 4.7 g protein

Green Tea Juice

1 SERVING • DF, GF, VEG, VGN

- 1 cup green tea, cooled
- ½ cup papaya
- ½ cup mango
- ½ banana
- ½ cup plain 2% Greek yogurt
- 1 teaspoon ground flaxseed

Place everything in a blender and mix until smooth.

Per serving: 257 calories, 1.4 g fat, 56.7 g carbs, 8.5 g fiber, 40.6 g sugars, 8.2 g protein

Oatmeal Shake

1 SERVING • DF, GF, VEG, VGN

- 1 small plain 2% Greek yogurt
- ½ cup peaches (fresh or frozen)
- ½ cup strawberries (fresh or frozen)
- 1 cup unsweetened almond or flax milk
- ¼ cup rolled oats
- ½ teaspoon cinnamon

Place everything in a blender and mix until smooth.

Per serving: 250 calories, 6.6 g fat, 33.1 g carbs, 5.8 g fiber, 15.5 g sugars, 16.4 g protein

Orange Zing

1 SERVING • DF, GF, NF, VEG, VGN

- 1 cup pineapple
- ½ banana
- 1 cup fresh-squeezed orange juice
- ⅓ cup cilantro
- ½ teaspoon ground flaxseed
- 1 scoop psyllium powder

Place everything in a blender and mix until smooth.

Per serving: 274 calories, 1.1 g fat, 66.8 g carbs, 8 g fiber, 23.3 g sugars, 3.6 g protein

Orange Lime

1 SERVING • DF, GF, VEG, VGN

- ½ banana
- 1 cup strawberries (fresh or frozen)
- ½ cup pineapple
- 1 cup orange juice
- 2 tablespoons lime juice
- ½ cup water
- ¼ cup sunflower seeds

Place everything in a blender and mix until smooth.

Per serving: 359 calories, 7.2 g fat, 77.5 g carbs, 11 g fiber, 45.5 g sugars, 7 g protein, 30% RDA for iron

Pineapple Punch

1 SERVING • DF, GF, NF, VEG, VGN

- 1 teaspoon chia seeds
- 1 cup red grapes
- ½ cup fresh pineapple
- ½ banana
- ½ cup water
- 1 teaspoon unsweetened coconut flakes
- 3 ice cubes

Soak chia seeds in water for a couple of minutes, then add all ingredients to blender and mix for 30 seconds or to desired consistency.

Per serving: 189 calories, 2.9 g fat, 42.4 g carbs, 5.9 g fiber, 30.3 g sugars, 3.2 g protein

Plum Punch

1 SERVING

- 1 plum, pitted
- 1 kiwi, peeled
- 10 blueberries (fresh or frozen)
- 1 cup unsweetened almond milk
- 1 teaspoon cinnamon
- 2 tablespoons hemp seeds

Place everything in a blender and mix until smooth.

Per serving: **269 calories, 13.6 g fat, 32.3 g carbs, 7.5 g fiber, 19.2 g sugars, 9.5 g protein**

Pomegranate Punch

1 SERVING • DF, GF, NF, VEG, VGN

- 1 cup pomegranate juice
- 1 tablespoon pistachios
- ½ cup papaya
- ½ banana
- 1 teaspoon chia seeds
- ½ cup coconut water

Place everything in a blender and mix until smooth.

Per serving: **393 calories, 7.9 g fat, 78 g carbs, 8.9 g fiber, 55.9 g sugars, 6.1 g protein**

Prune Shake

1 SERVING • DF, GF, VEG, VGN

- 4 prunes
- ½ banana
- 1 teaspoon chia seeds
- 1 small plain 2% Greek yogurt
- 1½ cups unsweetened almond milk

Place everything in a blender and mix until smooth.

Per serving: **283 calories, 7.2 g fat, 42.3 g carbs, 7.3 g fiber, 24.2 g sugars, 15.3 g protein**

Watermelon Juice

1 SERVING • DF, GF, NF, VEG, VGN

- 2 cups watermelon chunks
- 1 tablespoon lime juice
- pinch of mint

Place everything in a blender and mix until smooth.

Per serving: **202 calories, 0.5 g fat, 26.6 g carbs, 1.4 g fiber, 19.6 g sugars, 2 g protein**

Artichoke and Spinach Hummus

6 SERVINGS • DF, GF, VEG, VGN

  1 can (15 ounces) chickpeas, drained
  ½ cup fresh spinach
  1 can (15 ounces) artichoke hearts, packed in
    water, drained
  2 tablespoons olive oil
  2 tablespoons lemon juice
  2 tablespoons tahini
  1 clove garlic
  5 walnuts, chopped
  salt and pepper

Combine all ingredients in a blender or food processor and blend for 1 minute. Thin to desired consistency with about a tablespoon of water as needed. Season with salt and pepper, and serve with celery sticks, sliced cucumbers, snow peas, and baby carrots.

Per serving: 165 calories, 9 g fat, 17.7 g carbs, 3.7 g fiber, 4.8 g protein

Baba Ganoush

4 SERVINGS • DF, GF, VEG, VGN

  1 medium eggplant
  1 lemon
  2 garlic cloves
  ¼ teaspoon cumin
  2 tablespoons olive oil
  1 tablespoon fresh mint
  ½ cup pistachio nuts
  1 teaspoon ground flaxseed
  2 tablespoons tahini

1 Preheat oven to 375°.

2 Place eggplant on metal baking tray and prick with a fork a few times. Bake for 30 minutes or until soft. Remove eggplant from oven and set aside.

3 When cool enough to handle, scoop out eggplant flesh and put in blender or food processor with remaining ingredients. Blend until well combined, 15–30 seconds.

Per serving: 96 calories, 7.4 g fat, 8.6 g carbs, 4.5 g fiber, 3 g sugars, 1.5 g protein

Broccoli Pasta Salad

6 SERVINGS • GF, VEG, VGN

This is a great dish to double and take along to a picnic. It's delicious enough to share, and you'll know you have something on plan to eat.

   1 pound whole-wheat bow-tie pasta
   1 large head of broccoli
   2 cups cooked chicken, diced
   ½ cup plain 2% Greek yogurt
   ½ cup sliced almonds
   1 tablespoon apple cider vinegar
   1 teaspoon garlic powder
   salt and pepper
   1 tablespoon Parmesan cheese

Cook pasta according to directions on package. Chop broccoli into florets and lightly steam until it barely loses its crunch. Cut chicken into bite-size chunks. Place all ingredients in a bowl and mix.

Per serving: 300 calories, 7 g fat, 34.2 g carbs, 6.6 g fiber, 2.7 g sugars, 25.7 g protein

Mom's Meat Chili

6 SERVINGS • NF, FF

   1½ pounds lean ground beef
   1 large white onion, chopped
   1 can (15 ounces) pinto beans
   1 can (15 ounces) kidney beans
   1 can (15 ounces) chopped tomato
   1 can (15 ounces) hominy
   1 tablespoon garlic
   1 can (15 ounces) beef consommé
   1 teaspoon cumin
   1 teaspoon garlic, minced
   1 teaspoon paprika
   1 teaspoon cayenne pepper (optional)
   6 tablespoons grated cheddar cheese
   cilantro (optional)
   hot sauce (optional)

❶ Sauté ground meat and onion (reserve a bit of onion for step 3) in a large soup pot or Dutch oven until meat is browned, about 15 minutes.

❷ Add remaining ingredients, except cheese, cilantro, and hot sauce. Turn down heat and simmer, partially covered, for 30 minutes.

❸ Garnish each portion with 1 tablespoon cheese. Add a bit of chopped onion, cilantro, and hot sauce if desired.

Per serving: 529 calories, 13 g fat, 48.1 g carbs, 11.6 g fiber, 4 g sugars, 53.2 g protein

Quick Bean Salad

8 SERVINGS • DF, FF, GF

- 1 can (15 ounces) chickpeas
- 1 can (15 ounces) navy beans
- 1 can (15 ounces) cut green beans
- 1 can (15 ounces) kidney beans
- 1 white onion, finely chopped
- 1 stalk celery, finely chopped
- 1 red bell pepper, finely chopped
- ¼ cup sliced almonds
- ½ cup Italian dressing

Drain all canned vegetables. Place all ingredients in a large bowl and cover lightly with dressing. Stir in dressing, cover bowl, and let marinate overnight.

Per serving: 230 calories, 6.3 g fat, 35 g carbs, 10 g fiber, 3.5 g sugars, 9.3 g protein

Carrot Bran Muffins

12 SERVINGS • FF, NF, VEG

- coconut oil spray
- 2 eggs
- ¾ cup buttermilk
- 1 ripe banana, mashed
- ⅓ cup honey
- 2 tablespoons chia seeds
- 2 tablespoons coconut oil
- 1½ cups bran cereal
- ¾ cup spelt flour
- ½ teaspoon baking powder
- ½ teaspoon baking soda
- ½ teaspoon cinnamon
- ½ teaspoon ground ginger
- ½ cup raisins
- 1 carrot, shredded
- 1 teaspoon ground flaxseed

1. Preheat oven to 400°. Spray a 12-cup muffin pan with coconut oil spray.

2. In a bowl, combine eggs, buttermilk, banana, honey, chia seeds, and oil.

3. In another bowl, combine bran cereal, spelt flour, baking powder, baking soda, cinnamon, ginger, raisins, shredded carrot, and flaxseed.

4. Add flour mixture to wet mixture and stir until combined.

5. Place in coated muffin cups and bake for 20 minutes or until a toothpick comes out clean.

Per serving: 131 calories, 0.9 g fat, 2.5 g fiber, 13.6 g sugars, 3.4 g protein

Lemon Raspberry Muffins

12 SERVINGS • FF, GF, VEG

coconut oil spray
½ cup vanilla 2% Greek yogurt
3 tablespoons coconut oil
2 eggs
1½ cups spelt flour
½ cup honey
1 teaspoon vanilla extract
¼ cup coconut water
¼ teaspoon salt
½ teaspoon baking powder
½ teaspoon cinnamon
¼ cup walnuts, chopped fine
1 teaspoon chia seeds
½ cup raspberries
zest from 1 lemon

❶ Preheat oven to 400°. Spray a 12-cup muffin pan with coconut oil spray.

❷ Mix wet ingredients in a large bowl and dry ingredients in a second bowl, excluding the raspberries and lemon zest. Add the dry mixture to the wet one and stir until combined. Then stir in the lemon zest, then fold in the raspberries.

❸ Pour batter into muffin cups and bake for 20 minutes or until a toothpick comes out clean.

Per serving: 166 calories, 6.2 g fat, 5.2 g carbs, 2.7 g fiber, 13.2 g sugars, 4.6 g protein

Coconut Truffles

24 TRUFFLES • DF, FF, GF, VEG, VGN

1 cup cacao powder
¼ cup sunflower seed butter
1 cup unsweetened shredded coconut
¼ cup finely chopped pistachio nuts
½ cup honey
1 tablespoon vanilla extract
½ cup coconut oil, melted
1 teaspoon cinnamon
zest from 1 lemon
¼ teaspoon sea salt

Combine all ingredients in a bowl and mix thoroughly. Use a spoon to portion out 24 truffles onto a plate. Cover loosely with plastic wrap and chill in the refrigerator for at least an hour.

Per cookie: 158 calories, 13.1 g fat, 10.9 g carbs, 3.2 g fiber, 6.9 g sugars, 2.2 g protein

Gooey Chocolate Power Brownies

12 SERVINGS • DF, FF, GF, VEG

1 cup canned black beans
2 tablespoons coconut oil
2 tablespoons natural crunchy peanut butter
3 tablespoons unsweetened almond milk
½ cup coconut palm sugar
5 tablespoons cacao powder
2 tablespoons spelt flour
1 teaspoon cinnamon
1 teaspoon chia seeds
1 teaspoon baking powder
½ teaspoon sea salt
coconut oil spray
1 cup dark chocolate chips

1 Preheat oven to 350°.

2 Drain and rinse the beans in cold water. Place in a blender with oil, peanut butter, and milk. Blend until smooth. Add sugar, cacao powder, spelt flour, cinnamon, chia seeds, baking powder, and salt. Blend until smooth.

3 Spray a baking pan with coconut spray. Spread mixture evenly in pan, place chocolate chips evenly across the top, and bake for 20 minutes.

Per serving: 181 calories, 7.1 g fat, 27.7 g carbs, 3.7 g fiber, 11.8 g sugars, 5.7 g protein

Peanut Butter Avocado Cookies

30 COOKIES • DF, FF, GF, VEG

1 avocado
2 eggs, beaten
1 tablespoon chia seeds
3 tablespoons honey
⅔ cup natural crunchy peanut butter
¾ cup old-fashioned rolled oats
1 teaspoon cinnamon
½ teaspoon baking powder
½ cup dark chocolate chips
½ cup pistachio nuts, finely chopped

1 Preheat oven to 350°.

2 Mash avocado in a mixing bowl, then add eggs, chia seeds, and honey. Mix thoroughly.

3 Stir in peanut butter, oats, cinnamon, baking powder, chocolate chips, and pistachios. Mix until well combined.

4 Use a spoon to dollop cookies on a baking sheet, slightly pressing down with the back of the spoon. Bake for 12 minutes. Cool completely on a rack.

Per cookie: 93 calories, 6.3 g fat, 7 g carbs, 1.4 g fiber, 3.5 g sugars, 2.9 g protein

Vegan Chocolate Mousse

8 SERVINGS • DF, GF, VEG, VGN

2 cups dairy-free dark chocolate chips
⅓ cup brewed coffee
1 teaspoon vanilla extract
1 pound silken tofu, drained
1 tablespoon honey
½ cup pistachio nuts, chopped

1 In a medium pan, heat the chocolate chips, coffee, and vanilla over low heat, stirring constantly with a spatula until fully melted. Pour mixture into a blender. Add the remaining ingredients and blend until well combined.

2 Pour into 8 individual glass containers, cover with plastic wrap, and refrigerate for at least 1 hour until the mousse is firm.

Per serving: 229 calories, 13.1 g fat, 25.8 g carbs, 0.9 g fiber, 19.6 g sugars, 7.6 g protein

MOVES

Moves

Your 15-Minute Workouts

Abs (A, B, C, and D): insert (I) pages 9, 11, 13, and 15

Arms (A and B): insert pages 17 and 22

Back (A and B): insert pages 27 and 31

Buns (A and B): insert pages 36 and 40

Cardio (A and B): insert pages 46 and 49

Chest (A and B): insert pages 54 and 57

Legs (A and B): insert pages 60 and 65

Shoulders (A and B): insert pages 71 and 76

This chapter contains detailed instructions and pictures for the workouts prescribed in the 4-week plan. In addition, you'll find suggestions for pumping up the intensity, as well as modifications so you can adjust a move to your individual needs. All moves are organized by body part into two workouts, labeled A and B, except Abs, which has four shorter routines (A, B, C, and D) that are incorporated with the upper body workouts in the 4-week plan. This design allows you to have a different workout each week, targeting every muscle from every angle to give you fast results in minimal time.

The 1-to-10 Burn Scale

I told you back in chapter 3 how I love using a 1-to-10 scale; it's a fast way to get a read on just about anything, and exercise is no exception. During appointments with clients, I use a 1-to-10 scale to check effort and intensity throughout all parts of the workout, and you will learn to do this during the 15-minute routines you'll be doing.

The rating scale goes like this:

1–2: Very easy; don't really feel it.

3–4: Feels good; I could do this for a while.

5–6: Feeling it start to burn.

7–8: It is burning at an increasing rate.

9–10: It is very intense, with a deep burn; I'm not sure how much more I can do.

Let's say I'm having you do Triceps Push-Ups (page I-26). During the exercise, you rate the effort you're giving or how much the exercise is burning your arms. If you give it a 5, I will tell you to keep going until you feel the burn at a 9.5 or 10. So keep going until you reach this level. That's how you'll get results.

How to Do the Workouts

It's important that you do the exercises in the order they are prescribed. Alternating different strength and flexibility moves, as the workouts do, allows your muscles to rest, recover, and repair in between workouts. Rest does not mean kicking up your feet and watching your favorite TV show; it means doing the next day's workout, which will open and close your joints, bringing fresh synovial fluids to nourish, lubricate, and hydrate while expelling waste and scar tissue.

What You'll Need

If you spend most of your waking hours wearing shoes, I recommend doing these workouts barefoot. However, if you already do most of your workouts barefoot, switch it up and lace on some fitness shoes. When you alter your usual footwear, it triggers different stabilizing muscles and helps you achieve balance. Do all workouts on a flat surface with a yoga mat.

Warm Up Before Every Workout

Make sure you are warmed up before doing any exercises, especially if you work out first thing in the morning. If you slept on one side, which can increase muscle imbalance, these moves will help put you back in balance. Every workout starts with a warm-up move, but if you feel you need more, add Arm Rolls (page I-17), Hula Hoop (page I-27), Hippie (page I-49), or fifty jumping jacks.

The body can feel completely at ease and natural every moment. Just let it.

—EUGENE GENDLIN

How to Breathe Properly During Exercise

Many people run out of breath too early during exercise because they hold their breath, stutter, or strain unnecessarily, which can cause dangerous changes in blood pressure, interfere with performance and results, and leave you prematurely weak and depleted. When you breathe correctly, you fuel your body efficiently and effectively, which supplies you with energy and intensity—so you can take your workout to the next level and reach your goals faster. You should be able to calmly talk as you move. The quality of your voice should be as if you were talking normally to a person just outside the room, and that person would not be able to tell that you were working out. Aim to talk as if you weren't moving at all.

Stretching for Balance

Whenever you do a one-sided stretch, such as stretching each hamstring, rate each side separately (10 being super tight and tense, and 1 being extremely limber, loose, and flexible) and work toward full-body balance.

Often you will get different numbers. If the sides are imbalanced—let's say the first side is a 6 and the other side is a 9—this indicates muscle imbalance.

The goal is to get both sides even. You'd begin by shooting for a 5 on the first side and an 8 for the second side. Do both sides once, then concentrate on the tighter side, the 8, until it gradually loosens up. It won't happen immediately, so don't force it. If it doesn't happen the first time, move on to the next exercise and then come back to repeat this stretch.

By the end of every workout, you should feel balanced. If you notice that muscle tensing up later in the day, pause and do an appropriate stretch.

By focusing on the tighter areas of your body, you will gradually correct imbalances, reduce pain, and increase energy.

1-to-10 Scale for Rating Exercises

When I ask you to rate your exercise, use the following scale:

If it is a strength Move, Your Goal is a 10

Ask yourself, "How much is this move fatiguing my muscle, or how much am I feeling a burn on a scale of 1 to 10?" A 1 means you don't feel any effort or burn at all, while a 10 means it is burning *big time*. Your goal is to work in the 8–10 range. That's where you'll get results.

If it is a Stretch, Your Goal Is a 1

If you are really feeling the stretch because your muscle is tight, that is a 10. If you are not feeling it at all, it's a 1. Your goal is to get down to 1, which means you are very limber and have zero tension in this area being stretched. On that note, all stretches should feel good; you never want to force a stretch. Always relax into it. Sometimes a particular stretch won't change numbers or improve in one session; don't get frustrated. Each week you will get more and more limber. Flexibility takes time. Just keep melting and breathing into the tight area.

The 4-Week Plan Moves: Quick Reference Guide

This gives you a snapshot of the moves prescribed on the 4-week calendar in chapter 7.

WEEK 1

Day 1
Arms (A), page I-17
Abs (A), page I-9

Day 2
Legs (A), page I-60

Day 3
Back (A), page I-27

Day 4
Chest (A), page I-54
Abs (B), page I-11

Day 5
Buns (A), page I-36

Day 6
Cardio (A), page I-46

Day 7
Shoulders (A), page I-71
Abs (C), page I-13

WEEK 2

Day 8
Legs (B), page I-65

Day 9
Arms (B), page I-22
Abs (D), page I-15

Day 10
Back (B), page I-31

Day 11
Buns (B), page I-40

Day 12
Chest (B), page I-57
Abs (A), page I-9

Day 13
Cardio (B), page I-49

Day 14
Shoulders (B), page I-76
Abs (B), page I-11

WEEK 3	WEEK 4
Day 15 *Rest day: Get a massage or reward yourself with a special day off*	**Day 22** Chest (A), page I-54 Abs (A), page I-9
Day 16 Legs (A), page I-60	**Day 23** Legs (B), page I-65
Day 17 Arms (A), page I-17 Abs (C), page I-13	**Day 24** Back (B), page I-31
Day 18 Back (A), page I-27	**Day 25** Arms (B), page I-22 Abs (B), page I-11
Day 19 Buns (A), page I-36	**Day 26** Buns (B), page I-40
Day 20 Shoulders (A), page I-71 Abs (D), page I-15	**Day 27** Cardio (B), page I-49
Day 21 Cardio (A), page I-46	**Day 28** Shoulders (B), page I-76 Abs (C), page I-13

Your 15-Minute Workouts

Note: Don't just rely on the photographs. Make sure to read each exercise description carefully. While the photographs illustrate each exercise, they don't fully capture each moving part of your body as you move through the multiple sets included in most moves. That's what the written description is for. Once you've done the exercises a few times, the photographs can be used as a quick mental cue. But initially you'll want to follow the written word carefully, so you get the full impact of the modifications and of your 15-minute workout.

Ab Presses

STRENGTHENS AND TONES YOUR ABS

Get ready: Lie flat on your back and bring your knees up so they are in line with your belly button, making a right angle from your torso to your upper legs. Knees are bent with lower legs relaxed.

Go! Keeping your head relaxed on the mat, place your palms on your upper thighs and press as hard as you can while holding your stomach in and down toward the floor (imagine you are wearing a tight pair of jeans). Your thighs do not move; they resist your hands, causing your abdominal muscles to engage. Continue holding this contraction while you say the alphabet out loud backward (Z, Y, X, . . .), releasing when you reach A. *Make it harder:* Use both hands to push on one leg at a time.

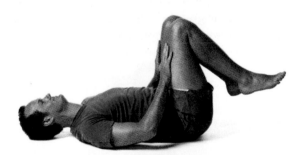

Ab Sways

STRENGTHENS YOUR ABS

Get ready: Lie on your back with knees bent and feet flat on the ground, hands interlaced behind your head. Pull in your abdominal muscles, and lift your head and shoulders as high as you comfortably can without putting pressure on your neck.

Go! Press your back into the ground. Lift your feet one inch off the ground and sway your feet side to side for one minute. Then, while continuing to sway your feet, do thirty crunches.

*Let your past make you
better, not bitter.*

Elastic Man

ELONGATES ENTIRE BODY

Get ready: Lie on your back with legs extended and feet pointed. Interlace your hands in front of you, palms facing out.

Go! Lift your arms above your head and stretch. Try to get the longest distance between your palms and your pointed feet. Hold and take five deep breaths.

No matter how "busy" you are, if you really care, you will always find a way and the time to do it.

Twisted Lifts

STRENGTHENS AND TONES OBLIQUES— OBLITERATES LOVE HANDLES

Get ready: Lie on your back with knees glued together and dropped halfway to one side, hands interlaced behind your head. During the entire exercise keep your chin a tennis balls' distance away from your chest to ensure you don't strain your neck.

Go! Engage and contract your abdominal muscles to lift your shoulders several inches off the mat. Keep your elbows out to the sides, gaze upward toward the ceiling, and focus on the effort coming from your obliques (the abdominal muscles that run down the sides of your torso), not from your neck. Pause for one second, then lower. Do twenty-five crunches on one side, then switch sides and repeat. *Make it harder:* Do the move with your legs and feet lifted one inch off the ground. *Even harder:* Crunch your upper and lower body simultaneously.

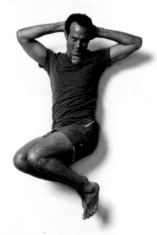

Repeat Elastic Man (see left).

Ab Circles

STRENGTHENS ABDOMINAL MUSCLES

Get ready: Lie on your back with legs fully extended, shoulder width apart, and feet flexed. Put your arms behind your head, each palm on the back of the opposite shoulder, making an X. Rest your head completely in the X.

Go! Engage and contract your abdominal muscles to lift your shoulders several inches off the mat and circle your torso to the left, then center, then right, and back to center. Do twenty-five clockwise circles, then repeat counterclockwise. *Make it harder:* Lift one foot off the ground and then when you switch directions, switch your legs.

Back Press

STRETCHES YOUR CHEST, HIPS, AND ABS

Get ready: Kneel upright (not resting on your calves), so that only your knees and shins rest on the mat, and put your hands on your lower back (fingertips pointing down). Or you can do it standing as pictured below if it is hard on your knees.

Go! Pull your stomach in and gently press your hips forward, arching your back and pulling your elbows back toward each other. If you want to go deeper, lift your chin and look up toward the ceiling for five deep breaths.

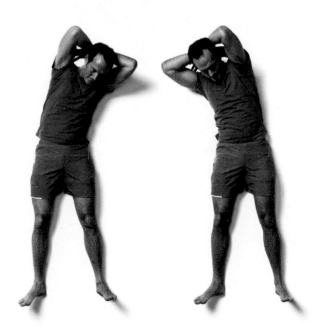

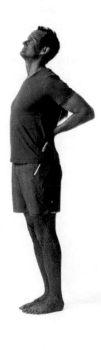

Seesaw Abs

STRENGTHENS CORE

Get ready: Sit on your mat with your legs bent to 90 degrees, ankles crossed, and hands behind your thighs for support. (More advanced exercisers can extend arms straight out to either side.)

Go! While keeping your spine straight, gently lean back to activate your abs and lift your ankles two inches off the ground. Use your abs to pull in your belly button. Hold for ten counts. Next, straighten your legs as best you can and pulse your upper and lower body in and away, one inch in each direction, thirty times. Return to the initial position, leaning back with ankles crossed and lifted, but this time reach your hands out to your sides, palms up, at shoulder height. Seesaw your arms in a straight line: your left arm lifts up about twelve inches as your right arm simultaneously comes down about twelve inches (arms move as one unit). Continue, holding your abs taut with legs lifted. Repeat thirty times. Bring your hands to prayer position; move your arms straight up and down thirty times.

Knee Drop

OPENS THE SPINE AND HIPS

Get ready: Lie on your back with knees bent and feet flat on the mat. Interlace hands behind your head to support your neck, with elbows out to the sides.

Go! Keeping your upper body in place, gently lower legs down to one side. Feel the stretch in your back as you relax and take five deep breaths, then repeat on the other side. Go deeper: Snake your legs around each other and use the weight of the lower leg to increase the stretch.

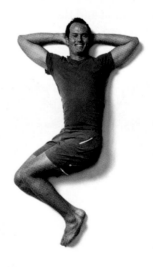

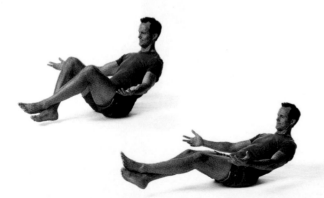

Butterfly Crunches

WORKS ABDOMINALS

Get ready: Lie on your back with knees bent and feet close to your tailbone. Bring the soles of your feet together, and let your knees fall out to either side. Interlace hands and place them behind your head for support, keeping your elbows out to either side.

Go! Looking up at the ceiling, contract your core muscles and lift your shoulders several inches off the floor, then lower. The effort should come from your abdominal muscles without pulling on your head or neck. Continue for thirty seconds. Next, lift your legs as a solid unit one inch up and down for thirty seconds. Finally, for the last thirty seconds, lift and lower both the upper and lower body together. *Make it harder:* Do the second set of the series at double time.

Cobra

STRENGTHENS BACK MUSCLES, OPENS YOUR CHEST, AND STRETCHES ABDOMINALS

Get ready: Lie facedown with palms down on either side of your chest, elbows bent and pointing back, fingertips pointing forward, and the tops of your feet and your forehead resting on the mat.

Go! Press into your palms, and imagine a string pulling from the top of your head, lifting your head and chest off the floor until you feel a nice stretch in your belly muscles. Relax into it. Don't force your arms straight. As you gaze straight ahead, hold for five deep breaths and release.

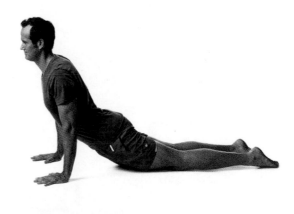

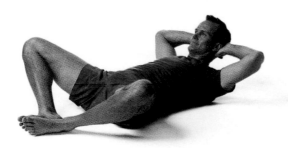

Straight Leg Twist

STRENGTHENS OBLIQUES

Get ready: Lie face up, knees up above your hips with your right hand behind your head holding it up. Put your left hand on your stomach and straighten and lift your left leg to point toward the ceiling. Keep your feet relaxed for the duration of the exercise.

Go! Lift and twist your right shoulder, keeping your elbow out of your line of vision and moving diagonally toward your left leg, with the effort coming from your obliques. Do thirty times; switch sides and repeat. Use the hand on your stomach to make sure your abs stay pulled in as you lift. *Make it harder:* Do the move with your bottom leg straight and hovering three feet off the floor.

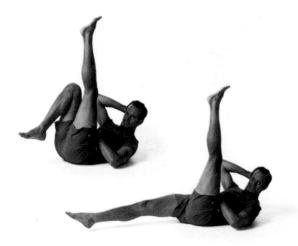

Straight Leg Ab Lift

SCULPTS YOUR ENTIRE CORE

Get ready: Lie face up with interlaced hands behind your head for support. Keep your elbows back on either side.

Go! Lift your shoulders, with the effort coming from your abs, and hold. Lift both legs straight up above your hips, then lift your tailbone one inch up and down thirty times, keeping your upper body lifted and your neck relaxed. Then, keeping legs up, crunch up, with the effort coming from your abs, thirty times. Finally, do upper and lower body simultaneously thirty times.

Repeat Cobra, but on this set lift your head and look straight ahead for three breaths, then look at your right foot over your right shoulder for three breaths, over your left shoulder for three breaths, and back to the center for three breaths.

---

*Trust your intuition. If it feels
wrong, it most likely is.*

I Dream of Jeannie

STRENGTHENS QUADS, ABS, AND SHOULDERS

Get ready: Kneel upright and cross your arms so hands are inside and just above opposite elbows. Lift your arms to just below shoulder height—like a genie.

Go! While keeping a straight line from the top of your head to your knees, lean back slightly (this engages your abs and thighs) and hold for thirty seconds. Then, maintaining the lean, use your torso to twist one foot back, leading with your right shoulder, then repeat to the left. Go back and forth thirty times. *Make it harder:* Lean back farther, pulling in your navel and squeezing your butt. Use a towel under your knees for cushion.

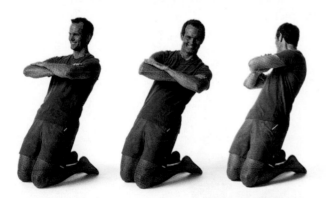

L-Crunches

STRENGTHENS ABS AND INNER THIGHS

Get ready: Lie face up with your head resting on your interlaced hands and lift your legs straight above your hips, feet pointed like a ballerina.

Go! Pull in your navel and press your lower back into the mat and lift your head up as high as you comfortably can. Drop your left leg down one foot off the ground. Now you are making an "L" with your legs. Do thirty one-inch-up pulses. Then switch legs and repeat on the other side. If it gets too hard don't bring your bottom leg down as low. Do thirty basketball-size clockwise circles with each leg, then repeat in the opposite direction. *Make it harder:* Do the exercise with your head and shoulders lifted as high as possible and your legs lowered to 45 degrees from the floor.

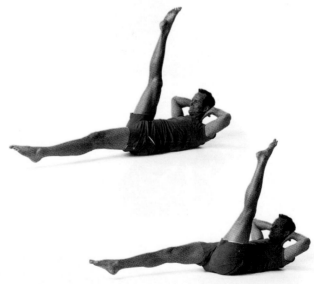

Thread the Needle

STRETCHES YOUR OUTER HIP AND HIGH HAMSTRING

Get ready: Lie on your back, knees bent and feet flat on mat, comfortably apart. Lift your right leg and cross it on top of your left thigh.

Go! Lift your head, reach your right hand between your legs, and bring your left hand to the front of your left leg, holding right below your knee. Gently lower and relax your upper body back to the mat as you pull your left knee in toward your shoulder. Go as far as it feels comfortable. If it feels too difficult, grasp behind your left quad instead. Hold for five deep breaths, then lift your forehead toward your knee and hold for five breaths. Then switch legs. Do both sides twice.

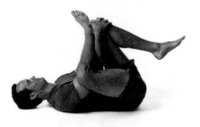

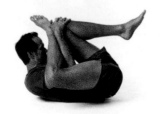

Reverse X Crunches

STRENGTHENS ENTIRE AB REGION

Get ready: Lie face up with legs together and keep knees bent at 90 degrees with lower legs parallel to the floor. Put your arms behind your head, each palm on the back of the opposite shoulder, making an X. Rest your head completely in the X. Crunch up, tightening your abs. Keep a tennis-ball width distance between chin and chest.

Go! Maintaining the right angle in your legs, drop your heels down to tap the mat, then bring them back up to 90 degrees. Do as many as you can while you count out loud until you are completely fatigued. *Make it harder:* Extend your legs straight up and tap down with straight legs (as shown in the picture below).

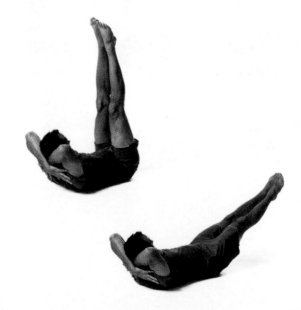

Back Walk

STRENGTHENS ENTIRE CORE AND ARMS

Get ready: Sit with your knees bent and feet flat on mat. Place your hands, elbows bent, on the mat behind you, palms down with fingertips pointing back toward you and slightly to the side. Gently bend your elbows farther, lean back and lift your legs off the ground, maintaining a 90-degree bend at the knees.

Go! Tap your left heel down to the mat, lift it back up, and then tap your right heel down. Continue in a fluid motion for thirty alternating heel taps. Second set: Pick up the pace and go double time. *Make it harder:* Do the move with straight legs, and lower each leg on a count of five. Still too easy? Do the move with straight legs, but this time hold your hands in prayer position out in front of you.

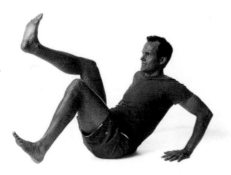

Repeat Cobra (page I-13).

Arm Rolls

WARMS UP SHOULDERS

Get ready: Stand with feet together and arms by your sides.

Go! Roll your shoulders forward five times and back five times as shown in the picture. Then use your entire arm to make circles, and "swim" shoulders, alternating your left arm, and then your right, rotating them as if they were bicycle pedals. Go backward for five on each side, and forward for five on each side. Your goal is to get full range of movement with your shoulders, so make the circles as big as possible. Notice any areas that don't move fluidly, and try to open them up by relaxing as you move. Get in the habit of rolling your shoulders five times forward and five times back between all the sets in this workout, as well as during the chest and shoulder workouts.

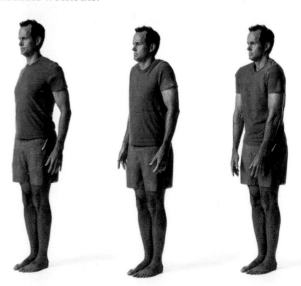

T-Circles

STRENGTHENS ARMS AND SHOULDERS

Get ready: Stand with your feet together and come up onto your toes. Bring your arms out to either side at shoulder height, so your body forms a T.

Go! Spread out the fingers of each hand, palms down, and begin making forward arm circles the size of a basketball. Count out loud backward from one hundred by threes (97, 94, 91, etc.). When you pass fifty, start to circle backward and keep counting until you get to zero. Then turn your palms up and continue making circles forward. This time count up by threes (1, 4, 7, 10, and so on) until you pass fifty, then circle backward until you reach 100.

Upper Cuts

STRENGTHENS AND TONES ARMS AND SHOULDERS, AS WELL AS CORE MUSCLES

Get ready: Stand with your feet shoulder width apart, knees slightly bent, arms at your sides with elbows bent and hands in fists, palms up.

Go! To begin, pull your right elbow slightly back and then punch your right fist up and slightly to the left with your palm toward your face, then bring your right arm back, and as you do, punch up your left fist. Imagine that two people are facing you, and you are aiming underneath their chins. Continue in a fast, fluid motion, throwing alternating uppercut punches for thirty seconds, then pick up the pace and go double time for thirty more seconds. Engage and contract your core muscles (in your abs and back) to stabilize your body, so your lower body remains stationary. Resist wiggling your knees.

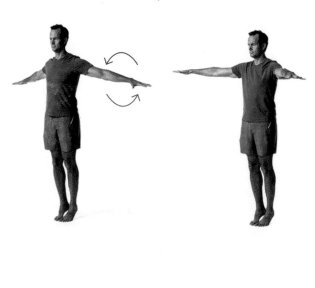

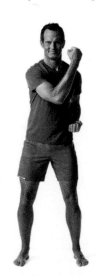
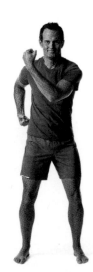

Rainbows

TONES ARMS AND SHOULDERS

Get ready: Balance on the balls of both feet and extend your arms as far as you can out to the sides, palms down and fingertips spread apart. Your body should form a T shape.

Go! Make small "rainbow" arcs with your hands by dipping your thumbs forward two inches, and then back with your pinkies two inches. Go back and forth for thirty seconds, and then go at double time for thirty seconds, and finally, at triple time for another thirty seconds. Repeat this series with your palms up, while balancing on your right foot and then switching to your left foot halfway. Keep your shoulders relaxed throughout the exercise.

Seaweed

STRENGTHENS ENTIRE ARM AND SHOULDER

Get ready: Stand with your feet together, toes pointing forward, and come up onto your toes. Bring your arms in front of you with elbows bent so your forearms are at right angles with palms facing each other, three inches apart. Your elbows are now shoulder height.

Go! Leading with your middle finger, sway your hands in and out like seaweed at the bottom of the ocean, switching the hand closest to your face each time. Your upper arms will move forward and back, maintaining the angle in your elbows but allowing your forearms and fingers to sway in and out. Do for one minute as fast as you can.

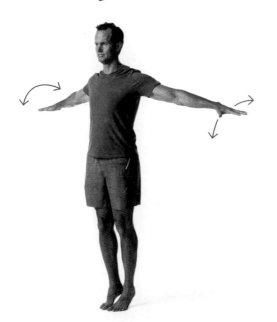

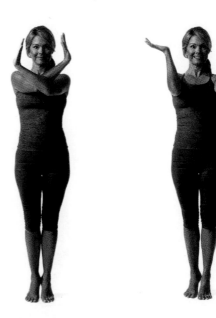

Arm Kickbacks

TONES TRICEPS

Get ready: Stand with your feet together, knees slightly bent. Bend your torso forward two feet, keeping a straight line from the top of your head to your tailbone. Keep your upper arms locked to your sides and drive your elbows back as far as you can, keeping your forearms forward at right angles, hands in loose fists facing each other. Your upper arms stay in this position for the duration of the exercise.

Go! From here, kick your forearms and hands back and up, while simultaneously twisting your forearms to press your palms up so they face the ceiling, then return to starting position. Make sure your arms stay in with elbows locked up and back the entire time. Focus on normal breathing throughout the exercise. Repeat fifty times. Advanced: Work up to one hundred times, while balancing on your toes.

Back Scratch

STRETCHES UPPER BACK AND TRICEPS

Get ready: Stand with your feet comfortably apart, hands at sides.

Go! Lift your arms up over your head, and bend both elbows so your forearms come toward each other. Grab just above your right elbow with your left hand, so your left hand is on the outside of your right upper arm. Use gentle pressure from your left hand to help your right hand slowly walk down between your shoulder blades to your upper back. When you feel the stretch, hold for three deep breaths. Relax your shoulders down away from your ears. To advance the stretch, lean to your left and push your right elbow to the left, so you can feel the stretch all the way down your right side. Repeat on the other side.

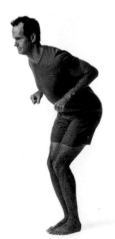
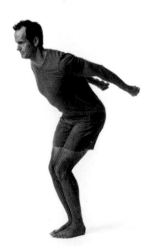
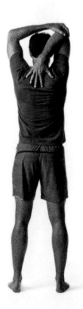

Jab/Cross

TONES ARMS, SHOULDERS, AND UPPER BACK

Get ready: Stand with feet hip width apart, knees slightly soft. Bend your elbows and bring both hands to your sides with fisted palms up.

Go! Twist your torso to the left as you punch your right arm and fist out in front of your left shoulder, then return arm to starting position. Immediately punch with the left arm to the right. Continue in a fast, fluid motion, alternating arms, for one minute. Punch as fast as you can. For a more advanced move, simultaneously kick the heel on the punching side up toward your butt as you punch.

Twelve to Six

STRETCHES ARMS AND CHEST
AND IMPROVES BALANCE

Get ready: Stand with your feet together, arms by your sides. Imagine that you are standing in the middle of a giant clock, with twelve o'clock directly in front of you and six directly behind you.

Go! Lift your right foot and wrap it behind your left ankle, reaching your right hand, palm up, in front of you to twelve o'clock, then swing your right arm horizontally in a half circle until you reach six o'clock behind you, leading with your thumb. Only go as far as feels comfortable. Do five times, then repeat with the other arm and leg.

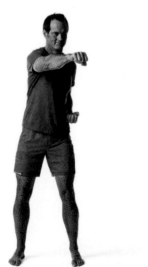 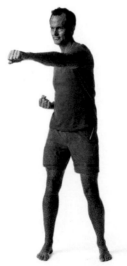 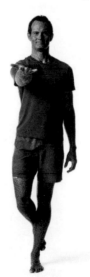 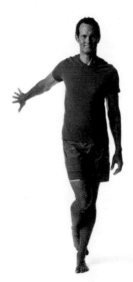

Repeat Arm Rolls (page I-17).

Field Goals

STRENGTHENS UPPER ARMS,
SHOULDERS, AND UPPER BACK

Get ready: Stand with your feet comfortably apart. Bring your arms out to the sides, palms forward and elbows in line with your shoulders. Bend your elbows to make a right angle with forearms pointing forward.

Go! Rotate your hands and forearms down until they are parallel to the floor, pause, then bring them back up. Repeat for thirty seconds. Alternate arms, repeating for an additional thirty seconds. Then bring your arms in front of you and tap your forearms all the way together and all the way back to the sides, repeating thirty times. *Make it harder:* Lift your heels and do the moves while standing on your toes. Raise the tempo to double time.

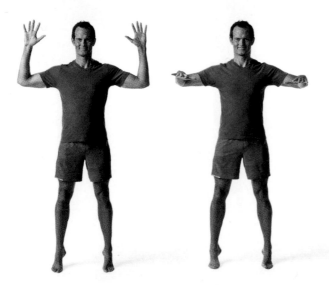

Arm Opener

STRETCHES ARMS, CHEST, AND SHOULDERS

Get ready: Stand with feet comfortably apart. Take your hands and interlace them behind your tailbone with knuckles down.

Go! Looking straight ahead and with soft arms, gently drive your arms up and as far away from your tailbone as you can. Go to where you feel a nice stretch and take five deep breaths into your chest. *Make it harder:* Lean all the way forward and drop your head.

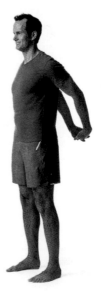

Punching Bag

STRENGTHENS ARMS AND SHOULDERS

Get ready: Stand with feet comfortably apart. Lift your right foot off the floor, bringing your arms out in front of you, elbows slightly bent with your knuckles facing away from your body and in line with the center of your chest.

Go! Circle your hands around each other vertically (up and over) as if you were hitting an imaginary punching bag. Go thirty seconds clockwise, then thirty seconds counterclockwise. To pump it up, do double time for thirty seconds in each direction, then an additional set at triple time. Don't stop, and resist lifting your shoulders; keep them away from your ears. Then do a second set with your left foot up.

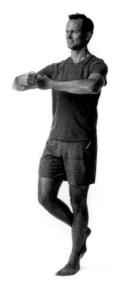 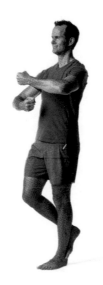 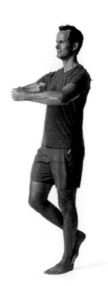 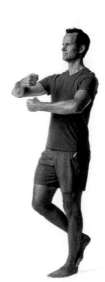

Twist and Reach

STRENGTHENS ARMS AND SHOULDERS

Get ready: Stand with your feet shoulder width apart, and reach your arms out to the sides, palms facing backward with thumbs pointing down.

Go! Bend your elbows and bring your arms down to your sides, rotating your wrists so your palms face up just as your upper arms reach your sides. Tap your elbows to your sides, then reverse the move to reach your arms all the way back out with your palms back and thumbs pointing down. Go back and forth for one minute. Then do double time for one minute. To pump it up, alternate kicking your heel up to your butt each time you reach your arms out.

Flabby Arm Evaporator

TONES TRICEPS

Get ready: Sit with your hands about a foot behind you, shoulder width apart, palms on the mat, and fingertips pointed toward your butt. Bend your knees with feet flat on the mat, about shoulder width apart.

Go! Use your arms to lift your butt off the ground until your elbows are one inch short of being fully straight, then bend your elbows and tap your tailbone forward toward your heels. Only your elbows move here, with the effort coming from your upper arms. Do twenty-five times. Once you have mastered this move, pump it up by simultaneously lifting your right leg off the mat and straightening it in the air above you, and do twenty-five dips. Then switch legs and repeat.

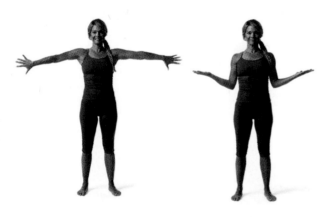

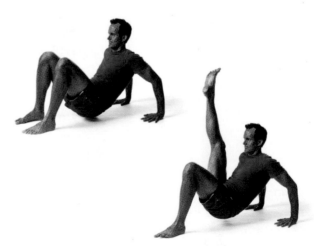

Forearm Stretch

STRETCHES FOREARMS

Get ready: Kneel upright, then place your hands down in front and right next to your knees with fingertips pointing back toward your knees.

Go! Keeping your elbows soft, gently drive the base of your palms forward until you feel a stretch in your forearms. Relax into the stretch and hold for five deep breaths. If you want a deeper stretch, keep your palms flat down and your elbows soft, and gently walk your knees and shoulders backward, away from your middle fingers.

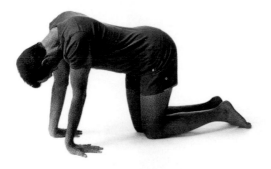

Overhead Eleven Punch

STRENGTHENS SHOULDERS AND ARMS

Get ready: Stand in a semilunge position, with your left leg stepped forward about three feet from your right, legs slightly bent. Bend your elbows to bring your arms out in front, making a number 11 with your forearms. Hold your arms one foot apart, elbows pointing down, palms in fists with knuckles facing each other.

Go! Punch both your arms straight up and then bring them back down. Your arms stay facing the same way the entire time. Punch for up to thirty seconds. Switch legs, right leg forward, left leg back, and repeat. If you want to work with balance, come up on your toes and do the entire exercise from the balls of your feet, adding a second set at double time.

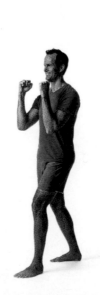
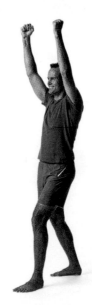

Triceps Push-Up

STRENGTHENS TRICEPS AND ARMS

Get ready: Lie facedown with your hands down underneath your shoulders, palms down and fingertips straight ahead. Your elbows should be flush against your sides and pointing straight up. For modified, do this on your knees; for advanced, do as pictured below.

Go! Relax your entire body and push your hands into your mat, using only your triceps to lift your upper body roughly two inches. Go up and down fifty times, keeping elbows locked in at your sides the entire time. To pump it up, do one hundred repetitions.

Two Things at Once

STRETCHES SHOULDERS AND UPPER BACK

Get ready: Stand with your feet shoulder width apart and knees slightly bent.

Go! Reach both arms to the left at shoulder height while turning your head to look over your right shoulder. Hold the stretch and take three deep breaths. Moving slowly, switch sides, reaching to the right while looking over your left shoulder. Do twice on each side. On the second set, look in the same direction as you are reaching and twist to where you feel a good stretch. Keep your shoulders relaxed and down.

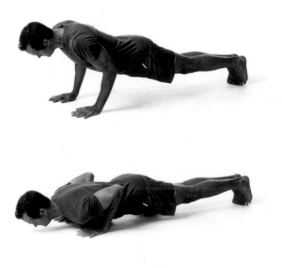

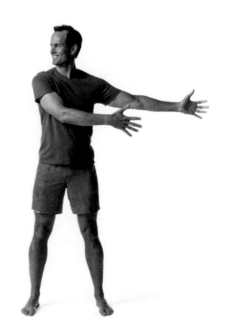

Hula Hoop

WARMS UP AND LOOSENS HIPS,
INCREASING MOBILITY

Get ready: Stand with your feet together and hands on your waist.

Go! Circle your hips five times clockwise and then five times counterclockwise. Pretend there is a string from the top of your head elongating your spine. Resist moving your shoulders, keep your stomach pulled in, and focus on moving your hips in as wide a circle as possible.

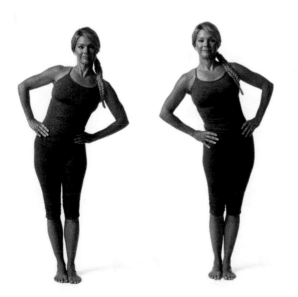

Flapper

STRENGTHENS ENTIRE BACK

Get ready: Stand with your feet together and your knees slightly bent. Lean forward from your waist until your back is flat and as parallel to the floor as possible (if you've got a bad back, stay up higher).

Go! Keeping your arms straight and your elbows unlocked, bring your arms out to the sides in line with your shoulders. Pause, then bring your hands together, as if clapping with straight arms. Do sixty times, then hold in the arm up position and pulse one inch up and down for sixty pulses. Then come up on your toes and do an additional sixty full-movement repetitions.

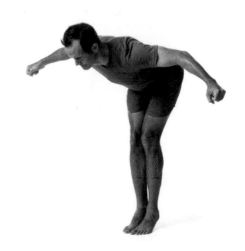

Single-Leg Windmill

STRENGTHENS ENTIRE BACK, AND
IMPROVES OVERALL STABILITY

Get ready: Balance on your left foot and reach your
right foot behind you for balance. Reach your arms
out to the sides at shoulder height with your palms
down. Keep your gaze fixed on the ground about
six feet in front of you throughout this exercise.

Go! Keep a straight line from the top of your head
to your tailbone, and lean forward two feet while
driving your hips back. Keeping your arms in the
same T position, rotate your torso to the left, so that
your left arm rotates back as your right arm rotates
down, then rotate to the other side, so that your
right arm goes back and your left arm comes down.
Continue, alternating, twenty-five times, then switch
legs and repeat. Do a total of two sets on each side.

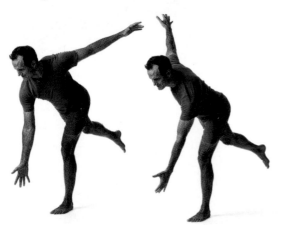

Yo-Yo

ALIGNS SPINE AND IMPROVES POSTURE

Get ready: Stand with your feet shoulder width
apart and toes angled slightly out. Interlace your
hands and bring them up to chest level, about six
inches in front of your chest, with palms facing away
from your body and elbows out to the sides.

Go! While keeping your lower body stationary,
twist your upper body from side to side as far as
it feels comfortable, leading with your elbows and
keeping your head in line with your torso, and look
in the direction you are twisting. If you feel dizzy
keep your gaze forward. Do ten times.

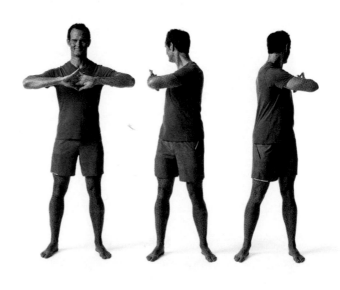

Rickety Table Pulses

STABILIZES AND STRENGTHENS
ENTIRE BACK AND GLUTES

Get ready: Come onto all fours (hands under shoulders and knees under hips). Extend your right arm out in front of you and your left leg behind you as far as you can in line with your back.

Go! Pulse your lifted arm and leg one inch up and down for twenty-five seconds. Then switch sides and repeat. When finished, go back to the first side and do side-to-side pulses, about one inch to each side for twenty-five seconds. Switch sides and repeat. For the third set, from the balanced position, punch your arm straight out above your head while holding your lifted leg steady, for twenty-five repetitions. Switch sides and repeat.

Superman

STRENGTHENS ENTIRE BACK AND GLUTES

Get ready: Lie facedown and rest your forehead on your hands, palms down and interlaced. With elbows pointing out to the sides and legs fully extended, squeeze your butt. Suck in and engage your abs for the duration of the exercise.

Go! Lift your upper body as much as you comfortably can, leading from your armpits. Leave your legs on the ground. Keep your eyes gazing down and don't overextend your neck. This exercise is not only about how long you can make your body but how high you can comfortably lift. Hold for a second, then lower. Repeat thirty times. Next, keep your upper body on the ground as you lift and lower your straight legs thirty times. For the third set, lift both your legs and your upper body thirty times without touching back down (as shown in the picture). Repeat the entire sequence once more. Do the Cat and Cow on page I-30 and then repeat Superman.

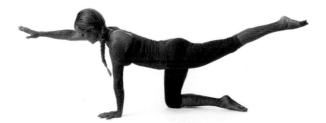

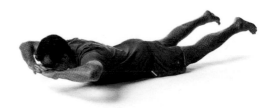

Cat and Cow

STRETCHES AND INCREASES
FLEXIBILITY IN THE SPINE

Get ready: Come onto all fours (knees under hips and hands under shoulders), with the tops of your feet flat on the mat and toes pointed back.

Go! Inhale, then as you exhale, round your back up like a cat, tucking your tailbone, bringing your chin toward your chest, and pulling in your abs. Then, as you inhale again, lift your tailbone and chin, arch your back, and let your belly drop toward the floor. Look straight ahead and bring your shoulders back and together as you inhale. Moving with your breath, go back and forth five times.

Superman Toe

STRENGTHENS LOWER BACK AND BUTT

Get ready: Lie facedown with your head turned to one side and resting on your palm-down hands.

Go! Squeeze your butt and lift your fully extended legs off the ground as high as you can; tap your toes together fifty times, then lower. Next, with your legs raised, lift your upper body; tap your toes for fifty more repetitions. *Make it harder:* Extend your arms out in front and lift both arms and legs, then scissor arms and legs while raised fifty times. Resist arching your neck; keep your gaze downward and focus on keeping your breath steady.

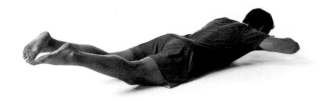

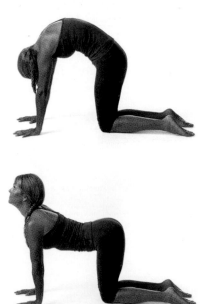

Knee Drop

STRETCHES THE BACK, CHEST, AND SPINE

Get ready: Lie on your back with your hands interlaced behind your head (use them like a pillow), knees bent, feet flat on the mat.

Go! Bring your knees up and gently drop them to the right. Resist lifting your left elbow. Relax into the pose and take five deep breaths. Repeat on the other side. Do a second set. Aim to get both knees resting on the ground on each side. If this is too easy take your upper leg up and over the bottom leg and use your opposite hand to gently pull your knee down toward your mat to where you feel a good stretch.

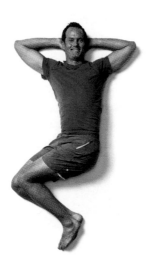

Palms Reach

STRETCHES THE BACK

Get ready: Stand with your feet together. Interlace your fingers and turn your palms away from your body so you're looking at your knuckles.

Go! Extend your arms and reach your palms out in front as far as you can at shoulder height. Simultaneously, hunch your back and curl your tailbone under, looking down at your toes. Take five deep breaths, expanding your rib cage as you do.

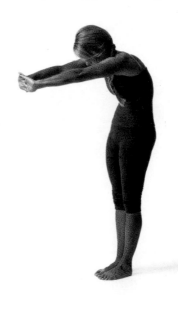

Waiter's Bow

STRENGTHENS LOWER BACK

Get ready: Stand with your feet shoulder width apart, knees slightly bent, on your toes, and hands interlaced behind your head.

Go! Gently lean forward in a straight line from the top of your head to your tailbone. Drop your torso as close to parallel as feels comfortable, pause for two seconds, then return to starting position. Do twenty-five times. *Make it easier:* Do this move with your hands crossed on your chest. Then do Hippie stretch (page I-49), and repeat for a second set.

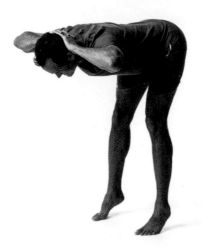

Airplane Press

STRENGTHENS ENTIRE BACK AND
GLUTES, IMPROVES BALANCE

Get ready: Stand with your feet together. Lift your right foot off the ground and bend your elbows, keeping them in at your sides, with your hands in fists in front of your shoulders.

Go! Gently lean forward and extend your right leg back, while pulling your abs in to prevent your back from arching. Go as far as you can, ultimately aiming to get your upper body parallel to the floor, so there is a straight line from your back pointed toe to the top of your head. From here, extend your arms up from your shoulders so they are in line with your torso and over your head, then bring them back. Do twenty-five presses on your left foot, then switch sides and repeat. On the next set, lift your right foot and alternate arms so that as one arm extends, the other comes in. Continue in this manner twenty-five times on each side. Then switch back to your right leg lifted. Extend both arms and pulse your hands one inch up and down, repeating twenty-five times. Switch legs and repeat arm pulses twenty-five times.

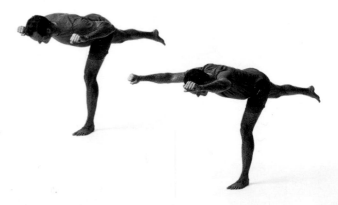

Inverted Balance

IMPROVES BALANCE, STRETCHES
BACK AND HAMSTRINGS

Get ready: Stand with your feet together. Slowly bend your torso forward until you are hanging down toward your toes. Turn your palms up and bring your hands up in line with your elbows so your forearms are parallel to the ground.

Go! While looking back at your legs and with a relaxed neck, slowly lift your heels off the ground. Hold for thirty seconds, balancing on your toes. Resist tightening your neck or lifting your head.

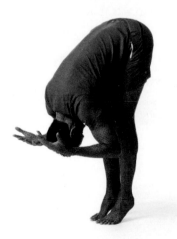

Rickety Table Touches

STRENGTHENS ENTIRE BACK

Get ready: Come onto all fours (hands below shoulders and knees below hips). Spread your fingers apart and point them forward. Keep your back flat and parallel to the floor. Look straight down at the floor.

Go! Reach your right hand forward and your left foot back, stretching them as far away from each other as possible, keeping your right hand higher than your head. The higher your arm goes up, the more work your back has to do and the more effective the exercise. Now bring your right elbow to your left knee. Do twenty-five times. Switch sides and repeat. If you are more advanced, you can move your arm and leg out at a right angle from your body, keeping them in line with your spine. Your stomach should be pulled in the entire time, supporting your lower back. Do two sets.

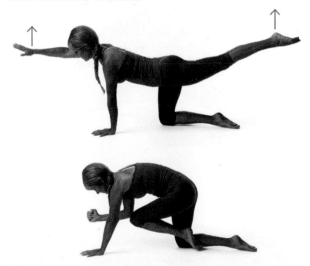

One Arm Half-Butterfly Stretch

STRETCHES BACK AND HAMSTRINGS

Get ready: Sit with straight legs extended out in front of you. Bend your left knee, bringing the sole of your left foot to your upper inner right thigh, in half butterfly.

Go! Place your right hand behind you and press your palm into the mat to propel yourself forward, reaching your left hand toward your pulled-back right toes. If this is easy for you, bring your right hand to the top of your left hand and pull your right toes back with both hands. Drop your head and relax your neck. Focus on gently pressing your lower left back toward your right quad. Hold for five breaths, then repeat on the other side.

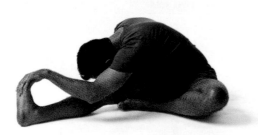

Upside-Down Angels

STRENGTHENS ENTIRE BACK, ARMS, GLUTES, AND HAMSTRINGS

Get ready: Lie facedown and reach your arms out above your head with thumbs touching, like Superman flying. Your head and neck should be lifted slightly. Tighten your abs, pull in your stomach, gaze down, and keep your face and neck relaxed throughout the exercise.

Go! Reach both arms back and touch the outside of your legs as you open your legs as wide as you can. Go back and forth thirty times, or until you have named out loud twenty airlines you could book a flight on today. Do two sets. Lift as high as you can.

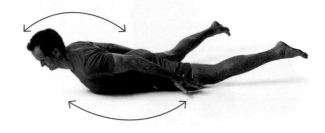

Seated Pretzel Stretch

STRETCHES BACK, ABS, AND HIPS

Get ready: Sit with your legs extended straight out in front of you. Bend your left knee and cross your left leg over the right, placing your left foot down on the outside of your right knee. For back support, put your left hand behind your left butt cheek. Flex your right foot so your toes point straight up.

Go! Reach your left hand up like a stop sign and twist your torso to the right, bringing your left triceps outside of your right thigh. To go deeper, twist more to apply pressure against your right thigh. Act like a string is pulling the top of your head up to elongate the spine. Take five deep breaths, expanding your rib cage on each inhale. *Make it harder:* Sit with your legs crossed in lotus position and reach your hands out and down on the mat in front of you. Switch sides and repeat.

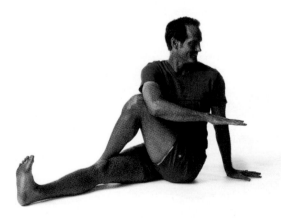

Super Reaches

STRENGTHENS ENTIRE BACK AND GLUTES

Get ready: Lie facedown and reach your hands all the way out in front of you.

Go! Lift your legs and arms off the ground as high as you can. Hold your legs there as you reach your arms back toward your feet, then reverse the move to stretch them out above your head. Do thirty times. Try keeping your arms close to your sides, bending your elbows to first bring your hands by your shoulders, then curl your fingers down and bring your hands and arms down by your sides so your arms are stretched straight down by your thighs, then reverse the move.

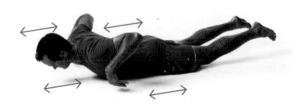

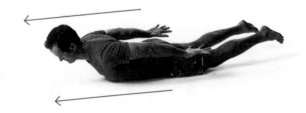

Upper Push-Up Reaches

STRENGTHENS ENTIRE BACK

Get ready: Come into an up push-up position with hands under your shoulders and feet a little wider than shoulder width.

Go! Lift your right hand off the ground and stretch it out to the right at shoulder height, then bring it back under your chest and tap the inside of your left arm. Do twenty-five times, then repeat with your left hand. *Make it harder:* Do the entire set with the opposite leg lifted. Your leg should be raised up straight and in line with your hips. Do two sets.

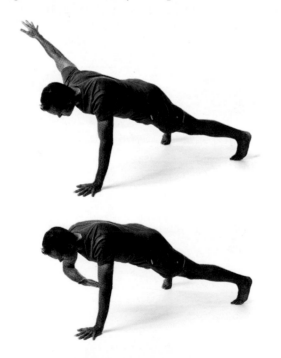

Repeat Knee Drop (page I-31).

Butt Lift

WARMS AND TONES HAMSTRINGS AND GLUTES

Get ready: Lie on your back with your knees bent and feet flat on the ground one foot apart. Cross your hands on your chest and lift your tailbone off the mat as high as you can, then lower it one inch—this is your highest point.

Go! Lower your butt and tap it on the mat, then bring it back up for one repetition. Each time make sure to really squeeze your butt and curl your tailbone up. Do twenty-five times. Then come back to the up position and hold, squeeze, and pulse twenty-five times. Then, staying in the up position, alternate squeezing your left butt-cheek, then your right, for thirty seconds. Finally, hold in the center up position and squeeze your butt as hard as you can for thirty seconds.

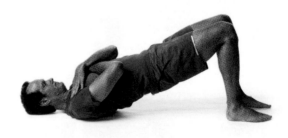

Kiss the Knee Stretch

STRETCHES GLUTES AND HAMSTRINGS

Get ready: Lie flat on your back.

Go! Using your hands, pull your right knee toward your right shoulder and lace your fingers around your right shin. Your left leg should be fully extended. Press your tailbone and lower back toward the ground. Hold for fifteen seconds, then switch sides.

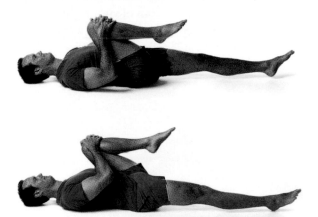

Leg Straighteners

STRENGTHENS THE GLUTES

Get ready: Lie on your back with knees bent and feet together flat on the ground. Cross your hands on your chest and lift your tailbone off the mat as high as you can, then lower one inch—this is your highest point.

Go! Press into the mat and extend your right leg out straight, keeping your knees together. From here, bend your right knee to tap your foot on the ground twenty-five times, keeping your butt lifted and your knees together the entire time. Switch sides. Do two sets.

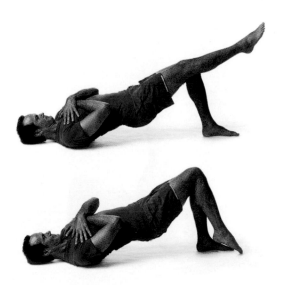

Ceiling Taps

STRENGTHENS THE BUNS

Get ready: Begin in the same position as the previous move, but this time lift your right leg so your toe points straight up toward the ceiling.

Go! Keeping your leg straight up, lift and lower your tailbone by one inch, repeating twenty-five times. Switch sides and repeat. Do each side twice. Then, with your right leg fully extended toward the ceiling and your butt lifted, lower your right leg, drawing an imaginary line from the ceiling down to where your knees are in line, then lift back up. Repeat twenty-five times, keeping your tailbone lifted throughout. Switch sides and repeat. Do two sets on each side.

Calf Reach

STRETCHES GLUTES AND HAMSTRINGS

Get ready: Lie on your back with your knees above your hips and extend your right leg straight up. Keeping your back flat and your neck relaxed on the ground, reach your hands up to hold your calf (if you can't reach this far, it's okay to hold lower on the hamstring).

Go! Gently pull your right leg back without lifting your tailbone. Flex your right foot toward your right shin, making sure the bottom of your right foot is flat. Hold for five deep breaths, then repeat on the other side. Do each side twice.

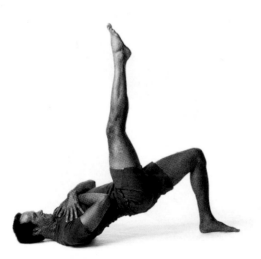

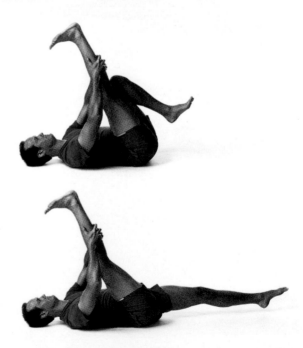

Horizontal Line

STRENGTHENS GLUTES AND OUTER THIGHS

Get ready: Lie on your back with knees bent and together, feet flat on the mat. Lift your butt and extend your left leg straight out, keeping your knees together.

Go! Use your left toe to draw an imaginary line out to the left side as far as you can go while opening your right knee to the side to maintain balance. Move your knees apart and together twenty-five times. Keep your butt lifted the entire time. Repeat on the other side. Do two sets on each side.

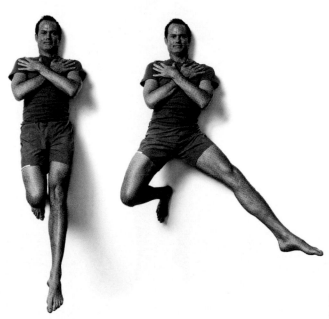

Repeat Calf Reach (page I-38), this time with the opposite foot on the ground during the stretch.

Leg Circles

TONES GLUTES

Get ready: Lie on your back with knees bent and together. Lift your butt up and extend your right leg straight up toward the ceiling.

Go! Circle your lifted leg clockwise in basketball-size circles twenty-five times, then repeat in the opposite direction. Switch sides and repeat with the right leg. Do two sets on each side.

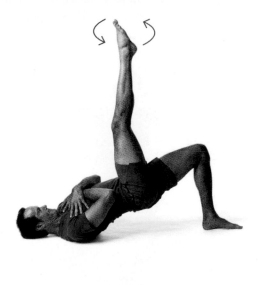

Repeat Calf Reach (page I-38), this time with the opposite leg straight out on the ground.

Knee Drops

STRETCHES HIPS, BACK, AND CHEST

Get ready: Lie on your back with knees bent and feet flat on the ground. Bring your hands behind your head and use them as a pillow.

Go! Drop your knees down to your right side. If this is easy, lift your left leg up and over your right leg. Still too easy? Use your right hand to gently pull your left knee down toward the mat. Pull your left elbow as far as you can away from your left knee. Take five deep breaths into the tightest area. Then repeat on the other side.

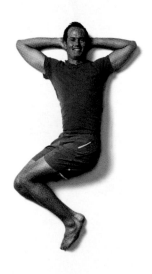

The Ballerina

STRENGTHENS GLUTES AND CALVES

Get ready: Stand with your legs and heels together, toes angled out diagonally (like first position in ballet) and hands on your waist.

Go! Lift your heels as high as you can. Squeeze your buns and calves as tight as you can and tap your heels back on the floor. Do forty repetitions.

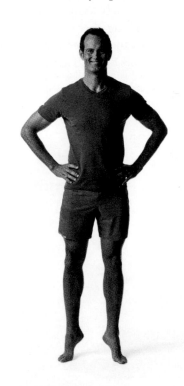

Knee Swivels

TONES BUTT, HIPS, AND CORE

Get ready: Stand with your feet together and your hands in prayer position in front of your chest. Bend your right knee and place the sole of your right foot on your left calf, right toes pointing toward your ankle and right knee pointing to the right.

Go! Swivel your right knee to the left while your torso and arms twist as one unit to the right. Keep your hands in prayer position. Go back and forth as far as you can in each direction twenty-five times, then switch feet and repeat. Do two times.

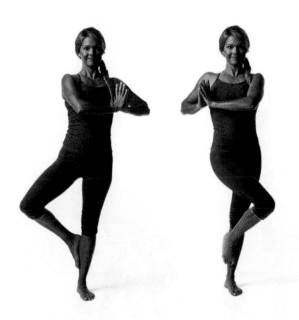

Hanging Blasters

STRENGTHENS HAMSTRINGS AND GLUTES

Get ready: Stand with your feet together, knees slightly bent. Walk your hands down your left leg, stopping wherever it feels most comfortable (either above or below your knee), ultimately working toward getting your fingertips on the floor on either side of your left foot, as in the picture below.

Go! Lift your right leg back, and kick your right foot behind you as high as you comfortably can. At the highest point, straighten your leg, squeeze your butt, then bend your right knee, bringing it down to the side of your left knee. Do twenty-five times. On the last repetition, hold your leg up, and do twenty-five one-inch pulses up and down. For more advanced exercisers, follow the pulses with some extra balance work by holding your left ankle and straightening your right leg as high up as you can, ultimately doing standing splits. Hold and balance on your left foot for thirty seconds. Then lower your leg, switch sides, and repeat the routine standing on your right leg. Keep your head down and your neck relaxed the entire time.

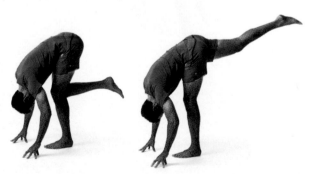

Crisscross Drop

STRETCHES HAMSTRINGS AND GLUTES

Get ready: Stand with your arms at your sides. Cross your right leg in front of the left, placing your right foot outside your left foot. Ideally, you want your feet and toes in line.

Go! Slowly walk your hands down your legs until you feel a stretch in your legs. If you can, walk your hands all the way down until they touch the mat. Completely relax your head and neck. Hold for fifteen seconds, then switch sides and repeat.

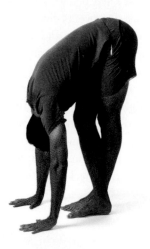

One-Legged Wood Chop

STRENGTHENS ENTIRE LEG WITH EMPHASIS ON GLUTES

Get ready: Stand on your right leg with arms lifted overhead, hands together in prayer position. Bend your left leg back in a right angle.

Go! Bend forward, driving your hips backward and your left leg up, and bringing your torso down with a straight back. Touch your hands to the ground in front of your right foot, then come back up. Do twenty-five repetitions, then switch sides and repeat. Keep your leg airborne the entire time. If this is too hard, only come halfway down.

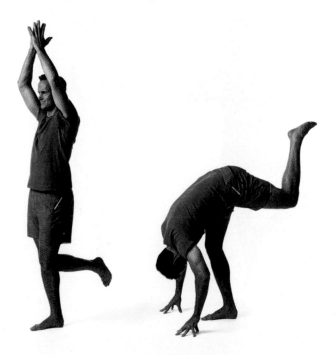

Bridge March

TONES GLUTES AND HAMSTRINGS

Get ready: Lie on your back with knees bent and feet flat on the mat.

Go! Push down through your heels, and squeeze and lift your buns so there is a straight line from your shoulders to your knees. Lift your left knee toward your chest, elevating your right heel, then set your left toes back down. Switch legs. Continue in a fluid motion, going back and forth for one minute.

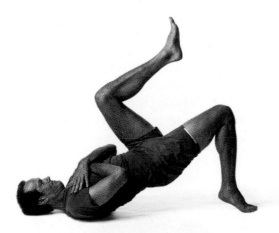

Lateral Leg Extension

STRENGTHENS OUTER LEG AND BUNS

Get ready: Lie on your right side with your knees in line with your spine and your right leg bent back at a right angle. Lean your upper body forward and prop yourself up on your right forearm.

Go! Squeeze your butt and lift your left leg, then kick your left leg straight out in front of you. Ultimately, you are aiming to kick in line with the top of your head. Return to the starting position. Do twenty-five repetitions, then hold your left leg up in front of you and do twenty-five one-inch pulses up and down. *Make it harder:* Lift your hip and balance on your right forearm and right knee. Do two sets on each side.

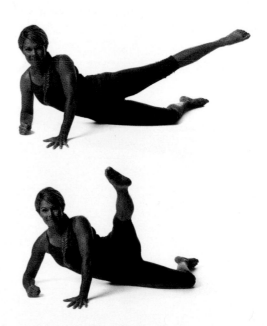

Kicking and Screaming

MAKES YOUR BUNS YELP FOR HELP

Get ready: Lie facedown on your mat with your head turned to the side and resting on your crossed arms. Extend your legs two feet apart. Keep your stomach pulled in and away from the mat for the duration of the exercise.

Go! Lift your legs as high as you can and flutter-kick them as if you were swimming for thirty seconds. Keep your legs perfectly straight throughout. Then hold your legs in the lifted position, turning your toes slightly toward each other. Tap your toes together, then two feet apart (moving horizontally) for thirty seconds. For a more advanced move, increase the duration of each phase of the exercise to one minute and/or lift and hold your upper body up one inch off the ground.

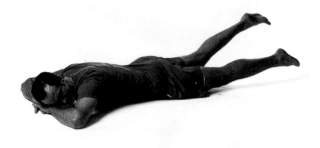

One Arm Half- and Full-Butterfly Stretch

OPENS HAMSTRINGS, CALVES, AND LOWER BACK

Get ready: Sit with your legs straight out in front of you. Fold your left leg into half butterfly (with the sole of your left foot against the inside of your right thigh).

Go! Reach your left hand forward over your extended right leg and pull your right foot back, keeping your foot perfectly flat. If you can't reach your foot, stretch as far as you can while flexing your right foot back. Relax, reaching only as far as it feels good. Remember, stretching is like massaging your body from the inside out. It should always feel good. Hold for five deep breaths, then switch sides. Then do full butterfly by bringing the soles of your feet together, holding for five deep breaths and gently using your arms to press your knees down toward your mat.

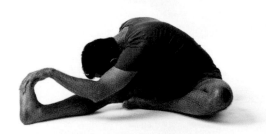

Butt Burner

STRENGTHENS GLUTES, HIPS, AND CORE

Get ready: Come onto all fours, with hands under shoulders and knees under hips.

Go! Extend your left leg straight out behind you. Open your hip to bring your left butt cheek above your right, keeping your left leg straight. Bend your left knee and bring it to your side in line with your right hip, then bring it back down in line with your right knee, in starting position. Continue in a fluid motion for twenty-five repetitions. Keep your upper body steady and your elbows soft for the duration of the exercise to work your core. Then repeat on your right leg. For a more advanced move, do a second set at double time.

Rock a Leg

STRETCHES GLUTES AND HIPS

Get ready: Sit upright with your legs extended straight out in front.

Go! Gently lean forward and bend your right leg up toward you. Grasp your right foot with your right hand and place it inside your left elbow. Wrap your right hand around your knee and clasp your hands. Rock your leg slowly from side to side eight times, then switch sides. Try to sit upright the entire time. If this is too hard for you, do Thread the Needle (page I-16).

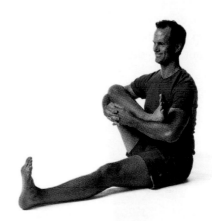

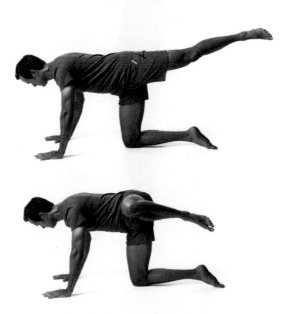

On cardio days, we will get your heart pumping and your blood circulating. I want you to think of your mat as a sheet of glass. You don't want to break it. Float, don't pound, and focus on using your knees and ankles as springs. Shoes are optional. Have a wide towel and two shoelace-length strings handy.

Frankensteins

Get ready: Reach your arms out straight in front of you like . . . yes, Frankenstein.

Go! Stand with straight legs. Lift your right knee up toward your right hand and bring it back down. Switch sides. Lift as high as you comfortably can without moving your hands. Resist leaning forward. Go side to side doing one hundred on each leg. To pump it up, get airborne with a bounce on the supporting foot, or do the move with straight legs.

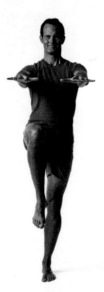

Leaning Tower

STRETCHES BACK AND OBLIQUES

Get ready: Stand with your feet together and reach your arms up above your head.

Go! Hold your left wrist with your right hand, pulling your wrist as you lean to the right. Elongate to achieve the greatest possible distance between your left pinky and your left heel. Hold for fifteen seconds, then switch sides. Do both sides twice.

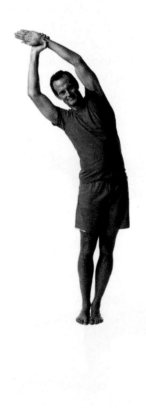

Knee Repeaters

Get ready: Make fists and raise your forearms to form a number 11, with fists a little higher than chin height.

Go! Lift your right knee while bringing your arms down until your knee is between your elbows, then raise your arms again and tap your foot down. Do two sets of twenty-five on each side, then one set of fifty on each side.

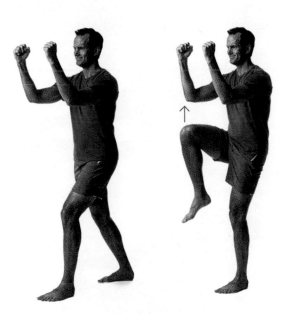

Quad Pull

STRETCHES THIGHS AND IMPROVES FLEXIBILITY

Get ready: Stand with your feet together and arms at your sides.

Go! Balance on your right leg and bend your left knee back, bringing up your left foot until you can grab the ankle with your left hand. Then bring your right hand back and interlace your fingers around your ankle. (If this is too difficult, do the move with just your left hand, and place your right hand on a chair or wall for balance.) Maintain a straight line from the top of your head to your tailbone. Keep your chest lifted and take five deep breaths, then switch sides. To mix it up slightly, soften your standing leg and move your left heel and interlaced fingers as far as you can away from your tailbone as you arch your back and pull in your stomach. Hold for five deep breaths. Then switch sides.

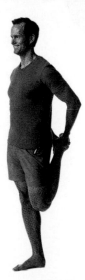

X-Rock

Get ready: Stand with your feet shoulder width apart and your knees barely bent. Cross your arms at the wrists in an X in front of you, like a shield, with palms facing you.

Go! Lift and lower your arms from side to side, so you are making a U movement with your elbows. As your arms go up to the left, kick your right heel toward your butt; as arms go right, kick left leg toward butt. Do fifty times. Then switch the front arm to the back and repeat with fifty more. *Make it harder:* Do the move on your toes. Do Quad Pull (page I-47) again, then repeat X-Rock two more times.

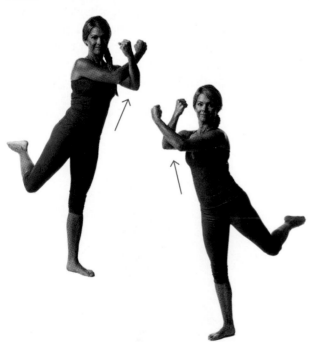

Towel Runs

Get ready: Grab a big towel and come into upper push-up position, with hands under shoulders and elbows slightly bent. Position your feet wide on either side of the towel, then bring your feet together, scrunching the towel between your feet.

Go! Slide your right foot up (on the towel) as you bend your right knee up toward your chest, then slide it back. Switch sides. Continue alternating legs for fifty repetitions. Keep your abs active and resist allowing your back to arch. Do four sets.

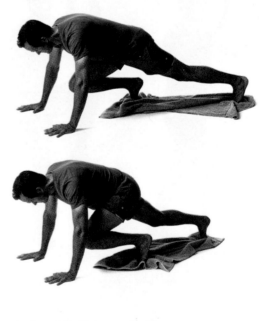

Repeat Quad Pull (page I-47).

Hippie

OPENS UP YOUR HIPS, BACK, AND HAMSTRINGS

Get ready: Stand with your feet together and cross your arms loosely with hands on biceps.

Go! Bend forward slowly at the waist and let your body melt down, releasing all tension. If this is too difficult, leave your arms on your legs for support (like brackets) and go to where you feel a comfortable stretch. Hold for ten seconds. Release your arms and let your head and arms relax down (okay to rest hands on floor if they can relax there) at an angle, while alternately bending one knee. (Keep your feet flat on the mat throughout.) Continue until you feel all tension release, about thirty seconds. You can also bend one knee and hold for five deep inhales. Then switch sides. If one side is tighter, hold for a few deep inhales longer.

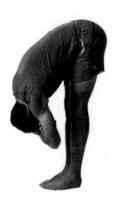 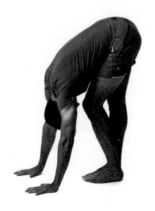

Ankle Circles

WARMS UP ANKLES AND OPENS SHOULDER BLADES

Get ready: Stand with your feet together. Lift your right knee waist high and, with straight arms, reach around and interlace your hands to hold just below the right knee.

Go! With your stomach pulled in and a long spine, gently lean back, opening your shoulder blades. Stay there and circle your foot five times in each direction. Switch sides and repeat.

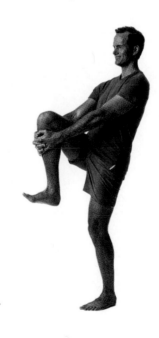

Marionette

Get ready: Stand with your legs and heels together, toes angled out diagonally (first position in ballet), then bring your hands above your head with palms facing each other.

Go! Bend your elbow and lower your right arm while bringing your right knee up to touch your elbow. Return to start. Do twenty-five times. Switch sides and repeat. Do two sets without stopping.

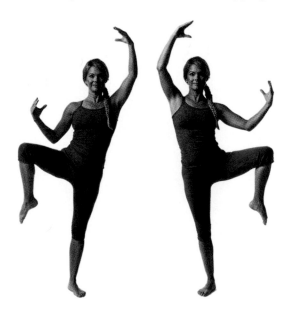

Towel Circles

Get ready: Grab a big towel and come into upper push-up position, hands under shoulders, elbows slightly bent. Position your feet wide on either side of the towel, then bring your feet together, scrunching the towel between your feet.

Go! Make as wide a circle as you can with your feet, starting with your feet in and together, then moving them up and apart. Do twenty-five circles, then switch directions and repeat. Do two sets.

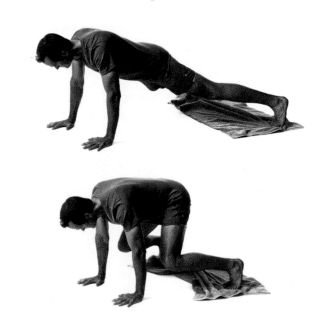

Down Dog

OPENS AND STRENGTHENS SHOULDERS AND UPPER
BODY, STRETCHES HAMSTRINGS AND CALVES

Get ready: Begin on hands and knees. Press into
your palms, lifting your knees and pressing your
thighs back until your body forms an inverted V.

Go! Look toward your waist. Lift your sitting bones
while you align your ears with your upper arms,
press your quadriceps toward your hamstrings, and
drive your heels down toward the mat. Hold for five
breaths, then first bend your left knee and then your
right knee. Go back and forth five times.

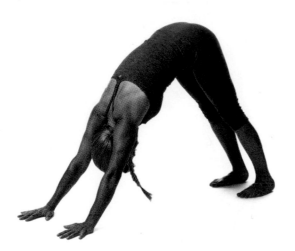

Squat Thrusts

Get ready: Stand with your feet together. Bend
at your knees and lower into a squat, placing your
palms outside your feet.

Go! Float one foot back and then the other until you
are in upper push-up position. (If this is easy for you,
do both feet simultaneously.) Then reverse the move
and come back to standing. Do fifty in a row. *Make it
harder:* You can do a Burpee by doing a push-up on
each jump back.

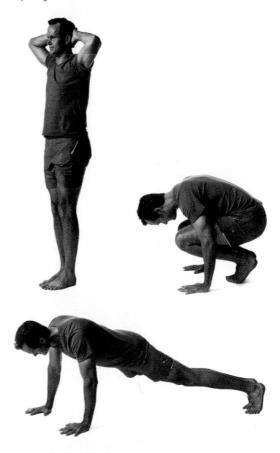

Sun in Your Eyes

STRETCHES ENTIRE SIDE FROM ANKLE TO ELBOW

Get ready: Stand with your left foot on the far side of the right, ideally with toes lined up. Take your interlaced hands and place them with knuckles to your forehead. Make sure your hips are lined up straight.

Go! Lift your left elbow toward the ceiling, stretching as far as possible from your left knee and pressing your right hip slightly forward. Hold for ten seconds, taking in deep breaths to release any tight muscles. Switch legs and repeat. Advanced variation: Try to look up toward the ceiling while in position.

Knee Slides

Get ready: Grab a big towel and come into upper push-up position, hands under shoulders, elbows slightly bent. Position your feet wide on either side of the towel, then bring your feet together, scrunching the towel between your feet. Keep your legs glued together.

Go! Bend both knees and move your legs forward and back fifty times, keeping your tailbone in line with your chin. Do fifty more repetitions keeping your legs straight and lifting your tailbone so you come into Down Dog (page I-51) each time.

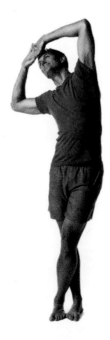

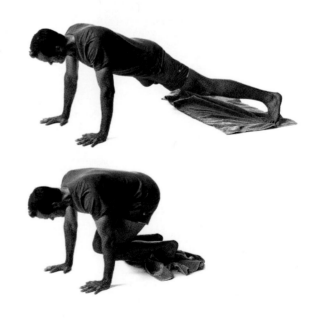

High Stepper

Get ready: Stand with feet comfortably apart and arms at your sides.

Go! Lift your right knee up in line with your hips (if you can) while lifting your left arm as high as you can, then switch sides. Continue alternating sides for one minute. To pump it up, get airborne with your feet, hopping side to side.

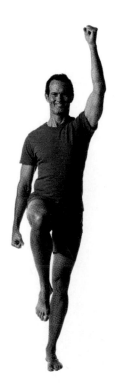

Hopscotch

Get ready: Place a shoelace or string in a straight line on the floor and stand straddling it.

Go! With soft knees, gently hop over and back twenty-five times. If this is too difficult, step over and back with one foot at a time. To pump it up, make a cross with a second string and gently hop for two minutes from one quadrant to another, making a square.

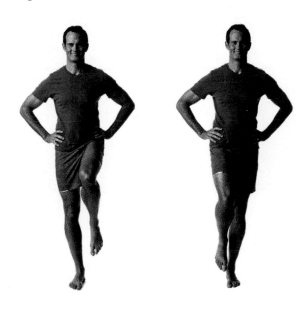

Repeat Quad Pull (page I-47).

Small Arm Rolls

WARMS UP SHOULDERS AND ARMS

Get ready: Stand with your feet comfortably apart and arms by your sides.

Go! Roll just your shoulders forward five times. Repeat in the opposite direction. Try to make as big a circle as possible while leaving your arms relaxed. Stand up straight the entire time.

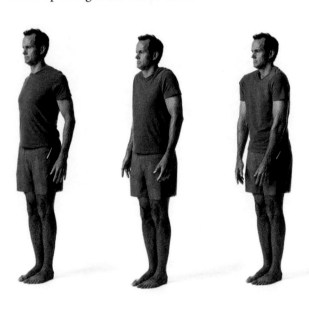

Every Others

WARMS UP CHEST AND ARMS

Get ready: Stand on your toes with feet together. Raise your arms in front to shoulder height, holding them a foot apart with palms up.

Go! Cross your right arm over the left, then your left over your right. Each time your arms cross, make fists; each time your arms come apart, open your palms. Continue going back and forth and do thirty seconds each of the following: palms up, palms facing, palms down, and palms out with thumbs down. Do four sets without stopping.

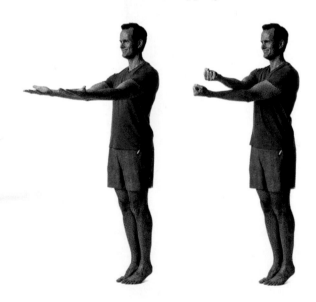

One-Legged Push-Ups

STRENGTHENS CHEST AND ARMS

Get ready: Come onto all fours with hands under shoulders and knees under hips. Lift your left leg straight back behind you in a modified one-knee push-up position. Keep your abs taut and sucked in for the duration of the exercise.

Go! Bend your elbows and lower your nose to the mat, bringing it to the far side of an imaginary line going between your middle fingers. Press back up, keeping your elbows slightly soft. Do twenty-five times. On the last push-up, pause one inch off the ground and pulse one inch up and down, repeating twenty-five times. Then pause and do a set of Small Arm Rolls (page I-54). Switch legs and repeat twenty-five push-ups, this time with your hands an inch wider than they were before. Then pause one inch off the ground and sway two inches side to side. Do twenty-five times. Do Pecs Flex (see right), then repeat the entire sequence for a second set. *Make it harder:* Do the move with knees off the mat so you are in a straight diagonal line from your head to your knees.

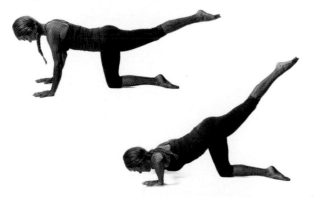

Pecs Flex

STRETCHES CHEST AND ARMS

Get ready: Kneel upright. Interlace your hands behind your head with elbows out to the sides.

Go! While looking straight forward, gently lift your chest and, without touching your head, drive your hands and elbows backward, feeling a good stretch across your chest. Take five deep breaths into your chest.

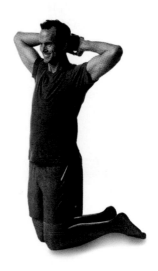

Snail Push-Ups

STRENGTHENS CHEST

Get ready: Come onto all fours with hands under shoulders and knees under hips. Lift your left leg straight back behind you. Make sure your nose is on the up side of your middle finger throughout the movement.

Go! Bend your elbows down slowly on a count of ten. Stop one inch from the mat, pause, then slowly press back up on a count of ten. Count out loud to normalize breathing. Do twenty-five times. Switch legs and repeat. Do Knuckle Lift (see right), then repeat on each side. *Make it harder:* Move your knees back to make a straight diagonal line from your knees to your shoulders, or lift your knees to make a straight line from your toes to your shoulders.

Knuckle Lift

STRETCHES ABS AND SHOULDERS

Get ready: You can do this stretch standing or sitting on your heels if it is comfortable for your knees. Interlace your hands behind your tailbone with knuckles down.

Go! With chest lifted and elbows soft, raise your hands back and up, away from the tailbone and as high as you can comfortably go. Hold the stretch for five deep breaths.

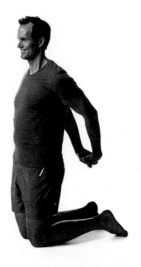

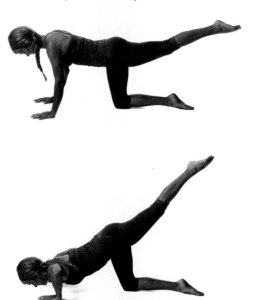

Wide Every Others

WARMS UP CHEST AND ARMS

Get ready: Stand on your toes with feet together and arms raised straight out to the sides, palms up.

Go! Cross your hands in front of your chest, putting a different arm on top each time, making fists when you cross and opening your hands when they are out to the side. Continue going back and forth, and do thirty seconds of each of the following: palms up, palms facing, palms down, and palms out with thumbs down. Do four sets. Pick up the pace on each set after the first one. At the end you will be sprinting with your arms.

Tilters

TONES ARMS AND CHEST

Get ready: Come onto all fours and lift your left leg behind you.

Go! Bend your right elbow. As you do, drop and turn your head to look to the left and lift and drive your left straight leg two feet up and to the right. Your left elbow will bend just a couple of inches. Do twenty-five repetitions, then switch sides and repeat. When you lower your head, make sure your chin is in line with your fingertips. Do two sets, pausing to do Pecs Flex (page I-55) in between.

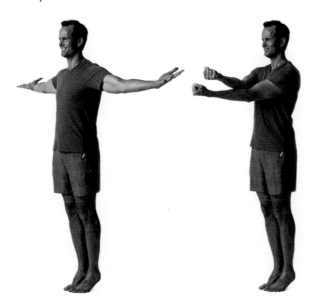

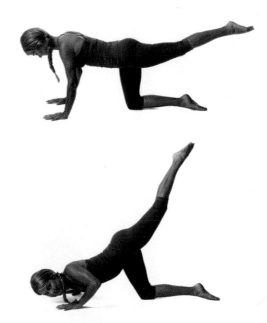

Repeat Hippie (page I-49).

Arm Swivels

STRETCHES CHEST, SHOULDERS, BACK, AND HIPS

Get ready: Lie on your right side with your knees bent in a right angle. Extend your arms out in front with palms together, so the side of your right arm is on the ground and your left arm is stacked on top.

Go! Keep your lower body still as you lift your left arm all the way up and over as far as you can, letting your chest open and turn. Try to touch your left forearm on the ground. Hold for three deep breaths. Do four more times, then switch sides and repeat.

Pyramid Push-Ups

TONES CHEST AND TRICEPS

Get ready: Choose full push-up position (your body in a straight line from head to toes, hands under shoulders) or modified push-up position (with knees down).

Go! Do ten push-ups, then hold in the up position with soft elbows for ten seconds. Then do nine push-ups and hold for nine seconds in the up position. Continue until you get to one. Keep your nose slightly up a few inches, hovering just in front of your fingertips. This forces you to use your chest and not overextend your neck.

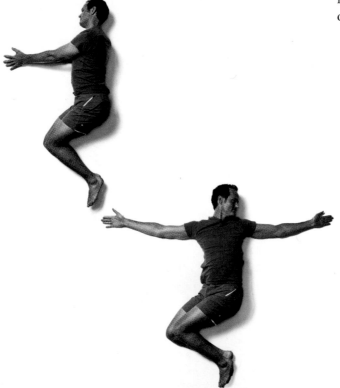

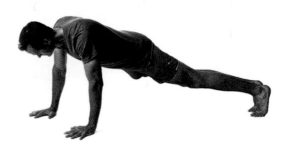

Shoulder Sways

STRETCHES SHOULDERS AND FOREARMS

Get ready: Sit on the floor with legs relaxed and extended straight out in front. Place your palms about two feet behind your hips with fingers pointing away from you. Bend your elbows and gently lean back as far as feels comfortable.

Go! Drop your chin toward your chest and let your back and chest naturally drop. Gently rock side to side five times. For a deeper stretch, lift your butt and slide it an inch farther from your hands. Pause on each side for two deep breaths, keeping both elbows bent.

Elbows Wide

STRENGTHENS CHEST

Get ready: Lie facedown with your forehead resting on the mat. Place your arms shoulder height on either side, with elbows bent and forearms out to the side up by your head, palms flat down.

Go! Press your arms into the mat and lift your chest up. Hold for thirty seconds. Do three sets of thirty seconds each, adding a set of Arm Rolls (page I-17) in between. *Make it harder:* Do the move with your hips, or hips and knees, lifted, so you are on your forearms and knees or forearms and toes.

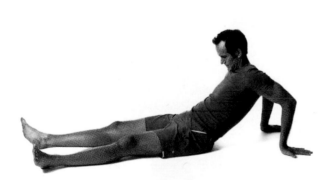

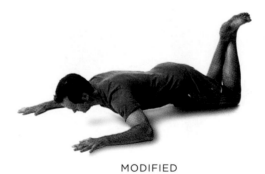

MODIFIED

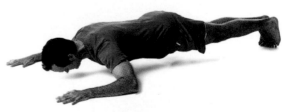

CHALLENGING

Hippie Twist

STRETCHES CHEST, ARMS, BACK, AND LEGS

Get ready: Stand with feet together and hands interlaced behind your tailbone with knuckles down.

Go! Gently drive your arms away from your tailbone and bend forward, driving your knuckles up and over as you drop down. Hold for three breaths. Then bend your left knee and drive your left shoulder toward your left knee as you look to the right, lifting your right butt cheek slightly. Take three deep breaths, then switch sides and repeat.

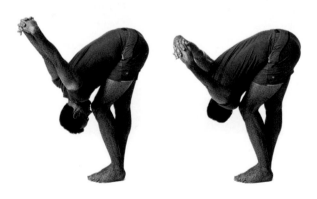

Ankle Sways

STRENGTHENS AND TONES FRONT OF THIGHS AND LOWER ABS

Get ready: Stand with your feet together. Place your left hand on your stomach and your right hand on your lower back. Balancing on your left leg, lift your right knee up as high as you can, aiming to ultimately get your right knee in line with your hips.

Go! While balancing and keeping your right knee stationary, sway your right ankle from left to right as far as you can twenty-five times. Repeat on the opposite side. Do two sets. To pump it up, on the second set do fifty repetitions on each side.

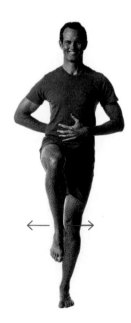

Repeat Quad Pull (page I-47).

Leg Pendulum

TONES ENTIRE LEG

Get ready: Standing with feet and knees together, stretch your arms out to the sides at shoulder height, palms up.

Go! Lift your right leg as far as you can out to the right (aim for two o'clock), and point your toe, then flex your foot and swoosh your right leg back down, swinging it as far as you can across in front of your left leg, pointing your toes again at the top (try to get to ten o'clock). Continue back and forth in a fluid swinging motion twenty-five times. Then switch sides. Do two sets on each side. To make it more advanced on the up movement, pause, flex, then point your foot before continuing.

Dog Lifts

STRENGTHENS BUTT AND OBLIQUES

Get ready: Come onto all fours, with a flat back, hands below your shoulders, and knees below your hips. If it feels more comfortable, you can do the move with your forearms on the ground and palms in prayer position.

Go! Lift your left leg to the side at hip height, maintaining a bent-knee position, then lower it back down. Continue lifting and lowering, leading with your knee rather than your ankle. Do twenty-five lifts, then repeat on the other side. Do a total of two sets on each side. *Make it harder:* Hold the lift at the top and stretch your leg straight out to the side at hip height, then bend and lower for two sets of twenty-five.

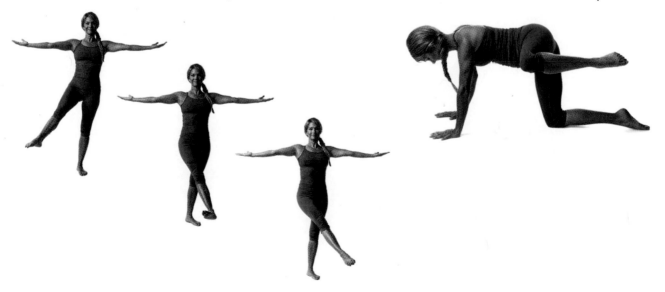

Repeat Quad Pull (page I-47) if you are feeling tight.

Butt Blaster

STRENGTHENS MUSCLES IN THE
BUTT AND BACK OF THIGHS

Get ready: Come onto your knees and forearms (elbows under shoulders and knees under hips). Lift your right leg up behind you, keeping the knee bent and the leg at a right angle.

Go! With your stomach muscles sucked in and contracted and your back flat, lower your leg back down until the right knee is in line with the left, but don't rest it on the ground. Repeat for twenty-five lifts, then hold your leg in the up position and pulse one inch up and down, twenty-five times. Then switch sides and repeat on the left. Do two sets on each side.

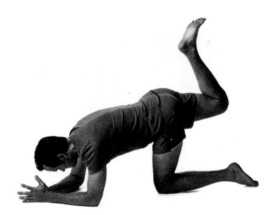

Hammock

STRETCHES HIPS

Get ready: Sit on the floor with knees bent and feet flat on the mat two feet from your tailbone. Rest your hands behind you with palms down, fingertips pointing away from you, and the heels of your hands about a foot from your butt.

Go! Keeping the soles of your feet flat on the mat, cross your left leg over the right, resting your left ankle just above your right knee. Sit up straight and focus on pressing your lower back toward your left calf. If you want to go deeper, press your left knee away from you. Hold for fifteen seconds, then switch sides. Do two times on each side. Keep your arms slightly bent throughout the stretch, so you work your muscles, not your joints.

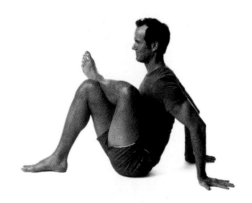

Knee Bounces

STRENGTHENS ENTIRE BODY, WITH
EMPHASIS ON QUADS

Get ready: Come onto all fours with hands under shoulders and knees under hips. Keep your elbows slightly bent and your back in a straight line from the top of your head to your tailbone the entire time; raise your knees one inch off the ground.

Go! Bounce your knees one inch up and down for two minutes. The effort should come from your quadriceps (the front of your thighs). Try to get 120 bounces in two minutes. *Make it harder:* Each time your knees come up, hop your toes one inch off the mat. Think floating, not pounding here. Imagine you are on a sheet of glass and you don't want to break it.

Side Circles

STRENGTHENS LEG AND BUTT MUSCLES

Get ready: While on all fours, lift your left leg out to the side (ideally at hip height), keeping the knee bent at a right angle, and hold it there.

Go! Turn your left ankle in a circle twenty-five times clockwise, then twenty-five times counterclockwise. Switch sides and repeat. Always keep your knee higher than your ankle. *Make it harder:* Reach your opposite arm straight out horizontally above your head and hold it there the entire time.

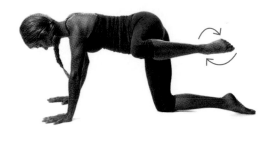

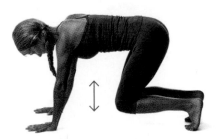

Crisscross Reach

STRETCHES HAMSTRINGS, CALVES, AND BACK

Get ready: While sitting on the ground, stretch your legs straight out in front of you. Place your left leg on top of your right and completely relax it there.

Go! Gently reach your right hand toward your right flexed foot. Use your left hand to propel yourself forward. Take notice of your flexed right foot. Pretend the sole of your right foot is flush against a board so you aren't favoring one side over the other. This is better for your knees, Achilles tendon, and calf. Pull your bottom foot straight back toward your knee. If this is easy, place your left hand on top of your right (as pictured). Focus on pressing your lower back toward your knees instead of seeing how far you can reach. Make sure you are flexing your foot back flat. Hold for five deep breaths and then switch to the right leg on top.

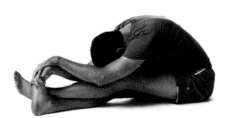

Squatting Lifts

STRENGTHENS ENTIRE LEG

Get ready: Stand with your feet a little more than shoulder width apart, toes slightly angled out. Lift your arms to the sides at shoulder height, palms up. Bend your knees and sit back as if you were lowering into a chair. Go as far as feels comfortable but no lower than quads parallel to the floor. Maintain this squatted position throughout the exercise.

Go! Lift your right heel, pause, then lower. Repeat with your left heel. Go back and forth, lifting each heel twenty-five times. *Make it harder:* Do the first set as directed, then lift both heels and balance on your toes for sixty seconds as you lift and lower your tailbone one inch up and down.

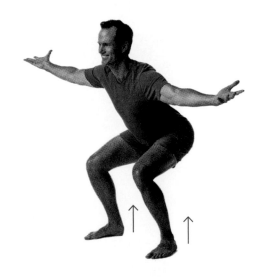

Repeat Hammock (page I-62) or Quad Pull (page I-47).

Knees Together Bounce

WARMS UP YOUR LEGS

Get ready: Stand with legs and feet flush, palms together in prayer position with your thumbs against your chest. Gently bend your knees and, while keeping your feet flat, drop down about one foot while continuing to look forward.

Go! Bounce sixty times, one inch up and down. Then, while holding in the lowest position, lift and lower your heels sixty times. Keep your chest lifted and shoulders relaxed, and look straight ahead the entire time.

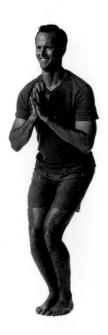

Repeat Hippie (page I-49).

Knee-Ups

TONES ENTIRE LEG AND IMPROVES BALANCE

Get ready: Stand with legs together and arms stretched out in front at chest level, palms together. Look straight ahead at eye level for the duration of the exercise.

Go! Kick your right heel up behind you at a right angle, then swing your leg up in front, maintaining that right angle, ideally until your knee is in line with your hip. Go back and forth twenty-five times without touching the ground, then switch sides. Do both sides twice. To make this move more advanced, on the second set, each time you lift your leg behind you, lean forward as far as you can, keeping your back knee in line with your nose. Ideally, lean forward until you are parallel to the ground, spreading your arms to the sides like a jet airplane.

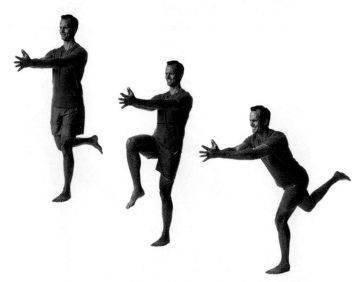

Standing Side Kick

TONES HIPS AND OBLIQUES, IMPROVES BALANCE

Get ready: Stand with feet together and hands in prayer position. Bend your right leg back at a right angle. Pull in your stomach and tighten your abs.

Go! In a fluid motion, lift your bent right leg to the side and simultaneously lean your torso slightly to the left. Using your obliques, straighten your leg to kick out, leading with your pointed toe. Then reverse the move to bring your right leg back to your side with bent knee. Hands remain in prayer position for the duration of the exercise. Do twenty-five repetitions, keeping your stomach tight and kicking as high as you can. Then switch to the left leg and repeat. To pump it up, do a second set of twenty-five, then hold your leg out in the straight kick position and, using your obliques, lean your torso to the side away from your lifted leg and hold it there. Pulse your foot one inch up and down twenty-five times or point and flex your foot twenty-five times.

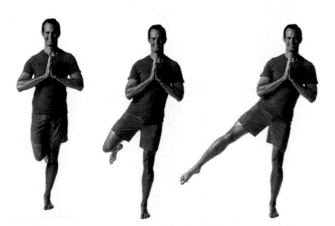

Airplane Stretch

STRETCHES HIPS

Get ready: Sit on the edge of a sturdy chair and cross your right leg on top of your left knee. Lean your right elbow on your right knee, while holding your right ankle.

Go! Lean forward and press your lower back toward your right calf while keeping your back straight. Gently drive your tailbone backward the entire time. Look straight ahead. To increase the stretch, use your left hand to gently twist your right foot so that you can see the sole of your foot. Hold for five deep breaths.

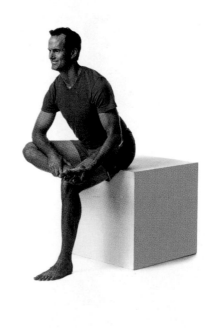

Ballet Squats

STRENGTHENS ENTIRE LEG AND GLUTES

Get ready: Assume an extreme version of second position in ballet—feet more than shoulder width apart, toes pointed to the sides. Keeping your arms straight, bring them out to the sides at shoulder height, palms up.

Go! Bend your knees and, keeping your chest lifted, lower down as far as you comfortably can, being sure to keep your knees over your ankles, not your toes. Stop when your thighs are parallel to the floor, gently pull your knees back, and squeeze your butt. Then press into your feet and use your thighs and butt to lift back up, keeping your knees slightly bent. Throughout the squats, maintain a straight line from the top of your head to your tailbone; resist leaning forward. As you come up, bring your arms into a V above your head. Work up to fifty repetitions. If you want to kick it up, hold at the bottom and sway from your torso, reaching your arms one inch left and one inch right for one minute.

Reverse Lunge Twist

WORKS ENTIRE LEG

Get ready: Stand with your feet hip width apart, knees soft, and hands in prayer position in front of your chest.

Go! Take a giant step back with your right leg and position it directly behind your left leg. Bend your knees and lower straight down, keeping your front knee over your ankle (not jutting out over your toes) and your back knee directly under your right hip. As you are lowering, drop your straight arms to the left side. Return to the start position with feet hip width apart and hands in prayer. Switch sides. Continue alternating sides for one minute. For a more advanced move, put a folded towel behind your back knee. Each time you step back, step over the towel and tap your knee to it. Each time you bring your leg back to standing, add a front kick before setting your foot down. *Make it harder:* Do twenty-five in a row before switching sides.

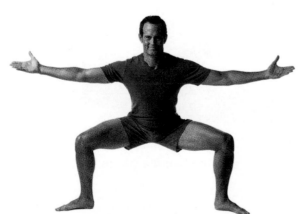

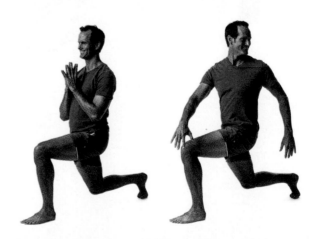

Weeping Willow Hamstring Stretch

STRETCHES HAMSTRINGS

Get ready: Assume an extreme version of second position in ballet—feet more than shoulder width apart, toes pointed forward.

Go! Bend forward from your waist and slowly drop both hands straight to the mat, relaxing your upper body and letting your head dangle loosely, releasing any tension in your neck. Then, keeping your legs straight, walk your hands (in the air if you can't touch the mat) to your left ankle. Hold for twenty seconds. Switch sides and repeat.

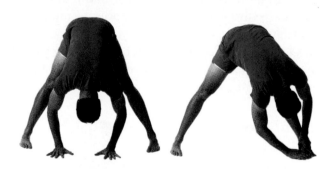

Resting Side Kick

TONES HIPS AND OBLIQUES

Get ready: Lie on your left side. Rest your left ear on your left arm or hand, and bend your stacked legs at right angles, your heels in line with your spine.

Go! Lift your right leg, flex your foot, then lower your leg, tapping your knee lightly on the ground in front of you in line with your belly button. Lift the leg back up, then kick it three feet in the air above your left foot. Do twenty-five times. Then lift your foot and hold it all the way up, pointing and flexing twenty-five times, then switch sides. Keep your stomach taut and resist rocking. Do two sets on each side.

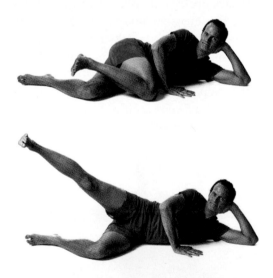

Repeat Thread the Needle (page I-16).

Knee Sways

STRENGTHENS ALL SIDES OF YOUR THIGHS

Get ready: Come onto all fours, hands under shoulders and knees under hips. Keep your elbows slightly bent and your back in a straight line from the top of your head to your tailbone; raise your knees one inch off the ground.

Go! Sway your knees two inches from side to side for one minute.

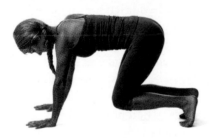

*The only bad workout
is the one that didn't happen.*

L Kicks

TONES HIPS

Get ready: Lie on your left side and bend your left knee in front of you so it forms a right angle to your torso. Place your right hand on the mat in front of you in line with your chest and gently lean forward. Straighten your right leg over your left thigh.

Go! Lift your right leg, keeping the toes pointed slightly down, twenty-five times. Move smoothly and consistently, avoiding any jagged movements or stuttering. Then hold at the highest spot, and point and flex your foot twenty-five times. Switch sides and repeat. For a more advanced move, do two sets of twenty-five on one side before switching and doing two sets on the other side.

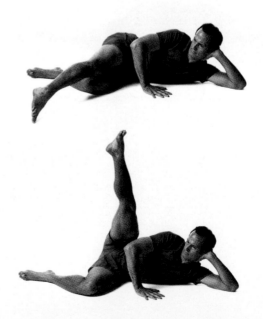

Half Pigeon

STRETCHES HIPS

Get ready: Come onto all fours, hands below shoulders and knees below hips.

Go! Using your arms for support, slide your right knee forward, bringing your right foot in front of your left knee with your shin resting on the mat. Slowly slide your left knee back, straightening the leg until you feel a comfortable stretch in your right hip. Interlace your hands and relax your arms with elbows out, resting your forehead on your hands. Hold for five deep breaths, then switch sides and repeat. To increase the stretch, bring your right heel up and, ultimately, perpendicular to your body, and gently press your lower back toward the mat.

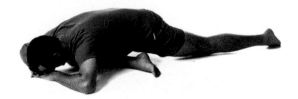

Hip Flexor Twist and Hamstring Reach

STRETCHES HIPS, QUADS, AND HAMSTRINGS

Get ready: Come onto your knees and step your left foot out in front of you. With your left heel lined up under your knee, put your left hand on your left thigh and your right hand to the right of your left foot for balance.

Go! Gently lean your entire body forward, driving your left knee over your left toe and gently twisting your right hip toward your left heel. Pull in your stomach and look straight ahead. To increase the stretch, lift your right hand and ballet it over your head to the left as you twist your right hip farther toward your left heel (not pictured). Hold for five deep breaths. Then move into Quad Pull by grabbing your right foot with your left hand and pull. Hold for five deep breaths, then repeat on the opposite side.

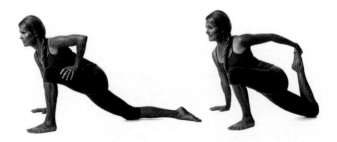

Torso Toner

WARMS UP ABS AND SHOULDERS

Get ready: Bring your feet together and stretch your arms out to the sides at shoulder height with palms facing forward.

Go! Keeping your arms in a straight line, lower your left arm as you raise your right. Keep your chest up and lean as far as you can to the left. Then bring your arms back to starting position and switch sides, bringing your right arm down and left arm up, and leaning to the right side. Each time you change directions, turn your palms to face the other direction. Continue alternating sides for fifty repetitions, keeping your stomach consistently taut and your hips stationary. *Make it harder:* Do the move while balancing on the balls of your feet.

Shoulder Presses

STRENGTHENS SHOULDERS

Get ready: Stand with your feet together. Bend your elbows to bring your hands up to your shoulders, hands in loose fists, knuckles up and palms forward. Tighten your stomach for the duration of this exercise to prevent arching your back.

Go! Exhale and press your arms straight up, then inhale as they return to shoulder height. Work up to one hundred repetitions in a row as fast as you can. *Make it harder:* Balance on your right foot for the first fifty, then on your left foot for the second fifty, or do alternating arms simultaneously.

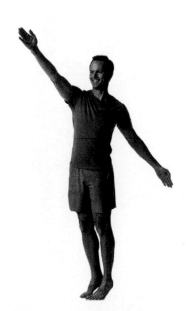

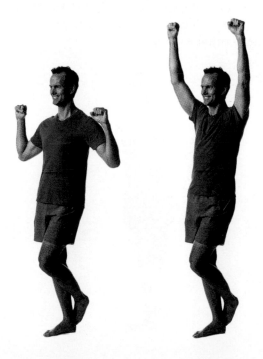

Hug Yourself

STRETCHES SHOULDERS, ARMS, AND UPPER BACK

Get ready: Stand with your feet together. Wrap your arms around your chest, crossing your right arm below your left. Reach your hands behind you toward the opposite shoulder.

Go! Walk your hands farther toward your shoulder blades. Relax your elbows in front of your chest and take five deep breaths into your upper back, breathing into your back muscles and expanding them as much as possible. To increase the stretch, reach your hands toward each other, seeing if you can place your palms fully flat on the shoulder blades. Release, shake your arms out, do arm rolls, and switch, putting your left arm below your right. Relax your shoulders away from your ears and melt into the position without forcing it.

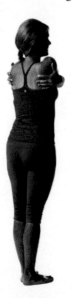

Shoulder Burner

STRENGTHENS SHOULDERS AND UPPER BACK

Get ready: Stand with your feet together and bring your hands to your stomach with middle fingertips touching.

Go! Hinging at your elbows, rotate your hands out away from each other until your palms face forward, then return to start. Repeat for one minute. Then alternate arms for an additional minute while balancing on your toes.

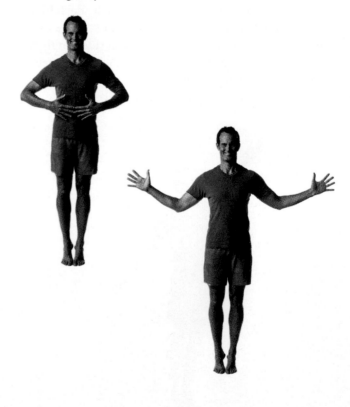

Over and Under

STRENGTHENS SHOULDERS AND ARMS

Get ready: Stand with your feet together, then lift your right foot behind you, bring your arms forward to shoulder height, holding them parallel with palms down and fingers together.

Go! Cross your arms over and under each other, going back and forth for thirty seconds. Next, rotate your arms so the palms face each other, and do the move again for thirty seconds. Now switch your feet so you are balancing on your right leg, and do the move again for thirty seconds, this time with your palms facing up. Continue balancing on your right leg and do one more set, this time with your palms facing out and thumbs pointing down, thirty seconds. For a more advanced move, try Over and Under with your eyes closed, balancing throughout. Keep your stomach taut and your shoulders relaxed for the duration of the exercise.

Chicken Wing

STRETCHES THE NECK AND SHOULDERS

Get ready: Stand with your feet hip width apart. Place the back of your left hand just above your left hip.

Go! Standing up straight, clasp your left elbow with your right hand (if you can't do this, slide your left hand behind your lower back until you can reach your elbow). Gently pull your elbow toward your stomach and take five deep breaths into your upper chest, opening the tightest area. On this stretch, go for only a 7 or 8 on a scale of 1 to 10. Keep your chest lifted and shoulders even. Repeat on the other side. If you want to go deeper, drop your opposite ear as the arm you have on your hip and drive your ear gently toward your shoulder.

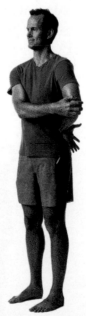

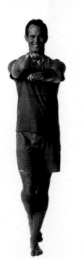 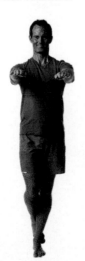 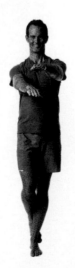

Praying Mantis

STRENGTHENS ARMS, SHOULDERS,
CHEST, AND BACK

Get ready: Stand with feet comfortably apart.
Bring your forearms together in front of you with
your hands in prayer position, elbows at shoulder
height. Your middle fingers should be directly above
your elbows.

Go! Pulse your arms one inch up and down
thirty times, then hold your elbows in the center
as you open and clap just your hands, keeping
your forearms glued together. Do thirty claps.
Then, keeping your forearms together and elbows
stationary, metronome your forearms side to side
thirty times. For a more advanced move, keep a
straight line from your palms to your elbows and,
keeping your elbows glued together, move your
hands as far apart as possible (your hands and
forearms should make a V), then clap your hands
and forearms. Do this thirty times. Balance on your
toes the whole time.

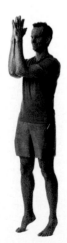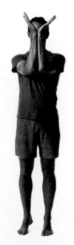

Ladybug Reach

LENGTHENS CHEST, NECK, AND ARM MUSCLES

Get ready: Stand with feet hip width apart.
Bring your arms to the sides at shoulder height,
then bend your elbows and touch your fingers to
your shoulders. Your elbows should point out to
either side.

Go! As you inhale, unbend your right arm and
reach out and back, making an arc with your hand.
Let your eyes follow the moving hand. Focus on
opening your chest. Exhale and return to the starting
point, then repeat on the opposite side. Continue
alternating sides, repeating five times with each arm.

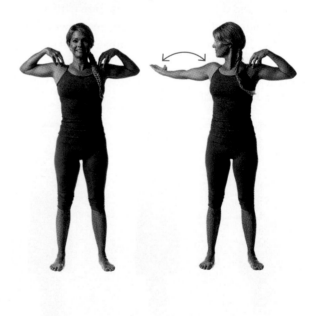

Modified Plank

STRENGTHENS ENTIRE CORE

Get ready: Come onto your knees and forearms so your body forms a straight line from your knees to your shoulders. Cross your ankles and lift them toward your tailbone.

Go! Pull in your stomach as tight as you can and hold the plank for thirty seconds. Do a second set, but this time, twist first your left hip one inch down toward the mat, then the right; continue alternating for one minute. *Make it harder:* Do your first set in full plank position, with knees lifted so you form a straight line from head to toes, and hold for one minute. For your second set, alternate bending your right and left knees to touch the mat or hop your feet in and out away from each other. Continue for one minute without moving your tailbone.

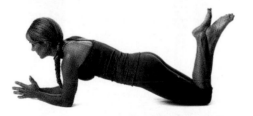

Titanic Reach

STRETCHES CHEST, SHOULDERS, AND ARMS

Get ready: Stand with your feet hip width apart and your arms out to the sides, two inches below shoulder height, palms facing forward.

Go! Keeping your torso upright and your arms straight, stretch your hands farther out and back and hold for twenty seconds. Breath into your chest as if it were a big balloon. For a deeper stretch, bend your wrists back (as pictured) and reach your fingers toward each other.

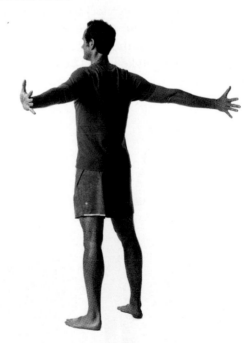

V Pulses

WARMS UP SHOULDERS

Get ready: Stand with your feet together. Straighten your arms above your head, making a narrow V, with palms facing each other.

Go! Pulse your arms toward each other one inch in and out for thirty seconds, then turn your palms away from each other and pulse for thirty seconds. Next, turn your palms to the front of the room, pulsing forward and back for one minute. Then do twenty-five synchronized basketball-size circles clockwise and then counterclockwise. Resist bending your elbows, stay upright, and breathe normally. *Make it harder:* Do half the time balancing on your right leg, with your left knee bent behind you at a right angle, then switch sides and repeat.

Elbow Circling

RELEASES TENSION IN THE SHOULDERS AND NECK

Get ready: Stand with feet hip width apart. Stretch out your arms to the sides at shoulder height, then bend your elbows and touch your shoulders. Your elbows should point out to the sides.

Go! Bring your elbows to touch in front, then start to make big circles. For the duration of the exercise, lightly rest your fingertips on your shoulders. Inhale on one complete circle and exhale on the next. Do ten circles in each direction, looking straight ahead the entire time.

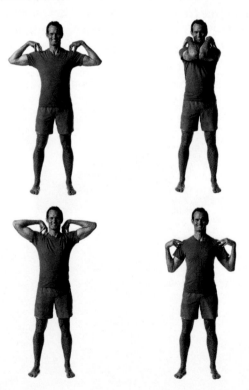

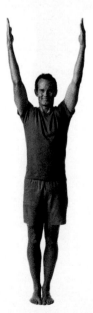

Sideways Cross

STRENGTHENS SHOULDERS AND CORE

Get ready: Come into upper push-up position, with your arms straight under your shoulders and your body forming a straight line from head to toes.

Go! Lift your right hand into the air, turning and lifting your torso to the right until your arms form one straight line. Hold for thirty seconds while you look down at your left hand. If this is hard for you, put your left knee down on the mat, keep your stomach taut, and stay there for thirty seconds, while you look down at your left hand. Switch sides and repeat. After you have done both sides, do a second set, but this time look up on each side for thirty seconds. Then switch back and do a third set. Starting with your left hand down again, arc your right hand up and over your head, palm facing down, while you look toward the inside of your armpit for thirty seconds, then switch sides and repeat. On your fourth and final set (yes, this is a long one), bend the knee on your up leg, and set that foot down flat in front of you. Press into your foot and lift your hips another inch or two up, as you reach your hand up over your head as you did in the last position. *Make it harder:* In the last two positions, lift your straight top leg two feet from your bottom leg for a count of thirty.

Listening to Your Ear

STRETCHES NECK AND TRAPS

Get ready: Sit on your heels and place your palms under your butt (this prevents you from raising your shoulders as you stretch).

Go! Slightly drop your right ear to your right shoulder, keeping your chin forward. Hold for five deep inhales, then switch sides. Do twice on each side, keeping your chest lifted and taking deep breaths into the tightest areas.

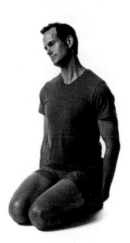

Plank

STRENGTHENS YOUR SHOULDERS,
ARMS, AND ENTIRE CORE

Get ready: Lie facedown, then push your body up
so you are resting on your forearms and your body
forms a straight line from shoulders to toes. If this
is too hard, leave your knees on the ground while
pushing the area between your shoulders toward the
ceiling and pulling in your stomach toward the lower
back for support.

Go! Keep your buttocks tight and look at the floor
(ignore the fact that you suddenly realize you have to
vacuum). Hold this position as long as you can. If you
can last more than one minute, make it more difficult
by lifting one foot up and down, toes pointed, twelve
inches or so, touching the mat thirty times. Then
switch legs and repeat.

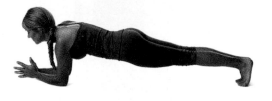

Wag Your Tail

LOOSENS BACK, HIPS, AND SHOULDERS

Get ready: Come onto hands and knees, hands
below shoulders, knees below hips, back flat, and
elbows slightly bent.

Go! Twist your shoulders toward your hip on one
side, then on the other, switching back and forth
ten times. Look at the ground two inches beyond
your fingers the whole time. If you want to loosen up
more, move your head with your shoulders. Pretend
you are wagging your tail.

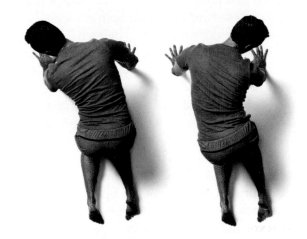

Horizontal Arm Lift

STRENGTHENS SHOULDERS AND OBLIQUES

Get ready: Come onto your elbows and assume a plank position with your feet shoulder width apart, so your body forms a straight line from head to feet.

Go! Reach your left arm straight out to the side, touch the ground, and then come back to center, repeating thirty times. Switch sides and repeat with your right arm. Try to keep your torso stable without twisting the entire time.

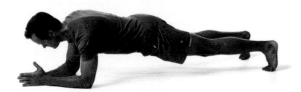

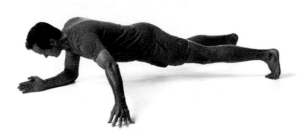

Repeat Shoulder Sways (page I-59).

Shoulder Push-Up

STRENGTHENS SHOULDERS AND CHEST

Get ready: Begin on hands and knees. Press into your palms, lifting your knees and pressing your thighs back until your body forms an inverted V. Look toward your waist. You are now in down dog position.

Go! Look at the area between your hands. Bend your elbows and bring your forehead to hover one inch over the space between your hands, then press back up. Do twenty times. Keep most of the weight in your arms rather than your legs. Stay in the down dog position the entire time, then hold one inch off the ground and do one-inch pulses twenty-five times. *Make it harder:* Lift your right leg straight up behind you for the first ten push-ups, then your left leg for the second ten.

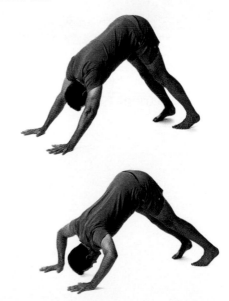

Shoulder Squeezer

STRETCHES SHOULDERS AND ARMS

Get ready: Lie on your right side. Bend your right arm to 90 degrees, holding your forearm straight up. Make sure your right elbow is slightly above your shoulder.

Go! Use your left arm to gently press your right arm down toward the mat without allowing your upper arm to lift. Press until you get a nice stretch (that would be around a 7 on a scale of 1 to 10 for stretching). Hold for five deep breaths. Repeat on the same side. Then switch sides and do two rounds.

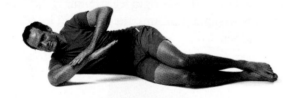

Repeat Arm Rolls (page I-17).

APPENDIX

Quick Solutions

Tips and Tricks

To make your life as simple as possible, I've designed this chapter as a reference guide for addressing common issues that you may encounter on your journey to better health. Included on the following pages are two charts of affirmations, along with other tips and exercises, to increase your awareness and help you move through your feelings, both mental and physical. Following these charts are suggestions for healthy snack options, finding health-friendly fast food when you are stuck with limited choices, and other important solutions.

Reading Your Body's Signals

You can't stop yawning, your muscles are sore, you have no energy, or you want to nosh on some nachos but you're trying to follow your eating plan. Sometimes a nap or a snack is your answer, but other times something less obvious might be going on. Look to your mind and body; both contain clues about what you really need. When you can name the emotion or physical symptom you are feeling, it raises your awareness, which is the first step to finding relief. Affirmations work. Repeat those suggested in the middle column a couple of times a day. Write them on sticky notes and put them in a place you frequently pass by. Then move to the third column and do the suggested exercises. Sometimes the exercises or affirmations might not make immediate sense or seem to fail to relate to the feeling or issue at hand. This is not a mistake. These exercises are meant to tap into your subconscious; they don't require a full explanation to work.

How to Read Your Body's Signals

Feeling	Affirmation	Exercise (mindset, move, or meal)
Angry, resentful, agitated, frustrated, irritated, annoyed	"I disengage from judging. I can't change others. I let go and experience life in the now. I deserve to enjoy this moment."	It's normal to be angry from time to time, but it's not healthy to hold on to it for long periods of time. Use the Punching Bag exercise (page I-23) to let it all out. Do for five minutes without stopping.
Anxious, stressed, tense	"I move forward in life with ease. My path opens up and is made clear."	Get in five minutes of cardio to burn excess energy. Do Towel Circles (page I-50) and Knee Bounces (page I-63).
Bored	"I am thankful for all the things I can do. Opportunities come to me from every direction. I am a very creative person."	Ask yourself, what do you want to see more of in your life? Then do something productive or helpful. Even cleaning out a drawer, taking a drive, or walking around the block will jolt you out of this feeling of self-pity.
Competitive	"I love to win, but it is also okay to let others win. Life is full of balance. I like to challenge myself and not others."	Pick an activity that you are not terribly skilled at, and do it with someone who is much better at it than you are. Practice being okay with that.
Controlled, manipulated	"I am my own being. I have boundaries, and I can do what I want whenever I want to do it."	Stand in front of a full-length mirror and say, "I am the boss of me. If I don't feel comfortable doing something, I don't have to do it, and I don't have to explain why."

Feeling	Affirmation	Exercise (mindset, move, or meal)
Confused, doubtful, unsure	*"I like what I see in the mirror. I have a perfectly working mind and body. I have clarity."*	Practice corpse pose: Lie on your back with your arms at your sides, palms up, and your legs extended. Look straight up and focus on your breathing. Scan your body and allow yourself to completely relax, letting gravity melt all tension. Focus on clarity.
Distracted, preoccupied	*"I think and act clearly in the present moment. Life happens at its own pace. I accept that I can only do what is in front of me now in this present moment."*	Say the alphabet out loud backward. Then start at 100 and keep subtracting 3 until you get to 1. Say the numbers out loud.
Fatigued, exhausted, sleepy	*"I sleep perfectly well. I wake up feeling refreshed and energized and with an abundance of energy to accomplish my many goals. I am motivated."*	Take a short power nap of no more than thirty minutes. If you haven't had coffee and you want some but also feel like a siesta is in order, drink your java right before your snooze. When you wake up, you'll be refreshed and the caffeine will just be kicking in.
Fearful, worried	*"Worry wastes my time unnecessarily. I am not the puppet master and I never will be. Everything works out according to divine order."*	Grab a pen and paper and write for five minutes without stopping. Don't worry about grammar or punctuation. Let it flow. Focus on getting all worry and fear out of your head and onto the paper. Leave it there.
Grieving	*"It is okay to feel loss. It is going to take time to feel better. I am going to allow myself to go through the stages. There is no time limit."*	Allow yourself to sit quietly and reflect on your life and on the connection that is no longer there. Breathe fully throughout. Remember how short life is and think of positive ways that you would like to move forward.
Hurt, wronged	*"Life is not meant to be fair. I am not the judge; I am only responsible for my own actions. I move forward as the loving person I am."*	Close your eyes, take a deep breath, and send love to all the children around the world who are looking for opportunities and trying to better their lives. Send them blessings.
Impatient, impulsive	*"Everything happens at the right time. I allow myself to relax and let go. It is okay not to have everything right when I need it. I am a very patient person."*	With your right index finger, start at the top middle of your head and run your finger down the left side along your entire body. Once you get to where you can't go any farther, switch to your left index finger. Do it once in each direction.

Feeling	Affirmation	Exercise (mindset, move, or meal)
Jealous, envious	*"I find new sources of positive energy within myself. I am enough just being me."*	Write down two goals and two action steps to better your life. Take those two steps even if you are afraid. Get out of your head and "just do it."
Lethargic, lazy	*"I exhibit dedication and diligence. I am going to put in the time and effort to accomplish the goals that are important to me."*	Practice Hippie (page I-49). It is best to put your head below your heart and get the blood flowing by hanging down. As long as you're not feeling ill or you don't have a fever, a brisk twenty-minute walk might be just the ticket to rev up your energy.
Lonely, alone, isolated	*"I will brighten my day by reaching out to someone, and I will also take pleasure when I have times of solitude. It is valuable time to self-reflect and explore my talents. The more I do this, the more I have to offer."*	Find a social event, book club, bowling league, or library event that you can join to get out and meet like-minded people. Everyone I know wants to make another friend.
Numb, lifeless, shut down	*"I have a sensitive palate. I taste and feel everything. I am alive and living my life to the fullest."*	It is time to let go. Treat yourself to a massage, even a foot massage if you don't have time for a full body massage.
Pitiful, self-pitying	*"People care about me in their own unique way. I accept responsibility for my choices and where I am in life. I move forward now with ease."*	No one likes to be around someone who is full of self-pity. It is time to attract different results. Be the person you want to meet. List two action steps you will take. Stop the pity party and implement.
Restless	*"I feel at ease in my body. I get stronger and stronger day by day."*	Drink a tall glass of water and sit in a comfortable chair. Take slow, long, deep breaths for five minutes. With each inhale and exhale, focus more on melting into the chair, and let gravity work to naturally help you relax.
Sad, unhappy, weepy	*"It is okay to be sad. I allow myself to fully experience the feeling. It will go away shortly."*	Use a timer and give the biggest smile you can for one minute without stopping. Then call someone you really care about but haven't talked to in a while and see how he or she is doing. Talk about them, not you.

Feeling	Affirmation	Exercise (mindset, move, or meal)
Self-centered, conceited, vain	*"I am filled with love and affection. I can learn from others, and they can learn from me. Life is a two-way street."*	Call two people and ask them about their lives. Ask what they are doing, and check in to see if they need help with anything.

Reading Your Body's Condition

Though the solutions here are extremely effective at releasing muscle tension and stress caused by muscle imbalance, they are not intended to fix all physical problems. If you don't find relief, make sure to schedule a medical appointment to pinpoint the issue and other possible solutions. Do only what feels comfortable and provides relief. If any move causes further discomfort, stop immediately and consult your physician.

How to Read Your Body's Condition

Condition	Affirmation	Exercise
Achy	*"I can slow down and still get ahead in life. I don't have to mentally push myself all the time."*	Grab a piece of paper and write for five minutes without stopping. Get it out. Ask yourself what is really bothering you and what you really want in life.
Ankle tightness	*"I am flexible. Tension serves no purpose whatsoever. I can allow my feet to take me wherever I want to go."*	Do ankle circles, five times in each direction. Lead with your toe and get as wide a range as possible.
Back tension	*"I am worthy of the best. I let go of unhealed injuries. I am supported by others and by the universe."*	*Lower back* Hippie, page I-49 Knee Drop, page I-12 Airplane Press, page I-32 *Middle back* Yo-Yo, page I-28 Wag Your Tail, page I-78 One Arm Half-Butterfly Stretch, page I-34 *Upper back* Seated Pretzel Stretch, page I-37 Hug Yourself, page I-72

Condition	Affirmation	Exercise
Calf tension	*"I can easily support myself. I lift others up easily. I believe in abundance."*	Down Dog, page I-51
Cough	*"I don't need to act out to be heard. Words flow out of my mouth with clarity and confidence."*	Yo-Yo, page I-28 Elbow Circling, page I-76
Fever	*"I allow my body to regulate and use its healing powers. I don't need to control everything all the time. I trust others. I can let go and allow them to take over."*	Allow yourself to relax and take a nap. Think of two nice things you can do for yourself. Do them after your nap.
Headache	*"My mind works perfectly and I think clearly. I create most of the tension in my life, and I can just as easily uncreate it. Tension is usually the result of thoughts. I easily throw all my unnecessary tension in the trash."*	Hippie Twist, page I-60 Weeping Willow Hamstring Stretch, page I-68 Drop your chin, taking both hands and putting them palm down on top of your head. Bring your elbows together in front of your face. Using the weight of your arms, gently drop your chin toward your chest and hold for five deep breaths.
Hip tightness	*"I am balanced and centered. I can easily move forward, backward, or side to side."*	Hippie, page I-49 Half Pigeon, page I-70 Hammock, page I-62
Knee tightness	*"I can reach higher than I ever thought possible. I spring forward without question."*	Quad Pull, page I-47 Airplane Stretch, page I-66
Nausea	*"It is okay to be unsettled. I find comfort in uncomfortable situations. I am relaxed and at ease."*	Write down what you have eaten in the past twelve hours. Analyze it and figure out what is bothering you. Learn from your food choices and use the knowledge to eat intelligently.
Neck tension	*"There are many roads in life. I see life from many angles and perspectives."*	Ladybug Reach, page I-74 Listening to Your Ear, page I-77 Chicken Wing, page I-73

Condition	Affirmation	Exercise
Shoulder tension	*"I can easily handle all the issues I carry around with me. After handling them one by one with divine guidance, I let them all go."*	Arm Rolls, page I-17 Chicken Wing, page I-73 Shoulder Sways, page I-59 Elbow Circling, page I-76 Shoulder Squeezer, page I-80
Sore muscles	*"I worked hard to get these sore muscles. I will give them the time they need to repair themselves."*	Do the stretches from the workouts insert that match the sore body part.
Sore throat	*"There are germs everywhere, but that is okay, because I don't pick them up. I am perfectly healthy."*	Practice restraint of pen and tongue. Don't feel the need to share every thought in your head. Speak only when necessary and use your words sparingly and intelligently.
Stomachache, indigestion	*"My digestive system works perfectly. I only eat what is right and healthy for my body. I process food easily and swiftly."*	How much water have you had in the past twenty-four hours? Fiber? On a scale from 1 to 10, how healthy has your eating been over the past day? You created this stomachache; now figure out a way to get rid of it.

Fast Food Dining Done Right

You are always better off making your own food at home over going out to eat, but I realize that there are times when you may not have that option, and there's no reason for your nutrition to suffer. Since you won't find many whole grains at these venues, plenty of fats and sugars, make an extra effort to ramp up your fiber and tone down fats and sugars for the remainder of the day. After reviewing the nutrient information at the following fast food restaurants, I've provided my take on what to order:

Restaurant	Item	Nutrient Information
Arby's	Roast chopped farmhouse salad with light Italian dressing	290 calories, 11g fat, 27g carbs, 2g fiber, 6g sugars, 22g protein
	Junior turkey and cheese sandwich (from kids' menu) and chopped side salad	250 calories, 14g fat, 10g carbs, 3g fiber, 6g sugars, 23g protein
Burger King	Tendergrill chicken sandwich (no mayo)	320 calories, 5g fat, 38g carbs, 2g fiber, 6g sugars, 31g protein
	BK veggie burger (no mayo)	320 calories, 8g fat, 43g carbs, 5g fiber, 9g sugars, 21g protein
Chipotle	3 soft corn tacos with barbacoa (braised beef), lettuce, and fresh tomato salsa	395 calories, 7g fat, 51g carbs, 7.5g fiber, sugars 3g, 28g protein
	Salad with black beans, brown rice, fajita vegetables, and fresh tomato salsa	370 calories, 8.5g fat, 64g carbs, 17g fiber, 7.5g sugars, 13.5g protein
Jack in the Box	*Breakfast:* Egg white and turkey sandwich Jr. Jack	324 calories, 15g fat, 33g carbs, 2g fiber, 6g sugars, 14g protein
	Lunch: Grilled chicken salad with low-fat balsamic vinaigrette dressing (without croutons)	274 calories, 11g fat, 18g carbs, 4g fiber, 9g sugars, 28g protein
KFC	Grilled chicken breast with green beans and corn on the cob	315 calories, 7.5g fat, 20g carbs, 4g fiber, 4g sugars, 43g protein
	Grilled thigh and coleslaw	340 calories, 20g fat, 19g carbs, 3g fiber, 14g sugars, 20g protein

Restaurant	Item	Nutrient Information
McDonald's	*Breakfast:* Egg white delight McMuffin (hold the margarine)	230 calories, 5g fat, 30g carbs, 4g fiber, 3g sugars, 18g protein
	Lunch: Grilled chicken classic sandwich (hold the mayo, ask for mustard, lettuce, and tomato), and a side salad, with low-fat balsamic vinaigrette	350 calories, 6g fat, 48g carbs, 4g fiber, 13g sugars, 28g protein
	Southwest salad with grilled chicken and lime (hold the tortilla strips)	250 calories, 7g fat, 24g carbs, 6g fiber, 10g sugars, 26g protein
Panera Bread	*Breakfast:* Steel cut oatmeal with summer blueberries and granola	350 calories, 9g fat, 62g carbs, 8g fiber, 22g sugars, 7g protein
	Lunch: Classic salad with chicken (half portion), reduced fat balsamic vinaigrette, and a cup of low-fat black bean soup	380 calories, 13g fat, 50g carbs, 8g fiber, 14g sugars, 23g protein
	Smoked turkey breast sandwich on wheat (half portion) with low-fat garden vegetable with pesto	360 calories, 7g fat, 58g carbs, 13g fiber, 7g sugars, 20g protein
Starbucks	*Breakfast:* 2 classic whole-grain oatmeals	320 calories, 5g fat, 56g carbs, 8g fiber, 0g sugars, 10g protein
	Spinach and feta breakfast wrap	290 calories, 10g fat, 33g carbs, 6g fiber, 4g sugars, 19g protein
	Lunch: Zesty chicken and black bean salad bowl	360 calories, 15g fat, 38g carbs, 8g fiber, 9g sugars, 19g protein
	Chicken and hummus bistro box	270 calories, 7g fat, 29g carbs, 4g fiber, 3g sugars, 20g protein
	Snack: Seasonal harvest fruit blend	90 calories, 0g fat, 24g carbs, 4g fiber, 19g sugars, 1g protein

Restaurant	Item	Nutrient Information
Starbucks	*Drinks:* Any Tazo tea, unsweetened	0 calories
	Black, passion or green iced tea, unsweetened	0 calories
	Iced or hot coffee, unsweetened	0 calories
	You can ask for a splash of soymilk (about 2 tablespoons) in your beverage, if you have no allergic reaction to soy.	16 calories, 0.5g fat, 2.1g carbs, 0g fiber, 1.5g sugars, 0.9g protein
Subway	6-inch oven-roasted chicken on nine-grain wheat, with mustard, cucumbers, green peppers, lettuce, red onions, spinach, and tomatoes	320 calories, 5g fat, 48g carbs, 6g fiber, 8g sugars, 23g protein
	6-inch turkey breast and provolone on nine-grain wheat, with mustard, cucumbers, green peppers, lettuce, red onions, spinach, and tomatoes	320 calories, 5g fat, 47g carbs, 5g fiber, 7g sugars, 22g protein
	Salad of lettuce, spinach, cucumbers, green peppers, red onions, and avocado, topped with turkey, or oven-roasted chicken and natural cheddar Dressing: vinegar, salt, and pepper	250 calories, 13g fat, 18g carbs, 8g fiber, 6g sugars, 18g protein
Taco Bell	2 fresco chicken soft tacos, and a side of black beans	360 calories, 8.5g fat, 44g carbs, 9g fiber, 5g sugars, 24g protein
	fresco burrito supreme—steak	350 calories, 9g fat, 48g carbs, 6g fiber, 4g sugars, 19g protein
Wendy's	Asian cashew chicken salad with light spicy Asian chili vinaigrette	255 calories, 5g fat, 21g carbs, 5g fiber, 11g sugars, 33g protein
	Grilled chicken sandwich on a regular bun with Asiago cheese, lettuce, tomato, and onion (no sauce)	330 calories, 6.5g fat, 27g carbs, 1g fiber, 4g sugars, 34g protein

Portion Guide

When it comes to proper portion sizes, a visual is worth a thousand words. Plus, lugging around a food scale, measuring cups, teaspoons, and tablespoons just isn't realistic. Here are some ideas to help you stick to proper portions.

Dividing Your Plate

When you are building lunches and dinners, load half your plate with vegetables and split the other half between protein and whole grains.

General Portions

1 cup: baseball

½ cup: lightbulb

2 tablespoons: Ping-Pong or golf ball

1 tablespoon: your whole thumb

1 teaspoon: tip of your thumb

Poultry, red meat, tofu: a 3-ounce serving is the size of a deck of cards

Fish: a 3-ounce serving is about the size of a checkbook

Lunch meat: a 1-ounce serving is about the size of a DVD (look for all-natural and nitrate-free)

Cheese: two dice equal about 1 ounce

Butter, mayo, or oil: bet on a poker chip for about 1 tablespoon (or use the thumb example above)

Peanut butter, hummus: a golf-ball-size serving equals 2 tablespoons

Instant portion control. Another good strategy is to use salad plates instead of dinner plates when sitting down for a meal. You can avoid seconds by serving proper portions (portion sizes are listed in chapter 10) and then putting the rest of the food away.

Snacking Right

The purpose of eating between meals is to keep your blood sugar, energy levels, and willpower running smoothly. Aim to eat snacks about two and a half to three hours after your last meal, and portion out 100 to 200 calories, which is just enough to keep you going but not so much that it will throw off your next meal. Best choices for snacks are fruit (to be eaten solo) or a small handful of nuts, which are extremely nutrient dense. Below you'll find a great list with suggested portion sizes within the 100–200 calorie range. Keep a fresh supply of some suggested snacks at work, in your car, and in your purse, bag, or briefcase. Print out this list and keep it with you. The next time you go to the store, you'll have plenty of handy ideas within reach, and you'll be able to choose items you haven't had in a while.

What Should I Eat When I Need a Little Healthy Pep?

Dried Fruit
Serving size: one small handful or ¼ cup

apple

apricot

banana

cranberries

dried goji berries

figs

mango

papaya

peach

raisins

Fresh Fruit

Fresh fruit makes a perfect snack for energy slumps.

apple, 1 medium

avocado, ½ medium

banana, 1 small

blackberries, 1 cup

blueberries, 1 cup

cantaloupe, ¼ wedge

figs, 4 small fresh

grapefruit, ½ medium

green or red grapes, 16

guava, ½ cup diced

honeydew, ¼ wedge

kiwi, 1 large

mango, ½ cup diced

nectarine, 1 medium

orange, 1 medium

peach, 1 medium

pear, 1 small

raspberries, 1 cup

strawberries, 1 cup

tangerines, 2 small

watermelon, 6 balls

What Should I Have After a Workout?

Nuts

A 1-ounce or 28-gram serving size per day (about the amount that fits in the palm of your hand).

Ounce for ounce, the protein content of nuts is comparable to meat. Go for raw nuts rather than salted, chocolate covered, honey roasted, or candy coated. Make sure the products you buy are all natural and don't contain any partially hydrogenated fats.

almonds

Brazil nuts

cashews

hazelnuts

macadamias*

pecans

pili nuts

pistachios

walnuts

*Keep in mind that macadamias have about 202 calories per ounce, so once you have your palm full, take off three or four nuts and put them back. And don't eat any nuts straight from the container. It's easy to eat too many, so portion out your snack, then put the container back in the cabinet—out of sight, out of mind.

Seeds

chia, 1 teaspoon

flax, 1–2 teaspoons ground

hemp, 1 tablespoon

pomegranate, ½ cup

pumpkin, ½ cup

sesame, ¼ cup

sunflower, ¼ cup

Edamame

½ cup shelled beans. A half cup is about 100 calories and provides 8 grams of protein and 4 grams of fiber.

Hard-boiled egg

An egg provides 70 calories and 6 grams protein.

String cheese

One stick provides 80 calories and 8 grams protein.

Simple Combination Snacks with Protein

These are some of my favorites, especially great on a day when you've had a lighter breakfast or lunch. These also contain protein, which helps your muscles recover after a workout.

1 cup low-fat cottage cheese, 1 teaspoon cinnamon, 1 teaspoon sunflower seeds

1 cup low-fat cottage cheese, 1 teaspoon chia seeds, 2 cherry tomatoes, 4 slices cucumber, salt and pepper to taste

1 cup low-fat cottage cheese with 2 slices tomato and a dash of paprika

1 celery stick with a heaping spoonful of almond butter

2 wedges jicama and 3 tablespoons Artichoke and Spinach Hummus (page 199) or Baba Ganoush (page 199)

½ cup part-skim ricotta cheese with half an avocado and 2 cherry tomatoes

4 pieces endive and half an avocado with string cheese, edamame, or boiled egg

What Should I Have If I'm Truly Not Hungry for a Snack?

Black or green tea, 1 cup. On days when you have a big breakfast or lunch and might not need the calories or nutrients from a food snack, tea is a great option. Both black and green varieties have been shown to rev up your calorie-burning engine, increase your energy, and help with weight loss.

SELECTED BIBLIOGRAPHY

Agarwal, G., A. Chatterjee, M. Saluja, and M. Alam. "Green Tea: A Boon for Periodontal and General Health." *Journal of Indian Society of Periodontology* 16(2) (2012): 161.

Agricultural Marketing Service—National Organic Program. http://www.ams.usda.gov/AMSv1.0/nop. Retrieved June 17, 2014.

Ai, A. L., P. Wink, T. N. Tice, S. F. Bolling, and M. Shearer. "Prayer and Reverence in Naturalistic, Aesthetic, and Socio-Moral Contexts Predicted Fewer Complications Following Coronary Artery Bypass." *Journal of Behavioral Medicine* 32(6) (2009): 570–81.

Allemand, M., I. Amberg, D. Zimprich, and F. D. Fincham. "The Role of Trait Forgiveness and Relationship Satisfaction in Episodic Forgiveness." *Journal of Social and Clinical Psychology* 26(2) (2007): 199–217.

Anderson, D. E., J. D. McNeely, and B. G. Windham. "Regular Slow-Breathing Exercise Effects on Blood Pressure and Breathing Patterns at Rest." *Journal of Human Hypertension* 24(12) (2010): 807–13.

Anderson, J. W., P. Baird, R. H. Davis Jr., S. Ferreri, M. Knudtson, A. Koraym, et al. "Health Benefits of Dietary Fiber." *Nutrition Reviews* 67(4) (2009): 188–205.

Andersson, E., and T. Moss. "Imagery and Implementation Intention: A Randomised Controlled Trial of Interventions to Increase Exercise Behaviour in the General Population." *Psychology of Sport and Exercise* 12(2) (2011): 63–70.

Apóstolo, J. L., and K. Kolcaba. "The Effects of Guided Imagery on Comfort, Depression, Anxiety, and Stress of Psychiatric Inpatients with Depressive Disorders." *Archives of Psychiatric Nursing* 23(6) (2009): 403–11.

Arch, J., and M. Craske. "Mechanisms of Mindfulness: Emotion Regulation Following a Focused Breathing Induction." *Behaviour Research and Therapy* 44(12) (2006): 1849–58.

Baikie, K. A. "Emotional and Physical Health Benefits of Expressive Writing." *Advances in Psychiatric Treatment* 11(5) (2005): 338–46.

Baird, C., and L. Sands. "A Pilot Study of the Effectiveness of Guided Imagery with Progressive Muscle Relaxation to Reduce Chronic Pain and Mobility Difficulties of Osteoarthritis." *Pain Management Nursing* 3 (2004): 97–104.

Baird, C., M. Murawski, and J. Wu. "Efficacy of Guided Imagery with Relaxation for Osteoarthritis Symptoms and Medication Intake." *Pain Management Nursing* 11(1) (2010): 56–65.

Bandura, A. "Self-efficacy Mechanism in Human Agency." *American Psychologist* 37(2) (1982): 122–47.

Barsky, A. J. "Nonspecific Medication Side Effects and the Nocebo Phenomenon." *JAMA: The Journal of the American Medical Association* 287(5) (2002): 622–27.

Baumeister, R. F., E. Bratslavsky, M. Muraven, and D. M. Tice. (1998). "Ego Depletion: Is the active Self a Limited Resource?" *Journal of Personality and Social Psychology* 74(5) (1998): 1252–65.

Baumeister, R. F., M. Gailliot, C. N. Dewall, and M. Oaten. (2006). "Self-Regulation and Personality: How Interventions Increase Regulatory Success, and How Depletion Moderates the Effects of Traits on Behavior." *Journal of Personality* 74(6) (2006): 1773–1802.

Benedetti, F., A. Pollo, L. Lopiano, M. Lanotte, S. Vighetti, and I. Rainero. "Conscious Expectation and Unconscious Conditioning in Analgesic, Motor, and Hormonal Placebo/Nocebo Responses." *The Journal of Neuroscience* 23(10) (2003), 4315–23.

Benson, H. *The Relaxation Response.* New York: Morrow, 1975.

Benyamini, Y., and O. Raz. (2007). "'I Can Tell You If I'll Really Lose All That Weight': Dispositional and Situated Optimism as Predictors of Weight Loss Following a Group Intervention." *Journal of Applied Social Psychology* 37(4): 844–61.

Benyamini, Y., R. Geron, D. M. Steinberg, N. Medini, L. Valinsky, and R. Endevelt. "A Structured Intentions and Action-Planning Intervention Improves Weight Loss Outcomes in a Group Weight Loss Program." *American Journal of Health Promotion* 28(2) (2013): 119–27.

Benzie, I. F. *Herbal Medicine Biomolecular and Clinical Aspects* (2nd ed.). Boca Raton: Taylor & Francis, 2011.

Benzie, I. F. "The Amazing and Mighty Ginger," in *Herbal Medicine Biomolecular and Clinical Aspects* (2nd ed.). Boca Raton: Taylor & Francis 2011.

Benzie, I. F. "Turmeric, the Golden Spice," in *Herbal Medicine Biomolecular and Clinical Aspects* (2nd ed., http://www.ncbi.nlm.nih.gov/books/NBK92752/). Boca Raton: Taylor & Francis, 2011.

Bernardi, L., G. Spadacini, J. Bellwon, R. Hajric, H. Roskamm, and A. Frey. "Effect of Breathing Rate on Oxygen Saturation and Exercise Performance in Chronic Heart Failure." *The Lancet* 351(9112) (1998): 1308–11.

Black Tea: MedlinePlus Supplements. U.S. National Library of Medicine. Retrieved June 17, 2014. http://www.nlm.nih.gov/medlineplus/druginfo/natural/997.html.

Blau, J. N. "Water Deprivation: A New Migraine Precipitant." *Headache: The Journal of Head and Face Pain* 45(6) (2005): 757–59.

Blau, J. N., C. A. Kell., and J. M. Sperling. "Water-Deprivation Headache: A New Headache with Two Variants." *Headache: The Journal of Head and Face Pain* 44(1) (2004): 79–83.

Boehm, J. K., D. R. Williams, E. B. Rimm, C. Ryff, and L. D. Kubzansky. "Relation Between Optimism and Lipids in Midlife." *The American Journal of Cardiology* 111(10) (2013): 1425–31.

Bowen, S., G. A. Parks, A. W. Blume, M. E. Larimer, B. D. Ostafin, T. L. Simpson, et al. "Mindfulness Meditation and Substance Use in an Incarcerated Population." *Psychology of Addictive Behaviors* 20(3) (2006): 343–47.

Brain Trivia | Laboratory of Neuro Imaging. Retrieved June 19, 2014. http://www.loni.usc.edu/about_loni/education/brain_trivia.php.

BrainFacts.org. Cell Communication. http://www.brainfacts.org/brain-basics/cell-communication/. Retrieved June 16, 2014.

Brefczynski-Lewis, J. A., A. Lutz, H. S. Schaefer, D. B. Levinson, and R. J. Davidson. "Neural Correlates of Attentional Expertise in Long-Term Meditation Practitioners." *Proceedings of the National Academy of Sciences* 104(27) (2007): 11483–88.

Bressan, R. A., and J. A. Crippa. "The Role of Dopamine in Reward and Pleasure Behaviour—Review of Data from Preclinical Research." *Acta Psychiatrica Scandinavica* 111(s427) (2005): 14–21.

Brown, R. P., and P. L. Gerbarg. "Yoga Breathing, Meditation, and Longevity." *Annals of the New York Academy of Sciences* 1172(1) (2009): 54–62.

Bufe, B., P. A. Breslin, C. Kuhn, D. R. Reed, C. D. Tharp, J. P. Slack, et al. "The Molecular Basis of Individual Differences in Phenylthiocarbamide and Propylthiouracil Bitterness Perception." *Current Biology* 15(4) (2005): 322–27.

Cahill, L. E., S. E. Chiuve, R. A. Mekary, M. K. Jensen, A. J. Flint, F. B. Hu, et al. "Prospective Study of Breakfast Eating and Incident Coronary Heart Disease in a Cohort of Male US Health Professionals." *Circulation* 128(4) (2013): 337–43.

Cameron, J. "Tarcher Talks: Julia Cameron—The Writing Diet." YouTube. https://www.youtube.com/watch?v=su_Z6A5FhcQ. Retrieved June 19, 2014.

Carmody, J., and R. A. Baer. "Relationships Between Mindfulness Practice and Levels of Mindfulness, Medical, and Psychological Symptoms and Well-Being in a Mindfulness-Based Stress Reduction Program." *Journal of Behavioral Medicine* 31(1) (2008): 23–33.

Castro, J. D. "The Time of Day of Food Intake Influences Overall Intake in Humans. *Journal of Nutrition* 134(1) (2004): 104–11.

Charney, D., S. Woods, W. Goodman, and G. Heninger. "Serotonin Function in Anxiety." *Psychopharmacology* 92(1) (1987): 14–24.

Charts by Topic: Leisure and Sports Activities. U.S. Bureau of Labor Statistics. Retrieved June 19, 2014. http://www.bls.gov/tus/charts/leisure.htm.

Choat, B. "What Are Your Thoughts Doing to You Each Day? Thoughts from Bob Choat." (June 24, 2013). Retrieved June 19, 2014. http://bobchoat.com/2013/06/24/what-are-your-thoughts-doing-to-you-each-day/.

Clarey, C. "Olympians Use Imagery as Mental Training." *The New York Times* (February 22, 2014). Retrieved June 19, 2014. http://www.nytimes.com/2014/02/23/sports/olympics/olympians-use-imagery-as-mental-training.html?_r=0.

Collingwood, J. "The Power of Music to Reduce Stress." *Psych Central*. Psych Central.com (January 30, 2013). Retrieved May 13, 2014. http://psychcentral.com/lib/the-power-of-music-to-reduce-stress/000930.

"Consequences of Insufficient Sleep." Harvard Medical School on Healthy Sleep. Retrieved May 11, 2014. http://healthysleep.med.harvard.edu/healthy/matters/consequences.

Cooke, M., W. Chaboyer, P. Schluter, and M. Hiratos. "The Effect of Music on Preoperative Anxiety in Day Surgery." *Journal of Advanced Nursing* 52(1) (2005): 47–55.

Creswell, J. D., J. M. Dutcher, W. M. Klein, P. R. Harris, J. M. Levine, and J. C. Perales. "Self-Affirmation Improves Problem-Solving Under Stress." *PLoS ONE* 8(5) (2013): e62593.

Culin, K. R., E. Tsukayama, and A. L. Duckworth. "Unpacking Grit: Motivational Correlates of Perseverance and Passion for Long-Term Goals." *The Journal of Positive Psychology* 9 (2014): 1–7.

Currier, J. American Society for Nutrition (March 19, 2012). Retrieved June 19, 2014. http://www.nutrition.org/asn-blog/2012/03/the-real-scoop-on-chia-seeds/.

Daniel, T. O., C. M. Stanton, and L. H. Epstein. "The Future Is Now: Comparing the Effect of Episodic Future Thinking on Impulsivity in Lean and Obese Individuals." *Appetite* 71 (2013): 120–25.

Daubenmier, J., L. Karan, M. Kemeny, R. H. Lustig, K. Jhaveri, M. Kuwata, et al. "Mindfulness Intervention for Stress Eating to Reduce Cortisol and Abdominal Fat Among Overweight and Obese Women: An Exploratory Randomized Controlled Study." *Journal of Obesity* (2011): 1–13.

Davidson, K. W., E. Mostofsky, and W. Whang. "Don't Worry, Be Happy: Positive Affect and Reduced Ten-Year Incident Coronary Heart Disease: The Canadian Nova Scotia Health Survey." *European Heart Journal* 31(9) (2010): 1065–70.

Davidson, R. J., and J. Kabat-Zinn. "Alterations in Brain and Immune Function Produced by Mindfulness Meditation." *Psychosomatic Medicine* 65(4) (2003): 564–70.

Davidson, R. J., and B. S. Mcewen. "Social Influences on Neuroplasticity: Stress and Interventions to Promote Well-Being." *Nature Neuroscience* 15(5) (2012): 689–95.

Davies, M., J. Judd, D. Baer, B. Clevidence, D. Paul, A. Edwards, et al. "Black Tea Consumption Reduces Total and LDL Cholesterol in Mildly Hypercholesterolemic Adults." *Journal of Nutrition* 133(10) (2003): 3298S–3302S.

Davis, P. A., and W. Yokoyama. "Cinnamon Intake Lowers Fasting Blood Glucose: Meta-Analysis." *Journal of Medicinal Food* 14(9) (2011): 884–89.

Diepvens, K., E. Kovacs, N. Vogels, and M. Westerterpplantenga. "Metabolic Effects of Green Tea and of Phases of Weight Loss." *Physiology & Behavior* 87(1) (2006): 185–91.

Dinges, D., F. Pack, K. Gillen, J. Powell, G. Ott, C. Aptowicz, et al. "Cumulative Sleepiness, Mood Disturbance, and Psychomotor Vigilance Performance Decrements During a Week of Sleep Restricted to 4–5 Hours Per Night." *Journal of Sleep Research and Sleep Medicine* 20(4) (1997): 267–77.

"Do Self-Affirmations Work? A Revisit." *Psychology Today: Health, Help, Happiness + Find a Therapist.* http://www.psychologytoday.com/blog/wired-success/201305/do-self-affirmations-work-revisit. Retrieved June 19, 2014.

"The Duckworth Lab." Retrieved June 19, 2014. https://sites.sas.upenn.edu/duckworth.

Duhigg, C. *The Power of Habit: Why We Do What We Do in Life and Business.* New York: Random House, 2012.

Ekman, I., B. Kjellstrom, K. Falk, J. Norman, and K. Swedberg. "Impact of Device-Guided Slow Breathing on Symptoms of Chronic Heart Failure: A Randomized, Controlled Feasibility Study." *European Journal of Heart Failure* 13(9) (2011): 1000–1005.

Elliott, W. J., J. L. Izzo, W. B. White, D. R. Rosing, C. S. Snyder, A. Alter, et al. "Graded Blood Pressure Reduction in Hypertensive Outpatients Associated with Use of a Device to Assist with Slow Breathing." *The Journal of Clinical Hypertension,* 6(10) (2004): 553–59.

Emmons, R. A., and M. E. Mccullough. "Counting Blessings Versus Burdens: An Experimental Investigation of Gratitude and Subjective Well-Being in Daily Life." *Journal of Personality and Social Psychology* 84(2) (2003): 377–89.

"Endocrinology Update." Mayo Clinic. Retrieved June 10, 2014. http://www.mayoclinic.org/documents/mc5810-0307-pdf/doc-20079082.

Epstein, L. H., N. Jankowiak, K. D. Fletcher, K. A. Carr, C. Nederkoorn, H. A. Raynor, et al. "Women Who Are Motivated to Eat and Discount the Future Are More Obese." *Obesity* 22(6) (2014): 1394–99.

Europe PubMed Central. Retrieved May 12, 2014. http://europepmc.org/abstract/MED/9921569/reload=0;jsessionid=MTRkHKGjh2nuKQ66lMx3.0.

Evans, J. F. *Wellness and Writing Connections: Writing for Better Physical, Mental, and Spiritual Health.* Enumclaw, WA: Idyll Arbor, 2010.

"Exercise in Cold Water May Increase Appetite, UF Study Finds." *ScienceDaily.* Retrieved June 19, 2014. http://www.sciencedaily.com/releases/2005/05/050504225732.htm.

"FAQ and Useful Links." Michael Pollan. Retrieved June 19, 2014. http://michaelpollan.com/resources/.

Feldman, G., J. Greeson, and J. Senville. "Differential Effects of Mindful Breathing, Progressive Muscle Relaxation, and Loving-kindness Meditation on Decentering and Negative Reactions to Repetitive Thoughts." *Behaviour Research and Therapy* 48(10) (2010): 1002–11.

"Flaxseed and Flaxseed Oil." NCCAM. Retrieved June 19, 2014. http://nccam.nih.gov/health/flaxseed/ataglance.htm.

Fontani, G., S. Migliorini, R. Benocci, A. Facchini, M. Casini, and F. Corradeschi. "Effect of Mental Imagery on the Development of Skilled Motor Actions." *Perceptual and Motor Skills* 105(3) (2007): 803–26.

Fritz, T. H., A. Villringer, J. Haynes, Y. Li, O. Giot, M. Demey, et al. "Musical Agency Reduces Perceived Exertion During Strenuous Physical Performance." Proceedings of the National Academy of Sciences 110(44) (2013): 17784–89.

Froh, J., W. Sefick, and R. Emmons. "Counting Blessings in Early Adolescents: An Experimental Study of Gratitude and Subjective Well-Being." *Journal of School Psychology* 46(2) (2008): 213–33.

"Functional Training." *ScienceDaily.* Retrieved June 19, 2014. http://www.sciencedaily.com/articles/f/functional_training.htm.

Garaulet, M., P. Gómez-Abellán, J. J. Alburquerque-Béjar, Y. Lee, J. M. Ordovás, and F. A. Scheer. "Timing of Food Intake Predicts Weight Loss Effectiveness." *International Journal of Obesity* 37(4) (2013): 604–11.

"Geneen Roth's Eating Guidelines." Oprah.com. Retrieved June 19, 2014. http://www.oprah.com/oprahshow/Author-Geneen-Roth-Shares-Her-Eating-Guidelines-Video.

"Goats Yelling Like Humans—Super Cut Compilation." YouTube (February 6, 2013). Retrieved May 12, 2014. http://www.youtube.com/watch?v=PpccpglnNf0.

Gore, C. J., and R. T. Withers. "The Effect of Exercise Intensity and Duration on the Oxygen Deficit and Excess Post-Exercise Oxygen Consumption." *European Journal of Applied Physiology and Occupational Physiology* 60(5) (1990): 169–74.

Gorgoni, M., A. D'atri, G. Lauri, P. M. Rossini, F. Ferlazzo, and L. D. Gennaro. "Is Sleep Essential for Neural Plasticity in Humans, and How Does It Affect Motor and Cognitive Recovery?" *Neural Plasticity* (2013): 1–13.

Gowin, J. "Why Your Brain Needs Water." *Psychology Today: Health, Help, Happiness + Find a Therapist* (October 15, 2010). Retrieved June 19, 2014. http://www.psychologytoday.com/blog/you-illuminated/201010/why-your-brain-needs-water.

Green Exercise/Research Findings. Retrieved June 19, 2014. http://www.greenexercise.org/Research_Findings.html.

Grossman, P., U. Tiefenthaler-Gilmer, A. Raysz, and U. Kesper. "Mindfulness Training as an Intervention for Fibromyalgia: Evidence of Postintervention and Three-Year Follow-Up Benefits in Well-Being." *Psychotherapy and Psychosomatics* 76(4) (2007): 226–33.

Haager, J. S., C. Kuhbandner, and R. Pekrun. "Overcoming Fixed Mindsets: The Role of Affect." *Cognition & Emotion* 28(4) (2014): 756–67.

Hagger, M. S., C. Wood, C. Stiff, and N. L. Chatzisarantis. "Ego Depletion and the Strength Model of Self-Control: A Meta-analysis." *Psychological Bulletin* 136(4) (2010): 495–525.

Hahn, R. "The Nocebo Phenomenon: Concept, Evidence, and Implications for Public Health." *Preventive Medicine* 26(5) (1997): 607–11.

Harvard Health Public New Releases. "The Health Benefits of Strong Relationships." Retrieved May 12, 2014. http://www.health.harvard.edu/press_releases/the-health-benefits-of-strong-relationships.

Harvard Medical School Health Reports. "4 Ways to Boost Your Energy with Breakfast" (March 14, 2013). Retrieved May 15, 2014. http://www.health.harvard.edu/healthbeat/4-ways-to-boost-your-energy-with-breakfast.

Haun, M., R. O. Mainous, and S. W. Looney. "Effect of Music on Anxiety of Women Awaiting Breast Biopsy." *Behavioral Medicine* 27(3) (2001): 127–32.

Heinrichs, M., T. Baumgartner, C. Kirschbaum, and U. Ehlert. "Social Support and Oxytocin Interact to Suppress Cortisol and Subjective Responses to Psychosocial Stress." *Biological Psychiatry* 54(12) (2003): 1389–98.

Hingle, M., B. Wertheim, H. Tindle, L. Tinker, R. Seguin, M. Rosai, et al. "Optimism and Diet Quality in the Women's Health Initiative." *Journal of the Academy of Nutrition and Dietetics* (2014): epub ahead of print, doi: 10.1016/j.jand.2013.12.018.

Hofmann, S. G., A. T. Sawyer, A. A. Witt, and D. Oh. "The Effect of Mindfulness-Based Therapy on Anxiety and Depression: A Meta-analytic Review." *Journal of Consulting and Clinical Psychology* 78(2) (2010): 169–83.

Holland, A., C. Hill, A. Jones, and C. McDonald. "Breathing Exercises for Chronic Obstructive Pulmonary Disease." *Cochrane Database System Review* 10 (2012): doi: 10.1002/14651858.CD008250.pub2.

Hollis, J., T. Erlinger, A. Dalcin, C. Champagne, J. Ard, L. Appel, et al. "Weight Loss During the Intensive Intervention Phase of the Weight-Loss Maintenance Trial." *American Journal of Preventive Medicine* 35(2) (2008): 118–26.

Holt, S. "The Effects of High-Carbohydrate vs. High-Fat Breakfasts on Feelings of Fullness and Alertness, and Subsequent Food Intake." *International Journal of Food Sciences and Nutrition* 50(1)(1999): 13–28.

Holt-Lunstad, J., T. B. Smith, J. B. Layton, and C. Brayne. "Social Relationships and Mortality Risk: A Meta-analytic Review." *PLoS Medicine* 7(7) (2010): e1000316.

Hölzel, B. K., J. Carmody, M. Vangel, C. Congleton, S. M. Yerramsetti, T. Gard, et al. "Mindfulness Practice Leads to Increases in Regional Brain Gray Matter Density." *Psychiatry Research: Neuroimaging* 191(1) (2011): 36–43.

Hoogwegt, M. T., H. Versteeg, T. B. Hansen, L. C. Thygesen, S. S. Pedersen, and A. Zwisler. "Exercise Mediates the Association Between Positive Affect and Five-Year Mortality in Patients with Ischemic Heart Disease." *Circulation: Cardiovascular Quality and Outcomes* 6(5) (2013): 559–66.

"How Does Writing Affect Your Brain?" *NeuroRelay* (August 7, 2013). *NeuroRelay*. Retrieved June 19, 2014. http://neurorelay.com/2013/08/07/how-does-writing-affect-your-brain/.

"How Stress Affects Your Health." Retrieved June 19, 2014. https://www.apa.org/helpcenter/stress.aspx.

Hoyland, A., L. Dye, and C. L. Lawton. "A Systematic Review of the Effect of Breakfast on the Cognitive Performance of Children and Adolescents." *Nutrition Research Reviews* 22(02) (2009): 220.

Hursel, R., W. Viechtbauer, and M. Westerterp-Plantenga. "Effects of Green Tea on Weight Loss and Weight Maintenance: A Meta-analysis." *Appetite* 52(3) (2009): 838.

"Insufficient Sleep Is a Public Health Epidemic." Centers for Disease Control and Prevention (January 13, 2014). Retrieved June 19, 2014. http://www.cdc.gov/features/dssleep/.

"Insulin Basics." American Diabetes Association. Retrieved June 17, 2014. http://www.diabetes.org/living-with-diabetes/treatment-and-care/medication/insulin/insulin-basics.html.

"Iron." University of Maryland Medical Center. Retrieved June 19, 2014. http://umm.edu/health/medical/altmed/supplement/iron.

"Iron Stores and Iron Deficiency." *BMJ* 1(5080) (1958): 1167–68.

Jakicic, J. M. "Effects of Intermittent Exercise and Use of Home Exercise Equipment on Adherence, Weight Loss, and Fitness in Overweight Women: A Randomized Trial." *JAMA: The Journal of the American Medical Association* 282(16) (1999): 1554–60.

Jamieson, J. P., W. B. Mendes, and M. K. Nock. "Improving Acute Stress Responses: The Power of Reappraisal." *Current Directions in Psychological Science* 22(1) (2013): 51–56.

Jamieson, J. P., M. K. Nock, and W. B. Mendes. "Mind Over Matter: Reappraising Arousal Improves Cardiovascular and Cognitive Responses to Stress. *Journal of Experimental Psychology: General* 141(3) (2011): 417–22.

Jeannerod, M. "Mental Imagery in the Motor Context." *Neuropsychologia* 33(11) (1995): 1419–32.

Johnstone, B., D. P. Yoon, D. Cohen, L. H. Schopp, G. Mccormack, J. Campbell, et al. "Relationships Among Spirituality, Religious Practices, Personality Factors, and Health for Five Different Faith Traditions." *Journal of Religion and Health* 51(4) (2012): 1017–41.

Jolij, J., M. Meurs, and J. Najbauer. "Music Alters Visual Perception." *PLoS ONE* 6(4) (2011): e18861.

Karageorghis, C. I., P. C. Terry, A. M. Lane, D. T. Bishop, and D. Priest. "The BASES Expert Statement on Use of Music in Exercise." *Journal of Sports Sciences* 30(9) (2012): 953–56.

Karremans, J. C., P. V. Lange, and R. Holland. "Forgiveness and Its Associations with Prosocial Thinking, Feeling, and Doing Beyond the Relationship with the Offender." *Personality and Social Psychology Bulletin* 31(10) (2005): 1315–26.

Keller, A., K. Litzelman, L. E. Wisk, T. Maddox, E. R. Cheng, P. D. Creswell, et al. "Does the Perception That Stress Affects Health Matter? The Association with Health and Mortality." *Health Psychology* 31(5) (2011): 677–84.

Klok, M. D., S. Jakobsdottir, and M. L. Drent. "The Role of Leptin and Ghrelin in the Regulation of Food Intake and Body Weight in Humans: A Review." *Obesity Reviews* 8(1) (2007): 21–34.

Knäuper, B., A. Mccollam, A. Rosen-Brown, J. Lacaille, E. Kelso, and M. Roseman. "Fruitful Plans: Adding Targeted Mental Imagery to Implementation Intentions Increases Fruit Consumption." *Psychology & Health* 26(5) (2011): 601–17.

Knäuper, B., R. Pillay, J. Lacaille, A. Mccollam, and E. Kelso. "Replacing Craving Imagery with Alternative Pleasant Imagery Reduces Craving Intensity." *Appetite* 57(1) (2011): 173–78.

Kolcaba, K., and C. Fox. "The Effects of Guided Imagery on Comfort of Women with Early Stage Breast Cancer Undergoing Radiation Therapy." *Oncology Nursing Forum* 26(1) (1999): 67–72.

Kosfeld, M., M. Heinrichs, P. J. Zak, U. Fischbacher, and E. Fehr. "Oxytocin Increases Trust in Humans." *Nature* 435(7042) (2005): 673–76.

Krulwich, R. "Born Wet, Human Babies Are 75 Percent Water. Then Comes the Drying." NPR. Retrieved June 19, 2014. http://www.npr.org/blogs/krulwich/2013/11/25/247212488/born-wet-human-babies-are-75-percent-water-then-comes-drying.

Labbé, E., N. Schmidt, and J. Babin. "Coping with Stress: The Effectiveness of Different Types of Music." *Applied Psychophysiology and Biofeedback* 32(3) (2007): 163–68. Retrieved March 12, 2012. http://dx.doi.org/10.1007/s10484-007-9043-9.

Lacaille, J., J. Ly, N. Zacchia, S. Bourkas, E. Glaser, and B. Knäuper. "The Effects of Three Mindfulness Skills on Chocolate Cravings." *Appetite* 76 (2014): 101–12.

Lai, H., and M. Good. "Music Improves Sleep Quality in Older Adults." *Journal of Advanced Nursing* 49(3) (2005): 234–44.

Lawler, K., J. Younger, R. Piferi, E. Billington, R. Jobe, K. Edmondson, et al. "A Change of Heart: Cardiovascular Correlates of Forgiveness in Response to Interpersonal Conflict." *The Journal of Behavioral Medicine* 26(5) (2003): 373–93.

Lawler, K. A., J. W. Younger, R. L. Piferi, R. L. Jobe, K. A. Edmondson, and W. H. Jones. "The Unique Effects of Forgiveness on Health: An Exploration of Pathways." *Journal of Behavioral Medicine* 28(2) (2005): 157–67.

Lawlerrow, K., and R. Piferi. "The Forgiving Personality: Describing a Life Well Lived?" *Personality and Individual Differences* 41(6) (2006): 1009–20.

Leche, E. "The Major Rule for Eating Fruit." *MindBodyGreen* (May 30, 2012). Retrieved May 15, 2014. http://www.mindbodygreen.com/0-4970/The-Major-Rule-for-Eating-Fruit.html.

Logel, C., and G. L. Cohen. "The Role of the Self in Physical Health: Testing the Effect of a Values-Affirmation Intervention on Weight Loss." *Psychological Science* 23(1) (2012): 53–55.

Low, J. A. "Air Travel in Older People." *Age and Ageing* 31(1) (2002): 17–22.

Luders, E., F. Kurth, E. A. Mayer, A. W. Toga, K. L. Narr, and C. Gaser. "The Unique Brain Anatomy of Meditation Practitioners: Alterations in Cortical Gyrification." *Frontiers in Human Neuroscience* 6 (2012).

Luszczynska, A., A. Sobczyk, and C. Abraham. "Planning to Lose Weight: Randomized Controlled Trial of an Implementation Intention Prompt to Enhance Weight Reduction Among Overweight and Obese Women." *Health Psychology* 26(4) (2007): 507–12.

Ma, Y. "Association Between Eating Patterns and Obesity in a Free-Living U.S. Adult Population." *American Journal of Epidemiology* 158(1) (2003): 85–92.

Macaskill, A. "Differentiating Dispositional Self-Forgiveness from Other-Forgiveness: Associations with Mental Health and Life Satisfaction." *Journal of Social and Clinical Psychology* 31(1) (2012): 28–50.

"Magnesium." University of Maryland Medical Center. Retrieved June 19, 2014. http://umm.edu/health/medical/altmed/supplement/magnesium.

Mahoney, M. J., and M. Avener. "Psychology of the Elite Athlete: An Exploratory Study." *Cognitive Therapy and Research* 1(2) (1977): 135–41.

Malhotra, S., G. Sawhney, and P. Pandhi. "The Therapeutic Potential of Melatonin: A Review of the Science." *MedScape General Medicine* 6(2) (2004): 46.

Mangen, A., and J. Velay. "Digitizing Literacy: Reflections on the Haptics of Writing." *Advances in Haptics*. Rijeka, Croatia: InTech, 2012.

Mangen, A., and J. Velay. "Digitizing Literacy: Reflections on the Haptics of Writing." *Advances in Haptics,* Mehrdad Hosseini Zadeh (ed.), InTech (2010), doi: 10.5772/8710. http://www.intechopen.com/books/advances-in-haptics/digitizing-literacy-reflections-on-the-haptics-of-writing.

Mann, T., A. J. Tomiyama, E. Westling, A. Lew, B. Samuels, and J. Chatman. "Medicare's Search for Effective Obesity Treatments: Diets Are Not the Answer." *American Psychologist* 62(3) (2007): 220–33.

Markwald, R. R., E. L. Melanson, M. R. Smith, J. Higgins, L. Perreault, R. H. Eckel, et al. "Impact of Insufficient Sleep on Total Daily Energy Expenditure, Food Intake, and Weight Gain." *Proceedings of the National Academy of Sciences* 110(14) (2013): 5695–5700.

Masand, P. S., and S. Gupta. "Selective Serotonin-Reuptake Inhibitors: An Update." *Harvard Review of Psychiatry* 7(2) (1999): 69–84.

Mayo Clinic. "Stress Management: Support Groups: Make Connections, Get Help" (August 1, 2012). Retrieved May 12, 2014. http://www.mayoclinic.org/healthy-living/stress-management/in-depth/support-groups/art-20044655.

Mayo Clinic Staff. "COPD." Mayo Clinic. Retrieved May 12, 2014. http://www.mayoclinic.org/diseases-conditions/copd/basics/definition/con-20032017.

Mayo Clinic Staff. "Stress Management: Chronic Stress Puts Your Health at Risk" (June 11, 2013). Retrieved June 18, 2014. http://www.mayoclinic.org/healthy-living/stress-management/in-depth/stress/art-20046037.

McGonigal, K. "How to Make Stress Your Friend." Retrieved June 19, 2014. https://www.ted.com/talks/kelly_mcgonigal_how_to_make_stress_your_friend#t-501242.

"More Sleep Would Make Most Americans Happier, Healthier and Safer." http://www.apa.org. Retrieved June 19, 2014. http://www.apa.org/research/action/sleep-deprivation.aspx.

Moritz, S., H. Quan, B. Rickhi, et al. "A Home Study-Based Spirituality Education Program Decreases Emotional Distress and Increases Quality of Life—A Randomized, Controlled Trial." *Alternative Therapy Health Medicine* 12(6) (2006): 26–35.

Moyer, C. A., M. P. Donnelly, J. C. Anderson, K. C. Valek, S. J. Huckaby, D. A. Wiederholt, et al. "Frontal Electroencephalographic Asymmetry Associated with Positive Emotion Is Produced by Very Brief Meditation Training." *Psychological Science* 22(10) (2011): 1277–79.

Muñoz-Sastre, M., G. Vinsonneau, and F. Neto. "Forgivingness and Satisfaction with Life." *Journal of Happiness Studies* 4 (2003): 323–35.

Muraven, M. "Building Self-Control Strength: Practicing Self-Control Leads to Improved Self-Control Performance." *Journal of Experimental Social Psychology* 46(2) (2010): 465–68.

Natelson, B. H. "Stress, Hormones and Disease." *Physiology & Behavior* 82(1) (2004): 139–43.

Neuhoff, C. C. "Effects of Laughing, Smiling, and Howling on Mood." *Psychological Reports* 91(7) (2002): 1079.

Oettingen, G., and T. A. Wadden. "Expectation, Fantasy, and Weight Loss: Is the Impact of Positive Thinking Always Positive?" *Cognitive Therapy and Research* 15(2) (1991): 167–75.

Oguntibeju, O., A. Esterhuyse, and E. Truter. "Red Palm Oil: Nutritional, Physiological and Therapeutic Roles in Improving Human Wellbeing and Quality of Life." *British Journal of Biomedical Science* 66(4) (2009): 216–22.

"Overview of Loving-kindness Meditation." Retrieved June 19, 2014. http://www.buddhanet.net/metta_in.htm.

Ozbay, F., H. Fitterling, D. Charney, and S. Southwick. "Social Support and Resilience to Stress Across the Life Span: A Neurobiologic Framework." *Current Psychiatry Reports* 10(4) (2008): 304–10.

"People Differ in Their Taste Senstivity." *The Taste Science Laboratory*. Retrieved June 19, 2014. http://www.tastescience.com/abouttaste3.html.

Peterson, D. "Music Benefits Exercise, Studies Show." *LiveScience* (October 21, 2009). Retrieved June 19, 2014. http://www.livescience.com/5799-music-benefits-exercise-studies-show.html.

Petry, N. M., D. Barry, L. Pescatello, and W. B. White. "A Low-Cost Reinforcement Procedure Improves Short-Term Weight Loss Outcomes." *The American Journal of Medicine* 124(11) (2011): 1082-85.

Pinto, A. M., J. L. Fava, D. A. Hoffmann, and R. R. Wing. "Combining Behavioral Weight Loss Treatment and a Commercial Program: A Randomized Clinical Trial." *Obesity* 21(4) (2013): 673–80.

Plessinger, A. "The Effects of Mental Imagery on Athletic Performance." Retrieved June 19, 2014. http://www.vanderbilt.edu/AnS/psychology/health_psychology/mentalimagery.html.

Popkin, B. M., K. E. D'Anci, and I. H. Rosenberg. "Water, Hydration, and Health." *Nutrition Reviews* 68(8) (2010): 439–58. Retrieved April 22, 2013. http://dx.doi.org/10.1111/j.1753-4887.2010.00304.x.

Poulin, M. J., S. L. Brown, A. J. Dillard, and D. M. Smith. "Giving to Others and the Association Between Stress and Mortality." *American Journal of Public Health* 103(9) (2013): 1649–55.

"Problems with Smell." NIHSeniorHealth. Retrieved June 19, 2014. http://nihseniorhealth.gov/problemswithsmell/aboutproblemswithsmell/01.html.

Qiu, Y., Y. Peng, and J. Wang. "Immunoregulatory Role of Neurotransmitters." *Advances in Neuroimmunology* 6(3) (1996): 223–31.

Ranganathan, V. "From Mental Power to Muscle Power—Gaining Strength by Using the Mind." *Neuropsychologia* 42(7) (2004): 944–56.

Rastogi, A., and S. Shukla. "Amaranth: A New Millennium Crop of Nutraceutical Values." *Critical Reviews in Food Science and Nutrition* 53(2) (2013): 109–25.

Raudenbush, B., R. Grayhem, T. Sears, and I. Wilson. "Effects of Peppermint and Cinnamon Odor Administration on Simulated Driving Alertness, Mood and Workload." *North American Journal of Psychology* 11(2) (2009): 245–56.

"Reducing Sedentary Behaviors: Sitting Less and Moving More." ACSM. Retrieved June 6, 2014. http://www.acsm.org/docs/brochures/reducing-sedentary-behaviors-sitting-less-and-moving-more.pdf.

"Relaxation Techniques: Breath Control Helps Quell Errant Stress Response." Retrieved June 18, 2014. http://www.health.harvard.edu/fhg/updates/update1006a.shtml.

Roberts, K. *Yoga for Golfers: A Unique Mind-Body Approach to Golf Fitness*. New York: McGraw-Hill, 2004.

Roemer, L., S. M. Orsillo, and K. Salters-Pedneault. "Efficacy of an Acceptance-Based Behavior Therapy For Generalized Anxiety Disorder: Evaluation in a Randomized Controlled Trial." *Journal of Consulting and Clinical Psychology* 76(6) (2008): 1083–89.

Rogers, P., A. Kainth, and H. Smit. "A Drink of Water Can Improve or Impair Mental Performance Depending on Small Differences in Thirst." *Appetite* 36(1) (2001): 57–58.

Roozendaal, B. "Stress and Memory: Opposing Effects of Gluco-corticoids on Memory Consolidation and Memory Retrieval." *Neurobiology of Learning and Memory* 78(3) (2002): 578–95.

Sawka, M., W. Latzka, R. Matott, and S. Montain. "Hydration Effects on Temperature Regulation." *International Journal of Sports Medicine* 19(S 2) (1998): S108–10.

Sawka, M. N., S. N. Cheuvront, and R. Carter. "Human Water Needs." *Nutrition Reviews* 63(6) (2005): 30–39.

Schroeder, C. "Water Drinking Acutely Improves Orthostatic Tolerance in Healthy Subjects." *Circulation* 106(22) (2002): 2806–11.

Schwartz, B. "The Tyranny of Choice." *Scientific American* 290(4) (2004): 70–75.

Sehati, N. "Craniotomy." Retrieved June 19, 2014. http://sehati.org/index/patientresources/neurosurgicalprocedures/craniotomy.html.

Shackell, E., and L. Standing. "Mind Over Matter: Mental Training Increases Physical Strength." *North American Journal of Psychology* 9(1) (2007): 189–200.

"Shelled Hemp Seed." UofMHealth homepage. Retrieved June 19, 2014. http://www.uofmhealth.org/health-library/hn-4393002#hn-4393002-uses.

Sherman, D. K. "Self-Affirmation: Understanding the Effects." *Social and Personality Psychology Compass* 7(11) (2013): 834–45.

Shirreffs, S. M., S. J. Merson, S. M. Fraser, and D. T. Archer. "The Effects of Fluid Restriction on Hydration Status and Subjective Feelings in Man." *British Journal of Nutrition* 91(06) (2004): 951.

Short, E. B., S. Kose, S. Q. Mu, J. Borckardt, A. Newberg, M. S. George, et al. "Regional Brain Activation During Meditation Shows Time and Practice Effects: An Exploratory FMRI Study." *Evidence-Based Complementary and Alternative Medicine* 7(1) (2010): 121–27.

Siedliecki, S. L., and M. Good. "Effect of Music on Power, Pain, Depression and Disability." *Journal of Advanced Nursing* 54(5) (2006): 553–62.

Silva, M. N., D. Markland, E. V. Carraça, P. N. Vieira, S. R. Coutinho, C. S. Minderico, et al. "Exercise Autonomous Motivation Predicts Three-Year Weight Loss in Women." *Medicine & Science in Sports & Exercise* 43(4) (2011): 1.

Silvers, W. S., and J. A. Poole. "Exercise-Induced Rhinitis: A Common Disorder T Adversely Affects Allergic and Nonallergic Athletes." *Annals of Allergy, Asthma & Immunology* 96(2) (2006): 334–40.

Sivertsen, B. "Cognitive Behavioral Therapy vs Zopiclone for Treatment of Chronic Primary Insomnia in Older Adults: A Randomized Controlled Trial." *JAMA: The Journal of the American Medical Association* 295(24) (2006): 2851–58.

"Sleep and Disease Risk." *Harvard Medical School: Healthy Sleep.* Retrieved May 9, 2014. http://healthysleep.med.harvard.edu/healthy/matters/consequences/sleep-and-disease-risk.

"Slide Show: See How Your Digestive System Works." Mayo Clinic. Retrieved May 16, 2014. http://www.mayoclinic.org/digestive-system/sls-20076373?s=2.

Smith, K. J., S. L. Gall, S. A. McNaughton, L. Blizzard, T. Dwyer, and A. J. Venn. "Skipping Breakfast: Longitudinal Associations with Cardiometabolic Risk Factors in the Childhood Determinants of Adult Health Study." *American Journal of Clinical Nutrition* 92(6) (2010): 1316–25.

Smith, K., and A. Graybiel. "Investigating Habits: Strategies, Technologies and Models." *Frontiers in Behavioral Neuroscience* 8 (2014): 39.

"Snack Size Nutrition." Hersheys.com. Retrieved June 19, 2014. http://www.hersheys.com/york/products/york-snack-size.aspx.

Southwick, S. M., M. Vythilingam, and D. S. Charney. "The Psychobiology of Depression and Resilience to Stress: Implications for Prevention and Treatment." *Annual Review of Clinical Psychology* 1(1) (2005): 255–91.

Sovndal, S., D. Barry, and M. Barry. "Overcoming Common Cycling Problems." *Human-Kinetics.* Retrieved June 19, 2014. http://www.humankinetics.com/excerpts/excerpts/overcoming-common-cycling-problems.

Spiegel, H. "Nocebo: The Power of Suggestibility." *Preventive Medicine* 26(5) (1997): 616–21.

"Spirituality." University of Maryland Medical Center (October 13, 2011). Retrieved May 12, 2014. http://umm.edu/health/medical/altmed/treatment/spirituality.

"Sport-Specific Training." Duke Raleigh Hospital. Retrieved June 19, 2014. http://www.dukeraleighhospital.org/healthservices/outpatient-rehabilitation/services/sports-specific-training.

"Sports Coach: Specific Respiratory Muscle Training for Athletic Performance." Retrieved June 19, 2014. http://www.ausport.gov.au/sportscoachmag/sports_sciences/specific_respiratory_muscle_training_for_athletic_performance.

Steptoe, A., E. L. Gibson, R. Vounonvirta, E. D. Williams, M. Hamer, J. A. Rycroft, et al. "The Effects of Tea on Psychophysiological Stress Responsivity and Post-Stress Recovery: A Randomised Double-Blind Trial." *Psychopharmacology* 190(1) (2007): 81–89.

Stiegler, P., S. Sparks, and A. Cunliffe. "Moderate Exercise, Postprandial Energy Expenditure, and Substrate Use in Varying Meals in Lean and Obese Men." *International Journal of Sports Nutrition & Exercise Metabolism* 18(1) (2008): 66–78.

Suhr, J. A., J. Hall, S. M. Patterson, and R. T. Niinistö. "The Relation of Hydration Status to Cognitive Performance in Healthy Older Adults." *International Journal of Psychophysiology* 53(2) (2004): 121–25.

"SURF TIP: Understanding Surfer's Aches and Pains." *SURFER Magazine.* Retrieved June 19, 2014. http://www.surfermag.com/features/surftip-body1107/.

"Survey: Americans Know How to Get Better Sleep—But Don't Act on It." Survey (April 1, 2013). Retrieved June 19, 2014. http://bettersleep.org/better-sleep/the-science-of-sleep/sleep-statistics-research/better-sleep-survey.

Tal, A., A. Musicus, and B. Wansink. "Eyes in the Aisles: Why Is Cap'N Crunch Looking Down at My Child?" (April 3, 2014). Retrieved June 19, 2014. http://papers.ssrn.com/sol3/papers.cfm?abstract_id=2419182.

Tal, A., and B. Wansink. "Fattening Fasting: Hungry Grocery Shoppers Buy More Calories, Not More Food." *JAMA Internal Medicine* 173(12) (2013): 1146.

Tapper, K., C. Shaw, J. Ilsley, A. Hill, F. W. Bond, and L. Moore. "Exploratory Randomised Controlled Trial of a Mindfulness-Based Weight Loss Intervention for Women." *Appetite* 52(2) (2009): 396–404.

"Tarcher Talks: Julia Cameron—The Writing Diet." YouTube (October 1, 2009). Retrieved June 19, 2014. https://www.youtube.com/watch?v=su_Z6A5FhcQ.

Teasdale, J. D., Z. V. Segal, J. M. Williams, V. A. Ridgeway, J. M. Soulsby, and M. A. Lau. "Prevention of Relapse/Recurrence in Major Depression by Mindfulness-Based Cognitive Therapy." *Journal of Consulting and Clinical Psychology* 68(4) (2000): 615–23.

Teitelbaum, J., and B. Gottlieb. *Real Cause, Real Cure: The 9 Root Causes of the Most Common Health Problems and How to Solve Them.* Emmaus, Pa.: Rodale, 2011.

Teixeira, P. J., M. N. Silva, J. Mata, A. L. Palmeira, and D. Markland. "Motivation, Self-Determination, and Long-Term Weight Control." *International Journal of Behavioral Nutrition and Physical Activity* 9(1) (2012): 22.

Tenenbaum, G. "The Effect of Music Type on Running Perseverance and Coping with Effort Sensations." *Psychology of Sport and Exercise* 5(2) (2004): 89–109.

"The 13 Best Food Combos on the Planet." Retrieved June 19, 2014. http://www.organicgardening.com/print/76424.

Tindle, H. A., Y. Chang, L. H. Kuller, J. E. Manson, J. G. Robinson, M. C. Rosal, et al. "Optimism, Cynical Hostility, and Incident Coronary Heart Disease and Mortality in the Women's Health Initiative." *Circulation* 120(8) (2009): 656–62.

Tinsley, H. E., J. D. Teaff, S. L. Colbs, and N. Kaufman. "A System of Classifying Leisure Activities in Terms of the Psychological Benefits of Participation Reported by Older Persons." *Journal of Gerontology* 40(2) (1985): 172–78.

Tinsley, H. E., and B. D. Eldredge. "Psychological Benefits of Leisure Participation: A Taxonomy of Leisure Activities Based on Their Need-Gratifying Properties." *Journal of Counseling Psychology* 42(2) (1995): 123–32.

Tononi, G., and C. Cirelli. "Sleep and the Price of Plasticity: From Synaptic and Cellular Homeostasis to Memory Consolidation and Integration." *Neuron* 81(1) (2014): 12–34.

Vohs, K. D., R. F. Baumeister, B. J. Schmeichel, J. M. Twenge, N. M. Nelson, and D. M. Tice. "Making Choices Impairs Subsequent Self-Control: A Limited-Resource Account of Decision Making, Self-Regulation, and Active Initiative." *Journal of Personality and Social Psychology* 94(5) (2008): 883–98.

Wallerius, S., R. Rosmond, T. Ljung, G. Holm, and P. Björntorp. "Rise in Morning Saliva Cortisol Is Associated with Abdominal Obesity in Men: A Preliminary Report." *Journal of Endocrinological Investigation* 26(7) (2003): 616–19.

Walling, E. "Drinking Water with Meals Can Impair Digestion." *NaturalNews* (September 30, 2011). Retrieved June 19, 2014. http://www.naturalnews.com/033731_digestion_drinking_water.html#.

Wang, J., Q. Huang, N. Li, G. Tan, L. Chen, and J. Zhou. "Triggers of Migraine and Tension-Type Headache in China: A Clinic-Based Survey." *European Journal of Neurology* 20(4) (2013): 689–96.

"The water in you." Water Properties: (Water Science for Schools) (March 17, 2014). Retrieved June 16, 2014. http://water.usgs.gov/edu/propertyyou.html.

Waterhouse, J., P. Hudson, and B. Edwards. "Effects of Music Tempo Upon Submaximal Cycling Performance." *Scandinavian Journal of Medicine & Science in Sports* 20(4) (2010): 662–69.

Watson, D. "Music Reduces Stress and Anxiety of Patients in the Surgical Holding Area." *AORN* 62(1) (1995): 113–14.

Webber, K. H., J. M. Gabriele, D. F. Tate, and M. B. Dignan. "The Effect of a Motivational Intervention on Weight Loss Is Moderated by Level of Baseline Controlled Motivation." *International Journal of Behavioral Nutrition and Physical Activity* 7(1) (2010): 4.

Werle, C. O., O. Trendel, and G. Ardito. "Unhealthy Food Is Not Tastier for Everybody: The 'Healthy=Tasty' French Intuition." *Food Quality and Preference* 28(1) (2013): 116–21.

"What Are the Health Benefits of Pili Nuts?" Pili Nuts (January 5, 2014). Retrieved June 19, 2014. http://pilinuts.org/what-are-the-health-benefits-of-pili-nuts/.

"What Is Organic Food and Why Should I Care?" www.organicconsumers.org. Retrieved June 15, 2014. http://www.organicconsumers.org/documents/OrganicFoodhandoutforwebv.2final.pdf.

"Why Do We Sleep, Anyway?" *Healthy Sleep* (December 18, 2007). Retrieved June 19, 2014. http://healthysleep.med.harvard.edu/healthy/matters/benefits-of-sleep/why-do-we-sleep.

"Why Do We Sleep, Anyway? Restorative Theories." *Healthy Sleep: Restorative Theories* (January 12, 2014). Retrieved May 12, 2014. http://healthysleep.med.harvard.edu/healthy/matters/benefits-of-sleep/why-do-we-sleep.

Wing, R. R., and R. W. Jeffery. "Benefits of Recruiting Participants with Friends and Increasing Social Support for Weight Loss and Maintenance." *Journal of Consulting and Clinical Psychology* 67(1) (1999): 132–38.

Wurtman, R. J., and J. J. Wurtman. "Brain Serotonin, Carbohydrate-Craving, Obesity and Depression." *Obesity Research* 3(S4) (1995): 477S–80S.

Yamashita, S., K. Iwai, T. Akimoto, J. Sugawara, and I. Kono. "Effects of Music During Exercise on RPE, Heart Rate and the Autonomic Nervous System." *Journal of Sports Medicine and Physical Fitness* 46(3) (2006): 425–30.

Ybarra, O., E. Burnstein, P. Winkielman, M. C. Keller, M. Manis, E. Chan, et al. (2007). "Mental Exercising Through Simple Socializing: Social Interaction Promotes General Cognitive Functioning." *Personality and Social Psychology Bulletin* 34(2): 248–59.

Zeratsky, K. "Does Ground Flaxseed Have More Health Benefits Than Whole Flaxseed?" *Healthy Lifestyle: Nutrition and Healthy Eating* (January 19, 2013). Retrieved June 19, 2014. http://www.mayoclinic.org/healthy-living/nutrition-and-healthy-eating/expert-answers/flaxseed/faq-20058354.

ACKNOWLEDGMENTS

I have spent most of my life in fitness—training clients, crafting the fitness sections of the YOU books, creating workout DVDs, designing home gyms, and crafting wellness programs for large companies. This work has given me the opportunity to meet thousands of hard-working people who are reaching for new heights, healthier bodies, and happier lives. These people inspired me to write this book and to continue my mission to spread the word about how much power the mind has over physical health.

My personal clients have helped me create a real-life "laboratory" out of my studio, and have assisted in formulating techniques to determine the most effective and efficient fitness programs. Thank you for your constant feedback and for your encouragement and friendship over the years.

This book was only an idea for a very long time, while I let everyday distractions get the better of me. I have to thank my inspiration—Lisa Oz—who taught me many lessons about reaching my own goals and gave me the kick in the butt that I needed to get started on this project. She is one of the most talented, laser-focused people I've ever met, and while I thought about my book idea, she led by example, writing her own book, *US: Transforming Ourselves and the Relationships That Matter Most*. This was the inspiration I needed to take action.

Though indebted to many, many people, this book would not be possible without patient support over the years from my agent, Eileen Cope, who was the true warrior in getting this book on the shelves. The dynamic and tireless HarperCollins team, especially my editor, Nancy Hancock, championed this project from the get-go and took a leap of faith by giving me the freedom to create something that wasn't "just another fitness book." To Gideon Weil, who graciously took the baton, and enthusiastically moved forward with the book. Suzanne Quist, who beautifully and patiently managed the inside. Adrian Morgan, who captured everything the book has to offer in the cover design. Amy VanLangen and Suzanne Wickham, who have done a fantastic job with marketing and publicity. I can't say enough good things about the focused and beyond-gifted Marianne McGinnis, who gave direction, support, and assistance that was invaluable, and masterfully shaped the final version.

I'd like to thank my family for their support over the years and especially my mother, Eileen, who has always taught me to reach for my dreams. Her natural optimism in life is something that I—thankfully—have inherited, and it has made all the difference. My mom has been an important partner in all my work, helping me shape my PBS Firming After 50 fitness regimen, appearing in numerous DVDs to model the "over 50" exercises, and helping to conceive the delicious and healthy recipes that appear in this book. She's always been an amazing cook, and I hope you all enjoy these creations as much as I and my clients do!

I'd also like to thank the family I have assembled over the years, those dearest friends and loved ones who have supported me in all my crazy ideas and adventures and helped me create a home here in New York City. I'd like to thank the best friend anyone could ask for, Potoula Chresomales, whom I met standing in line to register for classes my first year at NYU, and who has been my cheerleader, confidant, and titanium "rock" ever since. From helping with my one-man show twenty years ago to reading early drafts of this manuscript and providing excellent feedback, she has always been there for me. Dana and Andy Stone have gone far beyond being generous. They treat me like family 24/7, feeding my bottomless pit of an appetite so I had the energy to actually write this book. Carolyn Zonino has given me the gift of always saying yes whenever I asked for help. I will always be in her debt. Ashley Meece for being a very patient and perfect model for the poses in the exercise section. Clive Davis, Anthony and Becca Clemente, Elise Ballard, Jonathan Lewis, Marc Honaker, Amy Wollman, Kara Fisher, Sherri Brown, Stephanie Fields, Nick Brown, Debbie Kass, Sara Shenasky, Kara Leibowitz, Paige Nash, Greg Richman, Tammy Blake, Erin Schwitter, Victoria Holly, Johanna Mayer-Jones, and Susannah Shipman have enriched my life with their humor, generosity, warmth, spirit, and being there for me around the clock year after year. Lastly, I'd like to thank Dr. Mehmet Oz, who has changed our world for the better with his passion and devotion to health and fitness, and to helping people understand their bodies and take control of their lives. His funny way of demystifying things has given millions of people the vocabulary and tools to eat better, exercise better, and better understand their own health. When I think about the impact I want to have in life, Dr. Oz is my model. He helped me launch my career years ago, and I have learned something from him every day since.

INDEX

Note: page references leading with "I-," indicate color insert pages.

ABOUT THE AUTHOR

JOEL HARPER is a celebrity personal trainer who has developed custom workouts for countless clients for more than twenty years. He currently lives in New York City and Falls Village, Connecticut, but is originally from Dallas, Texas. He graduated from New York University. His great success is largely due to simple, no-nonsense, down-to-earth strategies that teach people how to harness the power of their minds to lose weight, get fit, and boost their moods. His exercise routines and eating plans are time-efficient and simple and produce immediate and impressive results. He is a favorite fitness expert among the media, online, and in print magazines, providing exercise tips, lifestyle advice, quotes, and commentary. His clients range from Dr. Oz to Olympic medalists as well as Hollywood elite, Broadway stars, and famous musicians.

Harper created all the personal workout chapters for the *New York Times* bestselling YOU book series as well as the accompanying workout videos. He makes regular appearances on *The Dr. Oz Show* and has been seen on ABC News, CBS News, FOX News, *Good Morning America, The Today Show,* CNN, Discovery Health, PBS, QVC, and *The Liza Oz Show.*

In addition to creating all of the accompanying workout videos for the bestselling YOU books series, Harper is the creator of the PBS bestselling DVDs *Firming After 50* and *Slim and Fit.* He has recently released the *Brain Fitness* DVD with Neal Barnard, M.D.

Harper is a regular contributor to Dr. Oz's magazine, *The Good Life,* and has written for *Esquire, O Magazine, Bottom Line,* and *Runner's World.*

Visit him online at http://www.joelharperfitness.com.